Hepatology

Editor

JONATHAN A. LIDBURY

VETERINARY CLINICS OF NORTH AMERICA: SMALL ANIMAL PRACTICE

www.vetsmall.theclinics.com

May 2017 • Volume 47 • Number 3

ELSEVIER

1600 John F. Kennedy Boulevard ● Suite 1800 ● Philadelphia, Pennsylvania, 19103-2899
http://www.vetsmall.theclinics.com

VETERINARY CLINICS OF NORTH AMERICA: SMALL ANIMAL PRACTICE Volume 47, Number 3
May 2017 ISSN 0195-5616, ISBN-13: 978-0-323-52868-9

Editor: Katie Pfaff
Developmental Editor: Meredith Madeira

Veterinary Clinics of North America: Small Animal Practice (ISSN 0195-5616) is published bimonthly by Elsevier Inc., 360 Park Avenue South, New York, NY 10010-1710. Months of issue are January, March, May, July, September, and November. Business and Editorial Offices: 1600 John F. Kennedy Blvd., Ste. 1800, Philadelphia, PA 19103-2899. Customer Service Office: 3251 Riverport Lane, Maryland Heights, MO 63043. Periodicals postage paid at New York, NY and additional mailing offices. Subscription prices are $319.00 per year (domestic individuals), $598.00 per year (domestic institutions), $100.00 per year (domestic students/residents), $422.00 per year (Canadian individuals), $743.00 per year (Canadian institutions), $469.00 per year (international individuals), $743.00 per year (international institutions), and $220.00 per year (international and Canadian students/residents). To receive student/resident rate, orders must be accompanied by name of affiliated institution, date of term, and the *signature* of program/residency coordinator on institution letterhead. Orders will be billed at individual rate until proof of status is received. Foreign air speed delivery is included in all *Clinics* subscription prices. All prices are subject to change without notice. **POSTMASTER:** Send address changes to *Veterinary Clinics of North America: Small Animal Practice*, Elsevier Health Sciences Division, Subscription Customer Service, 3251 Riverport Lane, Maryland Heights, MO 63043. Customer Service (orders, claims, online, change of address): Elsevier Periodicals Customer Service, Elsevier Health Sciences Division Subscription **Customer Service 3251 Riverport Lane Maryland Heights, MO 63043. Tel: 1-800-654-2452 (U.S. and Canada); 314-447-8871 (outside U.S. and Canada). Fax: 314-447-8029. E-mail: journalscustomerservice-usa@elsevier.com (for print support); journalsonlinesupport-usa@elsevier.com (for online support).**

Reprints. For copies of 100 or more of articles in this publication, please contact the Commercial Reprints Department, Elsevier Inc., 360 Park Avenue South, New York, NY 10010-1710. Tel.: 212-633-3874; Fax: 212-633-3820; E-mail: reprints@elsevier.com.

Veterinary Clinics of North America: Small Animal Practice is also published in Japanese by Inter Zoo Publishing Co., Ltd., Aoyama Crystal-Bldg 5F, 3-5-12 Kitaaoyama, Minato-ku, Tokyo 107-0061, Japan.

Veterinary Clinics of North America: Small Animal Practice is covered in *Current Contents/Agriculture, Biology and Environmental Sciences, Science Citation Index, ASCA, MEDLINE/PubMed (Index Medicus), Excerpta Medica,* and *BIOSIS.*

Contributors

EDITOR

JONATHAN A. LIDBURY, BVMS, PhD
Assistant Professor of Small Animal Internal Medicine, Gastrointestinal Laboratory, Department of Small Animal Clinical Sciences, College of Veterinary Medicine & Biomedical Sciences, Texas A&M University, College Station, Texas

AUTHORS

JULIA BEATTY, BSc (Hons), BVetMed, PhD, FANZCVS (Feline Medicine)
Professor of Feline Medicine, Faculty of Veterinary Science, Valentine Charlton Cat Centre, School of Life and Environmental Sciences, The University of Sydney, Sydney, New South Wales, Australia

NICK BEXFIELD, BVetMed, PhD, DSAM, FRSB, AFHEA, MRCVS
Diplomate, European College of Veterinary Internal Medicine-Companion Animals; Clinical Associate Professor, Small Animal Medicine and Oncology, School of Veterinary Medicine and Science, University of Nottingham, Leicestershire, United Kingdom

LARA BOLAND, BVSc (Hons I), MANZCVS (Feline Medicine)
Diplomate, European College of Veterinary Internal Medicine – Companion Animals; Specialist in Small Animal Medicine, Faculty of Veterinary Science, Valentine Charlton Cat Centre, School of Life and Environmental Sciences, The University of Sydney, Sydney, New South Wales, Australia

KAREN DIRKSEN, DVM, PhD
Department of Clinical Sciences of Companion Animals, Faculty of Veterinary Medicine, Utrecht University, Utrecht, The Netherlands

ROBERT P. FAVIER, DVM, PhD
Department of Clinical Sciences of Companion Animals, Faculty of Veterinary Medicine, Utrecht University, Utrecht, The Netherlands

HILLE FIETEN, DVM, PhD
Department of Clinical Sciences of Companion Animals, Faculty of Veterinary Medicine, Utrecht University, Utrecht, The Netherlands

ADAM G. GOW, BVM&S, PhD
Diplomate, European College of Veterinary Internal Medicine; Diplomate, Small Animal Medicine; Member of Royal College of Veterinary Surgeons, Head of Small Animal Medicine, Senior Lecturer in Small Animal Medicine, Hospital for Small Animals, Royal (Dick) School of Veterinary Studies, The University of Edinburgh, Easter Bush, Edinburgh, Scotland

YURI A. LAWRENCE, DVM, MA, MS
Professor, Gastrointestinal Laboratory, Department of Veterinary Small Animal Clinical Sciences, College of Veterinary Medicine & Biomedical Sciences, Texas A&M University, College Station, Texas

JONATHAN A. LIDBURY, BVMS, PhD
Assistant Professor of Small Animal Internal Medicine, Gastrointestinal Laboratory, Department of Small Animal Clinical Sciences, College of Veterinary Medicine & Biomedical Sciences, Texas A&M University, College Station, Texas

ANGELA J. MAROLF, DVM
Diplomate, American College of Veterinary Radiology; Associate Professor, Radiology, Department of Environmental and Radiological Health Sciences, College of Veterinary Medicine and Biomedical Sciences, Colorado State University, Fort Collins, Colorado

LAURA E. SELMIC, BVetMed (Hons), MPH
Assistant Professor, Department of Veterinary Clinical Medicine, College of Veterinary Medicine, University of Illinois Urbana-Champaign, Urbana, Illinois

JÖRG M. STEINER, medvet, DrMedVet, PhD
Gastrointestinal Laboratory, Department of Veterinary Small Animal Clinical Sciences, College of Veterinary Medicine & Biomedical Sciences, Texas A&M University, College Station, Texas

VINCENT THAWLEY, VMD
Diplomate, American College of Veterinary Emergency and Critical Care; Clinical Assistant Professor, Emergency and Critical Care Medicine, Department of Clinical Studies, Matthew J. Ryan Veterinary Hospital of the University of Pennsylvania, Philadelphia, Pennsylvania

CHIARA VALTOLINA, DVM
Diplomate, American College of Veterinary Emergency and Critical care; Diplomate, European College of Veterinary Emergency and Critical Care; Department of Clinical Sciences of Companion Animals, Faculty of Veterinary Medicine, Utrecht University, Utrecht, The Netherlands

PENNY WATSON, MA, VetMD, CertVR, DSAM, FRCVS
Diplomate, European College of Veterinary Internal Medicine; Department of Veterinary Medicine, Queen's Veterinary School Hospital, University of Cambridge, Cambridge, United Kingdom

CYNTHIA R.L. WEBSTER, DVM
Diplomate, American College of Veterinary Internal Medicine; Professor and Associate Chair, Department of Clinical Sciences, Cummings School of Veterinary Medicine at Tufts University, North Grafton, Massachusetts

Contents

> Laboratory evaluation of the hepatobiliary system has an important role in the diagnosis, monitoring, and assessment of patients with hepatobiliary diseases. Serum liver enzyme activities can be divided into markers of hepatocellular injury and cholestasis. Liver function can be assessed in several ways, including assessment of synthetic capacity, measurement of ammonia, and measurement of bile acids. It is essential to have an understanding of the performance characteristics and limitations of these tests in order to use them appropriately. This article reviews the laboratory parameters commonly used to aid diagnosing hepatobiliary disorders in dogs and cats.

> Recent advances in diagnostic imaging of the hepatobiliary system include MRI, computed tomography (CT), contrast-enhanced ultrasound, and ultrasound elastography. With the advent of multislice CT scanners, sedated examinations in veterinary patients are feasible, increasing the utility of this imaging modality. CT and MRI provide additional information for dogs and cats with hepatobiliary diseases due to lack of superimposition of structures, operator dependence, and through intravenous contrast administration. Advanced ultrasound methods can offer complementary information to standard ultrasound imaging. These newer imaging modalities assist clinicians by aiding diagnosis, prognostication, and surgical planning.

> Histopathologic evaluation of liver biopsy specimens yields information that is not otherwise obtainable and is frequently essential for diagnosing hepatic disease. Percutaneous needle biopsy, laparoscopic biopsy, and surgical biopsy each have their own set of advantages and disadvantages. Care should be taken to ensure an adequate amount of tissue is collected for meaningful histologic evaluation. Because sampling error is a limitation of hepatic biopsy, multiple liver lobes should be biopsied. This article discusses the indications for liver biopsy, associated risks, advantages and disadvantages of different biopsy techniques, and strategies to get the most useful information possible out of this process.

terriers and Labrador retrievers respectively. In the Labrador retriever, dietary copper intake contributes strongly to the disease phenotype.

hepatic histopathology and/or bile analysis is ideal but not always practical. Neutrophilic cholangitis is associated with bacterial cholecystitis, pancreatitis, and inflammatory bowel disease. The typical presentation is a short illness with lethargy, inappetence, pyrexia, and jaundice. Lymphocytic cholangitis, suspected to be immune-mediated, can have a prolonged clinical course with weight loss and ascites as the predominant features. The prevalence of liver fluke infestation in cats varies worldwide and clinical manifestations are uncommonly reported.

Laura E. Selmic

Older companion animals may be uncommonly affected with hepatobiliary neoplasia. If clinical signs are shown they are often nonspecific. Animals may have increased liver enzyme activities detected on serum biochemistry. Ultrasound imaging can help to characterize liver lesions and guide sampling with fine needle aspiration. Treatment for massive liver tumor morphology involves liver lobectomy. Prognosis depends on the tumor morphology, type, and stage, but can be good for cats and dogs with massive hepatocellular tumors, with animals experiencing prolonged survival and low recurrence rates.

VETERINARY CLINICS OF NORTH AMERICA: SMALL ANIMAL PRACTICE

THE CLINICS ARE NOW AVAILABLE ONLINE!
Access your subscription at:
www.theclinics.com

Preface

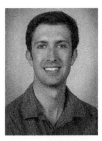

Jonathan A. Lidbury, BVMS, PhD
Editor

Canine and feline hepatology is an exciting and ever-changing field. Clinicians face a variety of challenges when diagnosing and treating companion animal hepatic diseases. First, much remains unknown about the etiopathogenesis of many of them, limiting the availability of treatments that target their underlying causes. Furthermore, despite the availability and widespread use of a variety of laboratory tests and imaging modalities paired with histopathologic assessment of the liver, clinicians face a variety of diagnostic challenges. Finally, because of the limited availability of high-quality evidence from clinical trials, even once an accurate diagnosis has been made, formulating a treatment plan can prove difficult. Some treatments that were previously dogmatically recommended have later been found to be contraindicated, while evidence supporting the efficacy of others is only just emerging. Despite these obstacles, due to the diligence and determination of researchers and clinicians working in the field, the veterinary profession's knowledge and upstanding of canine and feline hepatic disease are incrementally improving, allowing us to better serve our patients.

I am grateful to the staff at Elsevier for giving me the opportunity to guest edit this issue of *Veterinary Clinics of North America: Small Animal Practice*, and I am honored to have been fortunate enough to recruit a fantastic group of expert authors. This issue provides readers an update on a range of topics in small animal hepatology, including state-of-the-art discussions of hepatic encephalopathy, hemostatic disorders associated with hepatobiliary disease, and canine breed–specific hepatopathies as well as practical discussions regarding the diagnosis and management of canine chronic hepatitis, feline cholangitis, and hepatobiliary neoplasia. The authors have highlighted

Vet Clin Small Anim 47 (2017) xi–xii
http://dx.doi.org/10.1016/j.cvsm.2016.11.017
0195-5616/17/© 2016 Published by Elsevier Inc.

areas where recent research findings have a real-world impact on patient care and where further research is needed before definitive recommendations can be made.

Jonathan A. Lidbury, BVMS, PhD
Gastrointestinal Laboratory
Department of Small Animal Clinical Sciences
College of Veterinary Medicine &
Biomedical Sciences
Texas A&M University
College Station, TX 77843, USA

E-mail address:
jlidbury@cvm.tamu.edu

Laboratory Evaluation of the Liver

Yuri A. Lawrence, DVM, MA, MS*, Jörg M. Steiner, medvet, DrMedVet, PhD

KEYWORDS

- Hepatic enzymes • Bile acids • Bilirubin • Liver disease • Ammonia

KEY POINTS

- Laboratory tests can be used to determine whether hepatobiliary disease is present, if liver disease is primary or secondary, and to monitor response to therapy or disease progression.
- Chronic (>6 weeks) elevations in serum alanine aminotransferase (ALT) activity warrant further investigation.
- Extrahepatic disease should be ruled out when investigating patients with increased serum liver enzyme activities.
- Patients with normal laboratory tests can still have significant hepatobiliary disease.
- Knowledge of the biologic variation of analytes is important for accurate interpretation of laboratory tests.

INTRODUCTION

Laboratory evaluation of the hepatobiliary system has several objectives that include determining whether hepatobiliary disease is present, determining if liver disease is primary or secondary, determining the definitive type of liver disease, and monitoring response to therapy or disease progression. Reaching a diagnosis of hepatobiliary disease can present a challenge for several reasons. First, clinical signs are often nonspecific, and in some patients, the disease may in fact be subclinical. In addition, the large functional reserve of the liver requires a marked loss of functional hepatic tissue before clinical signs due to liver failure ensue. Rarely is a specific diagnosis possible without the aid of a biopsy. Despite these challenges, laboratory tests play an important role in the recognition and diagnosis of canine and feline hepatobiliary disease. This article reviews laboratory tests commonly used to evaluate the hepatobiliary system and discusses their utility as well as their limitations.

Dr Y.A. Lawrence and Dr J.M. Steiner are employed by the Gastrointestinal Laboratory at Texas A&M University, which offers hepatic function testing on a fee-for-service basis.
Gastrointestinal Laboratory, Department of Veterinary Small Animal Clinical Sciences, College of Veterinary Medicine & Biomedical Sciences, Texas A&M University, 4474 TAMU, College Station, TX 77843-4474, USA
* Corresponding author.
E-mail address: ylawrence@cvm.tamu.edu

REFERENCE INTERVALS AND BIOLOGICAL VARIATION

Comprehension of the limitations of diagnostic laboratory testing for hepatobiliary disease is important to avoid misinterpretation of results. Generally, these tests are quantitative assays performed on serum or plasma samples that are measured with a continuous scale. The clinical interpretation of these assays is guided by a reference interval and/or predetermined cutoff value. Reference intervals can be established by various methods, but most commonly comprise the central 95th percentile of a healthy reference population. Thus, values from 5% of this healthy population fall outside the reference interval. Determination of reference intervals varies based on the number of test subjects and the distribution of the data. A minimum of 40 test subjects is required according to guidelines established by the American Society for Veterinary Clinical Pathology.[1] Patients with significant hepatobiliary disease can have normal test results, and healthy patients can have abnormal test results. Not every value outside the reference interval is clinically relevant. To avoid misinterpretation, oftentimes cutoff values are used that trigger a certain diagnosis or response. For example, although a serum alanine aminotransferase (ALT) activity of 125 U/L may be greater than the upper limit of the reference interval, only a value higher than that would trigger further diagnostic testing.

Clinical biochemical parameters can vary due to intrinsic biological heterogeneity within a patient, but also can vary due to analytical imprecision. The magnitude of biological heterogeneity is also variable with some parameters having large changes over time and others being under more stringent homeostatic regulation. Comprehension of the presence and degree of intrinsic biological heterogeneity and determination of critical change values for biochemical parameters measured for assessment of canine and feline patients for possible hepatobiliary disease is important. A recent study in healthy dogs found that the critical change value for alanine transaminase was 47.7%.[2] Therefore, in a healthy dog, the alanine transaminase activity must change by at least 47.7% in order for that change to be considered statistically different. The biological variation that occurs in dogs with hepatobiliary disease and in healthy or diseased cats is currently unknown.

SERUM BIOMARKERS OF HEPATOBILIARY DISEASE

The specific laboratory tests used for the evaluation of patients with hepatobiliary disease can be classified into 3 groups: markers of hepatocellular damage, markers of cholestasis, and tests of various liver functions (uptake, conjugation, secretion, and synthesis).

Markers of Hepatocellular Damage

Alanine aminotransferase

ALT is found in high concentrations within the cytoplasm and mitochondria of canine and feline hepatocytes. The serum activity of this enzyme is used as a marker of hepatocellular injury in dogs and cats, and it is considered to be the gold-standard marker for hepatocellular injury.[3] Hepatocytes that are rapidly and irreversibly damaged release their cytoplasmic contents, including ALT, into the extracellular space from where it can enter the circulation. ALT release can also occur following reversible hepatocellular injury, which is thought to occur by cytoplasmic blebbing.[4] Distinguishing between irreversible and reversible damage is not possible based on assessment of serum or plasma ALT activity alone. However, reversible or less extensive injury is generally associated with changes of smaller magnitude than irreversible or widespread cellular injury.[5] ALT is predominantly found in the liver with lower enzyme activities found in skeletal and cardiac muscle. There are 2 isoenzymes of ALT (ie, ALT1, ALT2) that can be differentiated based on molecular structure and tissue specificity.[6] ALT1 immunohistochemical reactivity has been localized to hepatocytes, renal tubular epithelial cells, and salivary gland epithelial cells, whereas ALT2 has been localized to cardiac myocytes, skeletal muscle fibers, islets cells of the endocrine pancreas, and the adrenal cortex.[7] Serum/plasma ALT activity is considered to be relatively liver specific but can occasionally be increased due to muscle injury. Correlation with serum creatinine kinase activity is useful for differentiating ALT activity of muscle origin from that of hepatic origin. An assay that could discriminate among ALT activities of different cellular origin may add information to the measurement of serum total ALT activity.

An increased serum activity of ALT activity is generally associated with reversible or irreversible damage to the hepatocellular membrane. Potential causes of hepatocellular membrane damage include inflammatory diseases, hypoxia, toxins, drugs, and neoplasia (**Box 1**). Elevations of serum or plasma ALT activity associated with corticosteroid or phenobarbital therapy may be multifactorial due to an increased enzyme synthesis and cellular injury.[8] Although the degree of elevation of serum ALT activity is roughly proportional to disease severity and affected hepatic mass, abnormality can be present in the absence of elevated ALT activity due to a decrease in the number of hepatocytes (ie, advanced fibrosis, portosystemic shunting), in cases of noninflammatory primary or secondary neoplasia (eg, hepatocellular carcinoma or hemangiosarcoma), and potentially very early in the course of disease. Consequently, a single measurement does not provide an accurate prognosis. There are also several extrahepatic disorders and drugs that can result in elevated serum/plasma ALT activity

---

Box 1
Potential hepatobiliary causes for elevated serum or plasma activities of alanine aminotransferase and aspartate aminotransferase

Drug-induced liver injury: for example, acetaminophen, anesthetic agents, arsenical compounds, carprofen, diazepam/oxazepam, griseofulvin, itraconazole, ketoconazole, lomustine, phenobarbital, phenytoin, primidone, mebendazole, methimazole, oxibendazole-diethylcarbamazine, tetracycline, doxycycline, clindamycin, nitrofurantoin, trimethoprim-sulfadiazine, azathioprine

Hepatic lipidosis (cats)

Infectious: for example, ascending enteric bacterial infection, feline infectious peritonitis, schistosomiasis, leptospirosis

Inflammatory: copper-associated chronic hepatitis, idiopathic chronic hepatitis, cholangitis, gall bladder mucocele

Lysosomal storage disease

Neoplasia (primary or metastatic)

Nodular hyperplasia

Portosystemic shunt (congenital or acquired)

Toxin ingestion: for example, aflatoxin, amanita mushroom, blue-green algae, copper, herbicides, insecticides, iron, sago palm, zinc, xylitol

Trauma

Vacuolar hepatopathy (idiopathic)

early in the course of disease, and without the presence of significant primary hepatocellular disease (**Box 2**).

Activities of serum ALT activities increase within 12 hours of hepatocellular injury and reach peak levels after approximately 24 to 48 hours.[9] The time it takes for an increased serum ALT activity to return to baseline depends on the underlying disease process, for example, acute insult versus a chronic inflammatory or infectious process. Serum or plasma ALT activity has been reported to have a half-life of about 40 to 61 hours in dogs and 3.5 hours in cats.[10] Therefore, even mild elevations in the serum or plasma activity of this enzyme are often considered to be more clinically relevant in cats than in dogs.

The authors' general guidelines for increases in serum/plasma ALT activity are that increases up to 2-fold can be rechecked at 2-week intervals for up to 6 weeks and possibly treated with nutraceutical hepatoprotectants. Two- to 5-fold increases require more of a diagnostic workup that may include measurement of bile acids or ammonia as well as leptospirosis serology and/or polymerase chain reaction. For increases greater than 5-fold, an immediate diagnostic workup is recommended. Sustained smaller increases may also require a workup (**Fig. 1**).

Aspartate aminotransferase

Aspartate aminotransferase (AST) is another enzyme that is used as a marker of hepatocellular damage. This enzyme is present in significant quantities in skeletal muscle, brain, liver, kidney, erythrocytes, and cardiac tissue.[11,12] The extrahepatic sources tend to be more clinically significant than those of ALT because muscle damage and hemolysis can cause considerable increases in AST activity. AST is therefore considered less liver specific than ALT. The causes of an increased AST activity are similar to those of ALT (see **Box 1**). Nevertheless, evaluation of serum AST in conjunction with the activities of other hepatic enzymes and creatinine kinase generally allows the clinician to distinguish between increases due to hepatic damage and those due to muscle damage. AST has a half-life of approximately 12 hours in dogs and 1.5 hours in cats.[9] Increases of serum AST activity generally parallel those of ALT and are therefore considered to be a sensitive marker for hepatocellular injury.

Box 2
Potential extrahepatic causes for elevated serum or plasma activities of alanine aminotransferase and aspartate aminotransferase

Diabetes mellitus

Enteritis

Hemolysis (AST)

Hyperthyroidism (cats)

Hypoxia: cardiac disease, hepatic thrombosis, anemia

Hypothyroidism (dogs)

Myopathy (more likely AST)

Pancreatitis/pancreatic neoplasia

Peritonitis

Septicemia

Vacuolar hepatopathy (secondary to exogenous/endogenous glucocorticoids)

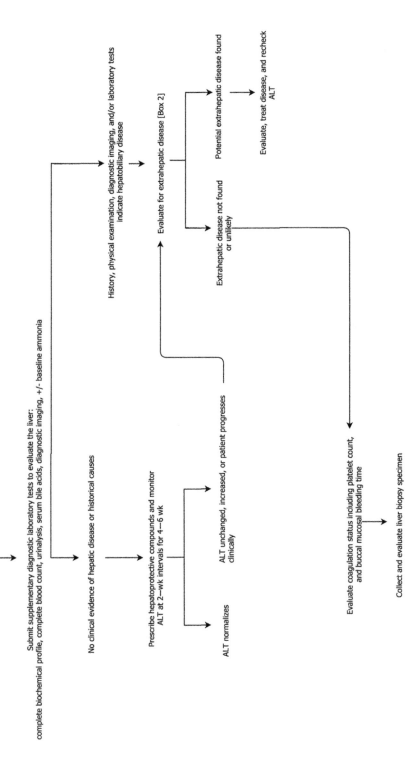

Fig. 1. Suggested diagnostic approach to dogs or cats with an increased serum/plasma ALT activity.

Markers of Cholestasis

Alkaline phosphatase

Alkaline phosphatase (ALP) is associated with the cell membrane in multiple tissues, including hepatocytes. There are several hepatic and nonhepatic processes that can lead to elevated serum ALP activity (**Box 3**). Several ALP isoenzymes have been identified in liver, bone, intestines, kidney, and placenta.[3] There is disagreement in the literature regarding the contributions to serum ALP activity from each of these tissues in cats. There are 2 genes encoding ALP in the dog and cat.[13] There are also different isoforms of ALP arising from the same gene due to posttranslational processing. Liver ALP, bone ALP, and kidney ALP are transcribed from the tissue nonspecific ALP gene.[13] Corticosteroid-induced ALP and intestinal ALP are isoforms of the intestinal ALP gene in the dog.[14] The serum half-lives of placental, kidney, and intestinal ALP are less than 6 minutes in the dog.[11] The serum half-life of intestinal ALP is less than 2 minutes in the cat and the half-lives of placental and kidney ALP in the cat are assumed to be short because of their similar structure to intestinal form.[11] The

---

Box 3
Potential causes of increased alkaline phosphatase activity

Biliary tract disease

Biliary neoplasia

Cholelithiasis

Cholecystitis

Gall bladder mucocele

Hepatic parenchymal disease

Cholangitis

Chronic hepatitis (idiopathic and copper associated)

Hepatic lipidosis (cats)

Hepatic neoplasia: primary or metastatic

Nodular hyperplasia

Toxin ingestion: for example, aflatoxin, amanita mushroom, blue-green algae, copper, herbicides, insecticides, iron, sago palm, zinc, xylitol

Vacuolar hepatopathy (idiopathic)

Extrahepatic disease

Bone neoplasia/osteolytic disease

Chronic passive congestion

Diabetes mellitus

Exogenous/endogenous glucocorticoids (glucocorticoid-induced isoenzyme in dogs, also cause vacuolar hepatopathy)

Growing animal

Hyperthyroidism (cats)

Hypothyroidism (dogs)

Pancreatitis/pancreatic neoplasia

Septicemia

serum half-life of liver ALP is approximately 70 hours in the dog and 6 hours in the cat.[11] Because of these characteristics, only liver and bone ALP in the cat and dog and corticosteroid-induced ALP in the dog contribute significantly to serum activity. An elevated serum ALP activity can indicate primary hepatobiliary disease, such as cholestasis, as well as canalicular cell necrosis, or alternatively increased hepatic synthesis. The membrane-bound liver ALP isoenzyme is released, becoming soluble, during cholestasis by phospholipase activity that is enhanced in the presence of bile acids.[15] Consequently, serum ALP activity is often markedly increased in patients with cholestatic disorders.

ALP is considered to be a sensitive marker for cholestasis with a reported sensitivity of 85%. The shorter half-life in cats means that increases in ALP are generally not as high as in dogs, and thus, this enzyme is a less sensitive marker of cholestasis in this species. An elevated serum ALP activity does not distinguish between intrahepatic and extrahepatic cholestasis. A wide variety of diseases can cause intrahepatic cholestasis through hepatocyte swelling, leading to obstruction of small bile canaliculi and extrahepatic cholestasis. The increase of ALP following hepatic injury is delayed compared with increases in markers of hepatocellular damage. The reason for this is that it takes time for the enzymes to be synthesized and released into systemic circulation.

Technically, it is possible to selectively measure the activity of glucocorticoid-induced ALP using techniques such as levamisole inhibition. Measurement of glucocorticoid-induced ALP has been investigated as a way to distinguish between increases due to corticosteroids versus cholestasis. Unfortunately, measuring glucocorticoid-induced ALP is not clinically useful because this enzyme can be increased in a variety of conditions, including hepatic disease, diabetes mellitus, hypothyroidism, and pancreatitis.

Gamma-glutamyltransferase

Gamma-glutamyltransferase (GGT) is another membrane-bound enzyme found in biliary epithelial cells and hepatocytes, as well as pancreatic, renal tubular, and mammary gland epithelial cells.[16] The results of electrophoretic studies indicate that the enzyme found in the serum of normal subjects originates from the liver.[16] Elevations of serum levels of GGT are attributed to cholestasis or biliary hyperplasia resulting in enzyme induction. GGT may be a more sensitive indicator of hepatobiliary disease in cats than ALP, owing to the shorter half-life of ALP in cats. A notable exception is hepatic lipidosis, as moderate to marked increases of ALP may be present with minimal, if any, increases of GGT. In dogs, GGT is often considered more specific but less sensitive than ALP for the detection of hepatobiliary disease. Corticosteroid administration or increased endogenous corticosteroid production may result in increased serum GGT activity in dogs, likely due to enzyme induction, but serum GGT is less influenced than ALP by secondary hepatic diseases or enzyme-inducing drugs. Mild to modest increases of serum GGT can also occur during anticonvulsant therapy (phenobarbital, phenytoin, primidone). GGT has a half-life of approximately 72 hours in dogs.[17]

Tests of Liver Function

Total serum bilirubin

Bilirubin is the oxidative product of the protoporphyrin portion of the heme group of proteins, such as hemoglobin, myoglobin, and cytochrome P-450.[18] Most bilirubin is generated during removal of senescent red blood cells through the mononuclear phagocyte system by the action of intracellular microsomal heme oxygenase. This enzyme catalyzes degradation of hemoglobin to iron, carbon monoxide, globin, and biliverdin. In turn, biliverdin is further reduced to bilirubin and released from the cell and transported to the liver bound to albumin.[18] Following transfer of bilirubin into hepatocytes, which is mediated by the transport proteins ligandin or fatty-acid binding protein, bilirubin is conjugated with glucuronide via the enzyme uridine diphosphate glucuronyl transferase.[18] The conjugated water-soluble form of bilirubin is actively transported from hepatocytes across the bile canalicular membrane, and following entry into the intestine as a component of bile, is subsequently degraded by colonic bacteria into urobilinogen. Hyperbilirubinemia can be caused by hemolysis, primary hepatic disease, or extrahepatic cholestasis.

Hemolysis is often distinguishable from other causes of hyperbilirubinemia due to the presence of concurrent anemia. Red blood cell morphology should be evaluated in all anemic hyperbilirubinemic patients for ghost cells, spherocytosis, autoagglutination, Heinz bodies, and hemotropic parasites. Common causes of hemolysis include immune-mediated hemolytic anemia, hemotropic parasites, drugs and toxins, or microangiopathic disease. Concurrent increases in ALT activity may occur due to hypoxic injury to hepatocytes.

Hepatic hyperbilirubinemia can be due to a concurrent decrease in hepatocyte function and intrahepatic cholestasis. These conditions lead to decreased bilirubin uptake, conjugation, and excretion. However, significant hepatic disease must be present to result in hyperbilirubinemia, and thus, total serum bilirubin is not a sensitive test for hepatic disease. There are numerous diseases associated with hyperbilirubinemia in dogs and cats, and the most common disease processes are listed in **Box 4**.

Posthepatic hyperbilirubinemia is secondary to obstruction of the extrahepatic bile duct. Common causes include pancreatitis, bacterial cholecystitis, biliary mucoceles, biliary neoplasia, and pancreatic neoplasia. Extrahepatic biliary duct obstruction often results in a disproportionate increase in cholestatic enzymes (ALP and GGT) in comparison with hepatocellular injury enzymes (ALT and AST). In addition, serum cholesterol concentrations are often increased with biliary obstruction. Hepatic ultrasonographic examination is often helpful in confirming the diagnosis and further directing therapy. Where available, magnetic resonance cholangiography may offer improved imaging of the biliary tract (see Jonathan A. Lidbury's article, "Getting the Most Out of Liver Biopsy," in this issue).

Measurement of the concentration of serum conjugated (direct) and unconjugated bilirubin (indirect) to distinguish between prehepatic, hepatic, or posthepatic hyperbilirubinemia has been found not to be clinically reliable and is thus rarely performed.

Bilirubin can bind irreversibly (covalently) to albumin.[19] This biliprotein cannot be cleared by the liver and consequently persists in the plasma.[19] Biliprotein has a serum half-life comparable to that of albumin, and this becomes clinically relevant because hyperbilirubinemia (and icterus) can persist for several weeks following resolution of the inciting cause.

Ammonia

Ammonia is predominantly produced in the intestines via catabolism of glutamine by enterocytes and bacterial deamination of dietary protein and gastrointestinal hemorrhage.[20,21] The ammonia in the intestinal lumen diffuses through the mucosa, reaches the splanchnic circulation, and is carried to the liver via the hepatic portal circulation where it is transported into hepatocytes in the form of ammonium. Because the liver has a large reserve capacity for the conversion of ammonia into urea, plasma ammonia measurement is a relatively insensitive marker for hepatic function,[22] and it has been suggested that a greater than 70% reduction of hepatic function is required for serum ammonia concentration to be increased.[23] Plasma ammonia concentrations are not influenced by cholestasis or hepatic disorders that do not alter the portosystemic circulation or significantly reduce hepatic

---

Box 4
Common hepatic causes of hyperbilirubinemia

Prehepatic (hemolysis)

Hemoparasites

Heinz-body hemolytic anemia

Hypophosphatemia-induced hemolytic anemia

Immune-mediated hemolytic anemia

Neonatal isoerythrolysis

Transfusion reaction

Zinc toxicity

Hepatic

Dogs
  Acute liver injury: drug-induced liver injury, hepatotoxins
  Chronic hepatitis (idiopathic and copper associated)
  Hepatic necrosis
  Infectious disease: for example, leptospirosis, hepatozoonosis
  Round cell neoplasia
  Septicemia

Cats
  Cholangitis
  Hepatic lipidosis
  Infectious disease: for example, feline infectious peritonitis, toxoplasmosis, cytauxzoonosis
  Round cell neoplasia
  Sepsis

Posthepatic

Bile duct neoplasia

Cholecystitis

Cholelithiasis

Gall bladder mucocele

Pancreatitis/pancreatic neoplasia

Traumatic rupture of bile duct or gallbladder

---

functional mass. The sensitivity of plasma ammonia for the detection of congenital portosystemic shunts has been reported to be 81% to 100% in dogs and 83% in cats.[23,24] Hyperammonemia is generally considered specific for hepatic insufficiency or portosystemic shunting. However, occasionally urea-cycle enzyme deficiencies can also cause increased blood ammonia concentrations. These enzyme deficiencies can be hereditary as a result of the absence of a particular enzyme or secondary to cobalamin or arginine deficiency.[25,26] Arginine deficiency may occur in cats with hepatic lipidosis and may contribute to hyperammonemia in this setting. Ammonia plays a central role in the pathogenesis of hepatic encephalopathy and thus is a useful marker for this condition. However, the plasma ammonia concentration of a patient with hepatic encephalopathy can be normal, and ammonia is not predictive of the severity of signs in individual patients.[27] In contrast, plasma ammonia concentration can be increased in patients without overt signs of hepatic encephalopathy, which in the opinion of the authors, should nonetheless be addressed therapeutically. Ammonia tolerance tests have been investigated in an attempt to increase the sensitivity of ammonia measurement for detecting hepatic insufficiency and portosystemic shunting. The oral administration of ammonium salts can cause vomiting and potentially worsen signs of hepatic encephalopathy. Ammonium chloride or sulfate can also be given rectally, which is less likely to produce adverse effects. However, ammonia tolerance testing is not commonly performed in the United States because there is a theoretic potential to induce worsening of hepatic encephalopathy.

It must be pointed out that ammonia is not very stable in plasma samples. Therefore, blood samples should be collected into prechilled tubes and analyzed within 30 minutes of collection. Thus, an in-house analyzer is needed to reliably measure plasma ammonia concentration.

Bile acids

Bile acids are amphipathic steroids synthesized from cholesterol in the liver and are the major constituent of bile. Through micelle formation, bile acids enhance solubilization of lipids within the intestine, facilitating digestion and absorption of fats and lipid-soluble vitamins. Serum bile acids often are used to assess hepatic function in dogs and cats. Serum bile acids are measured as a preprandial sample (after withholding food for 12 hours) or by collecting paired preprandial and 2-hour postprandial samples (provocative bile acids testing). Both of these tests are simple to perform and safe. The samples submitted for testing are stable at room temperature facilitating outside laboratory evaluation. However, lipemia or hemolysis can interfere with the assay. Patients that have had a cholecystectomy or have ileal disease may have unreliable results. Increases in fasting or postprandial serum bile acids concentrations are consistent with hepatic dysfunction, portosystemic shunting, or cholestasis. Thus, serum bile acids concentrations should not be evaluated in patients with other evidence of cholestasis, such as increased serum bilirubin concentrations. Spontaneous gallbladder contraction may occur during the fasting period and can result in a fasting value exceeding the postprandial sample; however, both values should be within the reference internal for the postprandial value in order to make this determination. The primary clinical use of serum bile acids measurement is to assess hepatic function in patients suspected to have hepatic disease with serum bilirubin concentrations that are within the reference interval. The measurement of postprandial serum bile acid concentrations does not have an advantage over fasting serum bile acid concentrations, but the sensitivity of the assay can be increased by collecting both paired preprandial and 2-hour postprandial samples.[22] Studies have shown that serum bile acid concentrations are useful for diagnosing hepatobiliary diseases, including portosystemic shunts in dogs and cats.[22,24] For diagnosis of hepatobiliary disease, the specificity of preprandial bile acids concentrations is 100% at values greater than 20 μmol/L and that of postprandial bile acids concentrations is 100% at values greater than 25 μmol/L.[22] A study found the sensitivity of fasting serum bile acids concentration for diagnosing portosystemic shunts (cutoff value of 20 μmol/L) to be 93% for dogs and 100% for cats. The sensitivity of serum bile acids concentrations for detecting hepatic insufficiency is lower than that for detecting portosystemic shunts. Because of different techniques and assays used, normal values must be established for each laboratory.

Markers of hepatic synthetic function

Hepatobiliary disease can result in decreased protein synthesis as well as altered glucose, urea, and lipid metabolism. A reduction of approximately 70% to 80% of hepatic function must be present before these biochemical abnormalities can be observed. Thus, these disturbances are not considered sensitive indicators for the diagnosis of hepatobiliary disease. Furthermore, changes in these analytes also occur due to other nonhepatic disease processes.

The liver plays a central role in lipid metabolism, including the synthesis of cholesterol. Serum cholesterol concentrations can be increased, normal, or decreased in patients with hepatobiliary disease. Decreases in serum cholesterol concentration can occur in patients with severe hepatic insufficiency and acquired or congenital portosystemic shunting due to impaired hepatic synthesis. Additional causes of hypocholesterolemia include gastrointestinal disease resulting in malabsorption or maldigestion, decreased dietary intake, and hypoadrenocorticism. Serum cholesterol concentrations within the reference interval are commonly observed in patients with various hepatobiliary disorders, and hypercholesterolemia may or may not be noted in patients with cholestasis. Abnormal serum cholesterol concentrations are not sensitive or specific for hepatobiliary disease in dogs or cats as increases or decreases can also occur with endocrinopathies, obesity, protein-losing nephropathy, protein-losing enteropathy, pancreatitis, or primary hyperlipidemias.

The liver also plays a central role in carbohydrate metabolism. The liver is responsible for glycogen storage, conversion of galactose and fructose to glucose, gluconeogenesis, and the synthesis of many compounds using carbohydrates as a substrate. Blood glucose measurement is not a sensitive or specific marker for liver disease. The liver has a large reserve capacity for gluconeogenesis. Consequently, hepatic insufficiency must be severe before hypoglycemia occurs. Also, hypoglycemia occurs in a subset of patients with congenital portosystemic shunts. Hypoglycemia can also occur as a paraneoplastic syndrome due to the release of insulin-like substances. A variety of extrahepatic conditions can also lead to hypoglycemia.

The liver plays a central role in protein metabolism and is responsible for the synthesis of plasma proteins, deamination of amino acids, conversion of ammonia to urea, and amino acid synthesis. These functions can be compromised in patients with hepatic disease. Albumin is a plasma protein synthesized exclusively by the liver. Serum albumin concentrations are maintained by an equal rate of hepatic synthesis and protein degradation. There are several disorders that can result in mild decreases in serum albumin concentrations, but severe hypoalbuminemia (<2 g/dL) occurs most commonly with hepatic insufficiency, protein-losing enteropathy, protein-losing nephropathy, and severe exudative skin disease. Because of the large synthetic reserve capacity of the liver for albumin, severe hypoalbuminemia is a relatively insensitive marker for hepatobiliary disease and is likely to be seen predominantly in cases with advanced hepatic failure or portosystemic shunts.

Coagulation factors (with the exception of factor VIII), anticoagulation factors, and the fibrinolytic protein plasminogen are all synthesized by the liver (see Karen Dirksen and Hille Fieten's article, "Canine Copper-Associated Hepatitis," in this issue). The liver is also the site of activation of the vitamin K–dependent clotting factors: II, VII, IX, X, and protein C. In addition, bile acids are needed to emulsify fat and aid in the absorption of fat-soluble vitamins, including vitamin K from the intestines. Vitamin K malabsorption may develop secondary to cholestasis, and thus, hepatobiliary disease can affect hemostasis along multiple pathways. Coagulation parameter abnormalities have been reported for specific clotting factor activities, prothrombin time, activated partial thromboplastin time, proteins induced in the absence of vitamin K, fibrin degradation products, fibrinogen, and/or protein C activity.[28–33] Coagulation abnormalities are not specific for or diagnostic of hepatobiliary disease, but disturbances in coagulation parameters can occur in hepatobiliary disorders. Disseminated intravascular coagulopathy is not uncommon in patients with liver disease and can be difficult to distinguish from a coagulopathy due to decreased hepatobiliary function. The assessment of a patient's coagulation status is considered the standard of care particularly when an invasive procedure such as a liver biopsy or esophageal feeding tube placement is being considered.

HEMATOLOGY

Patients with hepatobiliary disorders may exhibit erythrocyte morphologic abnormalities or anemia. There are no hematological abnormalities however that are specific for hepatobiliary disease.

Erythrocyte morphologic changes reported in patients with hepatobiliary disorders are characterized by poikilocytosis, which includes acanthocytes, echinocytes, target cells, and stomatocytes.[34] Phospholipid metabolism abnormalities and decreased tolerance to oxidative stress are thought to be responsible for most of these changes. The presence of schistocytes in patients with hepatic disease may result from microangiopathic changes that occur in the presence of disseminated intravascular coagulation or hepatic neoplasia.

Patients with hepatobiliary disease may develop an acute anemia secondary to blood loss that occurs following an invasive procedure or due to gastrointestinal hemorrhage. In addition, these patients are also susceptible to a nonregenerative normocytic normochromic anemia of chronic disease due to altered iron metabolism. Chronic blood loss can result in an iron-deficiency anemia characterized by microcytosis and hypochromia.

Changes in the thrombogram are occasionally observed in hepatobiliary disease. Thrombocytopenia may occur due to decreased production of thrombopoietin or a consumptive coagulopathy. In addition, infectious diseases affecting the liver, such as leptospirosis, may result in thrombocytopenia.[35]

URINALYSIS

The urine-specific gravity of patients with hepatic disease can be decreased due to an inability to fully concentrate urine. The decreased concentrating ability also leads to polyuria. In addition, hepatic encephalopathy can be associated with polydipsia.

Bilirubinuria and urate urolithiasis or crystalluria may also indicate the presence of hepatobiliary disease. Bilirubin is commonly measured semiquantitatively in canine and feline urine with a urine dipstick. Bilirubinuria (<2+ on a dipstick) can be a normal finding in dogs, especially male dogs. Bilirubinuria in dogs without hemolytic disease or hepatobiliary disease can occur as a consequence of the loss of unconjugated bilirubin that is bound to albumin in proteinuric patients or the conjugation and production of bilirubin in renal tubular cells. Cats have a much higher renal threshold for bilirubin than dogs, and any degree of bilirubinuria warrants investigation into hepatic or hemolytic disease in this species. Ammonium biurate crystalluria can be detected in the urine sediment of dog and cats with hepatobiliary disease. Allantoin is normally generated from uric acid due to the activity of hepatic urate oxidase. A deficiency of hepatic urate oxidase in patients with hepatobiliary disease may lead to increased serum concentrations of uric acid and with concurrent hyperammonemia, ammonium biurate crystalluria can occur. Ammonium biurate crystalluria has been detected in 40% to 70% of dogs and 15% of cats with portosystemic shunts.[36]

NOVEL BIOMARKERS OF HEPATIC DISEASE

Protein C is a vitamin K–dependent protein zymogen, synthesized in the liver with an important role in coagulation. Plasma protein C determination has been reported to aid in the diagnosis of liver disease.[32] Clinical studies of dogs with congenital portal vascular anomalies indicate that protein C is a noninvasive measure of portal blood flow with a role in distinguishing portosystemic shunting from microvascular dysplasia. Protein C activity greater than 70% of the pool is suggestive of microvascular dysplasia and not congenital portosystemic shunting. A protein C activity that increases to 70% or greater after corrective surgery for portosystemic shunting suggests restoration of portal blood flow.

MicroRNAs are a type of small noncoding RNAs that regulate posttranscriptional gene expression.[37] Various studies have demonstrated the ability of microRNAs of hepatic origin as stable and sensitive noninvasive biomarkers of hepatocellular injury in animal models and in human patients with normal or increased serum ALT concentrations. Several of these studies have indicated that hepatocyte-derived microRNAs have a higher sensitivity than serum ALT for hepatocellular injury.[38–40] A recent study in Labrador retrievers found microRNA-122 to be highly sensitive and specific for the detection of hepatocellular injury with the ability to identify more patients with hepatocellular injury than ALT activity.[41] MicroRNA-122 was also found to be able to identify patients will high hepatic copper concentrations but normal ALT activity.[41]

Hyaluronic acid is a nonsulfated glycosaminoglycan distributed in connective tissue and is one of the chief components of the extracellular matrix. Hyaluronic acid has been evaluated as a serologic biomarker for hepatic fibrosis with reported sensitivities for distinguishing patients with no to mild fibrosis from those with moderate to severe fibrosis of 75% to 87% and specificities of 80% to 100%.[42] Preliminary studies suggest that serum hyaluronic acid may also have utility for the diagnosis of canine hepatic fibrosis. A study in dogs with liver disease found dogs with cirrhotic liver disease to have higher serum concentrations of hyaluronic acid than those with noncirrhotic liver disease, healthy dogs, or dogs with extrahepatic disease.[43]

The FibroVet test has recently been developed (Echosens). This index combines patient age, sex, and several biochemical parameters in a proprietary algorithm. A study reported as a research abstract reported this index to have a negative predictive value for the diagnosis of moderate fibrosis of 90% to 100%, and the ability to differentiate dogs with fibrosis with a positive predictive value of 90% to 100%.[44]

REFERENCES

1. Friedrichs KR, Harr KE, Freeman KP, et al. ASVCP reference interval guidelines: determination of de novo reference intervals in veterinary species and other related topics. Vet Clin Pathol 2012;41(4):441–53.

2. Ruaux CG, Carney PC, Suchodolski JS, et al. Estimates of biological variation in routinely measured biochemical analytes in clinically healthy dogs. Vet Clin Pathol 2012;41(4):541–7.

3. Ozer J, Ratner M, Shaw M, et al. The current state of serum biomarkers of hepatotoxicity. Toxicology 2008;245(3):194–205.

4. Lemasters JJ, Gores GJ, Nieminen AL, et al. Multiparameter digitized video microscopy of toxic and hypoxic injury in single cells. Environ Health Perspect 1990;84:83–94.

5. Solter PF. Clinical pathology approaches to hepatic injury. Toxicol Pathol 2005; 33(1):9–16.

6. Yang RZ, Blaileanu G, Hansen BC, et al. cDNA cloning, genomic structure, chromosomal mapping, and functional expression of a novel human alanine aminotransferase. Genomics 2002;79(3):445–50.

7. Lindblom P, Rafter I, Copley C, et al. Isoforms of alanine aminotransferases in human tissues and serum-differential tissue expression using novel antibodies. Arch Biochem Biophys 2007;466(1):66–77.

8. Ennulat D, Walker D, Clemo F, et al. Effects of hepatic drug-metabolizing enzyme induction on clinical pathology parameters in animals and man. Toxicol Pathol 2010;38(5):810–28.

9. Stockham SL, Scott MA. Enzymes. In: Thrall MA, editor. Fundamentals of veterinary clinical pathology. 2nd edition. Ames (IA): Iowa State Press; 2002. p. 639–75. Chapter 12.

10. Comazzi S, Pieralisi C, Bertazzolo W. Haematological and biochemical abnormalities in canine blood: frequency and associations in 1022 samples. J Small Anim Pract 2004;45(7):343–9.

11. Lidbury JA, Steiner JM. Liver-diagnostic evaluation. In: Washabau RJ, Day MJ, editors. Canine & feline gastroenterology. St Louis (MO): Elsevier; 2013. p. 863–75. Chapter 61.

12. Chapman SE, Hostutler RA. A laboratory diagnostic approach to hepatobiliary disease in small animals. Vet Clin North Am Small Anim Pract 2013;43(6): 1209–25.

13. Kutzler MA, Solter PF, Hoffman WE, et al. Characterization and localization of alkaline phosphatase in canine seminal plasma and gonadal tissues. Theriogenology 2003;60(2):299–306.

14. Sanecki RK, Hoffmann WE, Dorner JL, et al. Purification and comparison of corticosteroid-induced and intestinal isoenzymes of alkaline phosphatase in dogs. Am J Vet Res 1990;51(12):1964–8.

15. Solter PF, Hoffmann WE. Solubilization of liver alkaline phosphatase isoenzyme during cholestasis in dogs. Am J Vet Res 1999;60(8):1010–5.

16. Penn R, Worthington DJ. Is serum gamma-glutamyltransferase a misleading test? Br Med J (Clin Res Ed) 1983;286(6364):531–5.

17. Chapman SE, Hostutler RA. A laboratory diagnostic approach to hepatobiliary disease in small animals. Clin Lab Med 2015;35(3):503–19.

18. Iyanagi T, Emi Y, Ikushiro S. Biochemical and molecular aspects of genetic disorders of bilirubin metabolism. Biochim Biophys Acta 1998;1407(3):173–84.

19. Gautam A, Seligson H, Gordon ER, et al. Irreversible binding of conjugated bilirubin to albumin in cholestatic rats. J Clin Invest 1984;73(3):873–7.

20. Summerskill WH, Wolpert E. Ammonia metabolism in the gut. Am J Clin Nutr 1970;23(5):633–9.

21. Souba WW, Smith RJ, Wilmore DW. Glutamine metabolism by the intestinal tract. JPEN J Parenter Enteral Nutr 1985;9(5):608–17.

22. Center SA, ManWarren T, Slater MR, et al. Evaluation of twelve-hour preprandial and two-hour postprandial serum bile acids concentrations for diagnosis of hepatobiliary disease in dogs. J Am Vet Med Assoc 1991;199(2):217–26.

23. Gerritzen-Bruning MJ, van den Ingh TS, Rothuizen J. Diagnostic value of fasting plasma ammonia and bile acid concentrations in the identification of portosystemic shunting in dogs. J Vet Intern Med 2006;20(1):13–9.

24. Ruland K, Fischer A, Hartmann K. Sensitivity and specificity of fasting ammonia and serum bile acids in the diagnosis of portosystemic shunts in dogs and cats. Vet Clin Pathol 2010;39(1):57–64.

25. Battersby IA, Giger U, Hall EJ. Hyperammonaemic encephalopathy secondary to selective cobalamin deficiency in a juvenile Border collie. J Small Anim Pract 2005;46(7):339–44.

26. Morris JG, Rogers QR. Ammonia intoxication in the near-adult cat as a result of a dietary deficiency of arginine. Science 1978;199(4327):431–2.

27. Rothuizen J, van den Ingh TS. Arterial and venous ammonia concentrations in the diagnosis of canine hepato-encephalopathy. Res Vet Sci 1982;33(1):17–21.

28. Badylak SF, Dodds WJ, Van Vleet JF. Plasma coagulation factor abnormalities in dogs with naturally occurring hepatic disease. Am J Vet Res 1983;44(12): 2336–40.

29. Lisciandro SC, Hohenhaus A, Brooks M. Coagulation abnormalities in 22 cats with naturally occurring liver disease. J Vet Intern Med 1998;12(2):71–5.

30. Prins M, Schellens CJ, van Leeuwen MW, et al. Coagulation disorders in dogs with hepatic disease. Vet J 2010;185(2):163–8.

31. Mount ME, Kim BU, Kass PH. Use of a test for proteins induced by vitamin K absence or antagonism in diagnosis of anticoagulant poisoning in dogs: 325 cases (1987-1997). J Am Vet Med Assoc 2003;222(2):194–8.

32. Toulza O, Center SA, Brooks MB, et al. Evaluation of plasma protein C activity for detection of hepatobiliary disease and portosystemic shunting in dogs. J Am Vet Med Assoc 2006;229(11):1761–71.

33. Center SA, Warner K, Corbett J, et al. Proteins invoked by vitamin K absence and clotting times in clinically ill cats. J Vet Intern Med 2000;14(3):292–7.

34. Christopher MM, Lee SE. Red cell morphologic alterations in cats with hepatic disease. Vet Clin Pathol 1994;23(1):7–12.

35. Goldstein RE, Lin RC, Langston CE, et al. Influence of infecting serogroup on clinical features of leptospirosis in dogs. J Vet Intern Med 2006;20(3):489–94.

36. Center SA, Magne ML. Historical, physical examination, and clinicopathologic features of portosystemic vascular anomalies in the dog and cat. Semin Vet Med Surg (Small Anim) 1990;5(2):83–93.

37. Bartel DP. MicroRNAs: target recognition and regulatory functions. Cell 2009; 136(2):215–33.

38. Wang K, Zhang S, Marzolf B, et al. Circulating microRNAs, potential biomarkers for drug-induced liver injury. Proc Natl Acad Sci U S A 2009;106(11):4402–7.

39. Laterza OF, Lim L, Garrett-Engele PW, et al. Plasma microRNAs as sensitive and specific biomarkers of tissue injury. Clin Chem 2009;55(11):1977–83.

40. van der Meer AJ, Farid WR, Sonneveld MJ, et al. Sensitive detection of hepatocellular injury in chronic hepatitis C patients with circulating hepatocyte-derived microRNA-122. J Viral Hepat 2013;20(3):158–66.

41. Dirksen K, Verzijl T, van den Ingh TS, et al. Hepatocyte-derived microRNAs as sensitive serum biomarkers of hepatocellular injury in Labrador retrievers. Vet J 2016;211:75–81.

42. Plebani M, Basso D. Non-invasive assessment of chronic liver and gastric diseases. Clin Chim Acta 2007;381(1):39–49.

43. Kanemoto H, Ohno K, Nakashima K, et al. Characterization of canine focal liver lesions with contrast-enhanced ultrasound using a novel contrast agent-sonazoid. Vet Radiol Ultrasound 2009;50(2):188–94.

44. Lecoindre A, Lecoindre P, Chevallier M, et al. A new combination of blood parameters for accurate non-invasive diagnosis of liver fibrosis in dogs. J Vet Intern Med 2016;29:1197.

Diagnostic Imaging of the Hepatobiliary System
An Update

Angela J. Marolf, DVM

KEYWORDS

- Computed tomography • CT • Magnetic resonance imaging • MRI
- Contrast-enhanced ultrasound • Elastography • Liver • Biliary

KEY POINTS

- Computed tomography (CT) and MRI are useful in the evaluation of liver and biliary tract disorders.
- The use of intravenous contrast with CT and MRI provides additional information that can aid in distinguishing different disease processes.
- The lack of superimposition of adjacent stomach and bowel gas, as well as decreased operator dependence of these imaging modalities, leads to more accurate assessments of the cranial abdomen.
- Advanced techniques in ultrasound of the hepatobiliary system may be useful in the evaluation of liver and biliary tract disorders.

INTRODUCTION

Abdominal radiography and ultrasound have been performed in dogs and cats for evaluation of liver and biliary abnormalities for many years in veterinary medicine. Abdominal ultrasound, in particular, has been used for diagnosis of biliary tract and parenchymal liver diseases. Ultrasound imaging is very sensitive at identifying liver and biliary abnormalities but often lacks specificity, and cytology or histology are required for definitive diagnosis. Advantages to abdominal ultrasound include the ability to perform the study on awake or sedated patients, use of nonionizing sound waves, and the ability of ultrasound to distinguish fluid and soft tissue changes. Disadvantages to sonographically evaluating the liver and biliary system include similarity in the appearance of different disease processes, incomplete assessment of the organs due to deep-chested body conformation or overlying stomach and bowel gas,

Disclosure Statement: The author has nothing to disclose.
Department of Environmental and Radiological Health Sciences, College of Veterinary Medicine and Biomedical Sciences, Colorado State University, 300 West Drake Road, Fort Collins, CO 80523-1620, USA
E-mail address: angela.marolf@colostate.edu

Vet Clin Small Anim 47 (2017) 555–568
http://dx.doi.org/10.1016/j.cvsm.2016.11.006
0195-5616/17/© 2016 Elsevier Inc. All rights reserved.

vetsmall.theclinics.com

or poor patient compliance during the study. Additionally, ultrasound is highly operator dependent, and thorough evaluation of these organs can be limited due to the experience level of the sonographer.

Newer techniques in ultrasound imaging include use of contrast agents and elastography for evaluation of the liver parenchyma. Contrast agents use microbubbles that resonate with appropriate ultrasound settings and create changes in organ parenchymal echogenicity, increasing the conspicuity of lesions.[1-4] Elastography evaluates the firmness of tissues and can detect differences in normal and abnormal tissue.[5,6] These 2 advances can be used to differentiate benign from malignant lesions. Disadvantages of ultrasound contrast agents include increased cost and short half-life; elastography requires special software that needs to be purchased.

MRI and computed tomography (CT) of the abdomen have been performed in people for years to assess the hepatobiliary system. These 2 imaging modalities are considered the preferred method to diagnose many conditions, including biliary tract abnormalities and various liver and pancreatic disorders, including inflammation and neoplasia.[7-13]

With the increased availability of CT and MR scanners in veterinary hospitals, these imaging modalities are more readily available for diagnosis of abdominal diseases in dogs and cats. The ability to image veterinary patients without superimposition of other organs or bowel gas, as well as to perform a complete assessment of the biliary tree and liver, offer distinct advantages over current imaging methods. With the advent and increased availability of multislice CT scanners, the speed at which CT studies can be performed has increased and sedating rather than anesthetizing animals for some studies is now a possibility. Both CT and MRI use intravenous contrast to better evaluate the blood flow to organs and adjacent tissues. CT imaging uses iodinated contrast agents and MRI uses gadolinium contrast agents.

MRI offers excellent contrast resolution of the soft tissues and provides multiple anatomic planes to visualize organs in the abdomen. The term "intensity" is used to describe tissue characteristics and appearance on various sequences. Tissues that are bright are hyperintense, dark tissues are hypointense, and tissues of a similar intensity are isointense.

Standard imaging sequences obtained in MRI include T1-weighted and T2-weighted sequences, which demonstrate the molecular differences in various tissues and can detect abnormalities due to differences in tissue appearance in the sequences. Fluids are typically hypointense on T1-weighted images and hyperintense on T2-weighted images. An additional technique often used in MR abdominal imaging is called "fat saturation." This technique makes fat appear hypointense on T1-weighted and T2-weighted images and can highlight inflammation and edema in tissues. Disadvantages to MRI are the need for general anesthesia, added expense, and decreased availability compared with ultrasound and CT.

CT imaging provides excellent contrast resolution of soft tissues and bones. Multiple planes can be reconstructed with CT imaging, allowing for visualization of all anatomic structures in the abdomen. With the ability to perform multiplanar reconstructions (a commercially available software imaging tool), the liver and biliary tract can be evaluated in dorsal and sagittal imaging planes in unlimited angles for thorough assessment.

CT terminology uses the term "attenuation" to describe tissue characteristics. Tissues that are bright will be hyperattenuating, dark tissues will be hypoattenuating, and similar tissues will be isoattenuating to each other. Fluids are typically hypoattenuating. Disadvantages to CT imaging include the use of ionizing radiation, added expense, need for anesthesia or sedation, and decreased availability compared with ultrasound.

This article familiarizes readers with current uses of MRI, CT, and advanced ultra-sound techniques for the liver and biliary system in dogs and cats.

MRI AND COMPUTED TOMOGRAPHY OF THE NORMAL LIVER AND BILIARY SYSTEM

On MRI, the normal liver is uniformly hypointense relative to the spleen on T1-weighted and T2-weighted sequences with homogeneous contrast enhancement of the parenchyma. The gallbladder and common bile duct are homogeneously hyperintense on T2-weighted images and hypointense on T1-weighted images due to bile being stored within the gallbladder and coursing through the common bile duct (**Fig. 1**). The normal common bile duct may not be identified because of its small size, but the gallbladder wall and evidence of internal contents can be assessed. Additionally, the margins of the liver and subjective size should be evaluated. Normal liver margins are smooth.

On CT imaging, the normal liver is isoattenuating to the spleen with a hypoattenuating gallbladder due to storage of bile. The liver parenchyma uniformly contrast enhances. The normal common bile duct may not be seen due to its small size and lack of enhancement; however, the gallbladder wall thickness and intraluminal biliary contents can be evaluated as in MRI. The bile should be hypoattenuating with no evidence of internal contents, such as debris or calculi. To specifically evaluate the hepatic arteries and portal veins, CT angiography must be performed, which is a timed bolus of intravenous contrast followed by multiple specifically timed scans to capture the arterial, venous, and delayed phases of contrast passage through the organ.[14,15] When all 3 phases are captured, this is termed a 3-phase angiogram (**Fig. 2**). With the ability to perform multiplanar reconstructions, the liver and biliary tract can be evaluated in multiple imaging planes (**Fig. 3**).

ABNORMAL CONDITIONS OF THE LIVER AND BILIARY SYSTEM
Neoplasia of the Liver and Biliary Tract

Primary liver neoplasia is relatively uncommon in dogs and cats; metastatic liver nodules and masses from other organ neoplasia are more common.[16] In cats, bile duct adenoma/cystadenoma and bile duct carcinoma/cystadenocarcinoma are more common than in dogs, and these masses are often benign in older cats.[17] Ultrasound is usually performed for initial imaging of the liver; however, there is overlap in the appearance of different neoplastic and inflammatory processes.[18,19] Further

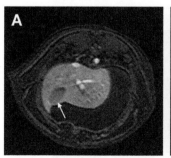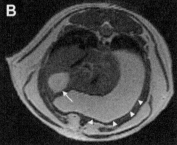

Fig. 1. (*A*) Transverse postcontrast T1-weighted MRI of a feline normal liver. Note the hypointense fluid within the gallbladder (*arrow*). Contrast is present in the aorta, caudal vena cava, and hepatic veins. (*B*) Transverse T2-weighted image of a normal liver. Note the hyperintense fluid within the gallbladder (*arrow*). A large amount of hyperintense falciform fat is ventral to the liver (*arrowheads*).

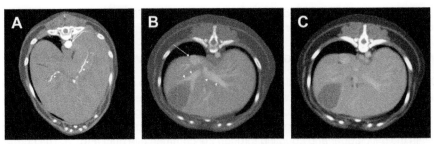

Fig. 2. (*A*) Transverse CT angiographic images of a normal canine liver. Arterial phase image shows thin, linear contrast enhancement of the hepatic arteries (*arrowheads*) and aorta (*arrow*). The liver parenchyma is fairly homogeneous in appearance. (*B*) Venous phase image shows contrast enhancement of the hepatic veins (*arrowheads*) and caudal vena cava (*arrow*). Note the hypoattenuating bile in the gallbladder. (*C*) Delayed phase image. There is still contrast filling the hepatic veins and caudal vena cava but there is less than in the venous phase. There is mild diffuse increased attenuation of the liver parenchyma.

characterization of liver masses, staging, and surgical planning are reasons to perform cross-sectional imaging with either CT or MRI for suspected liver masses based on abdominal ultrasound or radiographs. Establishing imaging characteristics of primary liver tumors, such as adenocarcinoma, carcinoma, hemangiosarcoma, and biliary carcinomas compared with benign conditions, such as nodular hyperplasia or adenomas, could assist in making diagnoses noninvasively. Also, evaluation of the liver for metastasis, and the appearance of these lesions is important. In people, CT and MRI are preferred for diagnosis and staging of liver tumors.[20]

Size, shape, and margination of masses and nodules should be noted; however, these characteristics cannot definitively differentiate tumor types. Several studies in dogs have looked at the CT characteristics of liver masses.[21–24] Two of these studies used CT angiographic methods to evaluate the arterial, venous, and delayed phases to assess tumor type.[22,24] Both studies evaluated hepatocellular carcinomas and nodular hyperplasia. The hepatocellular carcinomas had different enhancement patterns compared with benign lesions, including hypoattenuation in the later phases

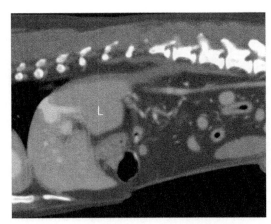

Fig. 3. Sagittal plane reconstruction of the normal canine liver (L) in venous phase of the angiographic study.

and heterogeneous, marginal, or central arterial contrast enhancement (**Fig. 4**). Nodular hyperplasia had a diffuse enhancement pattern in the arterial phase and was isoattenuating to normal liver in the delayed phase. Liver metastatic lesions were also reviewed in one of the studies and were found to be hypoattenuating in both arterial and delayed phases (**Fig. 5**).[24] These differences can potentially be used to distinguish liver masses and metastases noninvasively and assist in therapeutic planning.

A more recent retrospective study evaluated dual-phase CT imaging in dogs with liver and splenic masses.[21] Dual-phase CT examinations acquired images in early (<30 seconds) and delayed phases (>60 seconds) after intravenous contrast administration.[21] This study did not find any significant differences in enhancement patterns of malignant and benign liver lesions with this imaging technique.

MRI of the liver and liver masses also has been performed in dogs and cats. MRI of hepatic lesions using standard gadolinium contrast has shown good sensitivity and

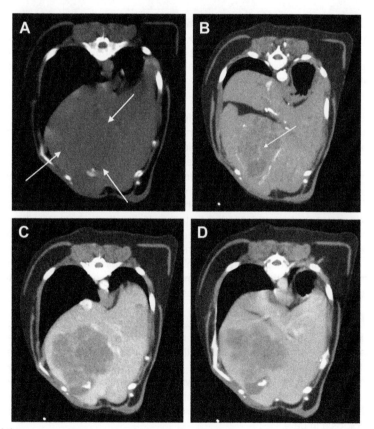

Fig. 4. (*A*) Transverse CT precontrast image of a canine liver with a confirmed hepatocellular carcinoma. Note the ill-defined hypoattenuating region in the right ventral liver (*arrows*). (*B*) Arterial phase. Note the heterogeneous contrast enhancement internally within the poorly defined mass (*arrow*). (*C*) Venous phase. Note that the mass is becoming more hypoattenuating as the surrounding liver parenchyma shows increased enhancement. (*D*) Delayed phase. The liver mass shows further hypoattenuation consistent with hepatocellular adenocarcinoma CT characteristics.

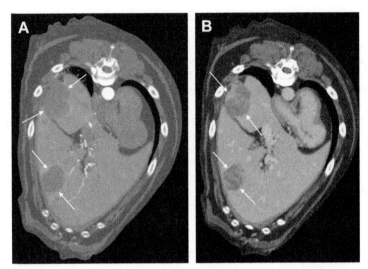

Fig. 5. (*A*) Transverse CT images of a liver with metastasis from a dog with a known adrenal adenocarcinoma. Arterial phase. Note the hypoattenuating nodules in the liver (*arrows*). (*B*) Delayed phase. Note the hypoattenuating nodules in the liver (*arrows*). These lesions have consistent CT features of metastasis.

specificity for differentiating malignant from benign lesions.[25] Malignant lesions tended to be more heterogeneous and have different enhancement patterns than the surrounding normal liver or benign lesions.[25]

Newer contrast agents that target the hepatobiliary system have been evaluated in dogs.[26–28] These contrast agents are administered intravenously, have a vascular phase, and then concentrate in normal hepatocytes during the later hepatobiliary phase.[29] This allows for normal liver to enhance while lesions that lack normal hepatocytes do not enhance and are hypointense. Using these liver-specific contrast agents, malignant liver masses are characterized by hypointensity in the hepatobiliary phase, enabling tumor characterization noninvasively.[27,28] With the use of newer contrast agents, the conspicuity and number of liver metastases have been shown to increase compared with other imaging methods.[28] This would allow for better staging of patients with primary tumors diagnosed elsewhere in the body.

Hepatic Lipidosis

Hepatic lipidosis is the most common liver disorder in cats.[30] Ultrasound is frequently performed to evaluate the liver in cats with suspected hepatic lipidosis. The liver is often diffusely hyperechoic and can look similar to other disease processes, such as lymphoma and diabetes mellitus. CT evaluation of the liver in cats has been evaluated to determine normal fat content within the liver and in livers with hepatic lipidosis.[31,32] Mixed results have been shown, and CT is not currently used for diagnosis of hepatic lipidosis in cats.

Inflammation of the Liver and Biliary Tract

Inflammation of the biliary tract is more common in cats than in dogs. This may be due to the unique ductal anatomy of cats in which the common bile duct and pancreatic duct both open onto the major duodenal papilla.[33] This relationship may allow for infection or inflammation to spread from one area, such as the intestinal tract, into the pancreas and biliary system. As such, cholangitis is second only to hepatic lipidosis as the most common liver disease in cats.[30] Ultrasound is typically performed to evaluate dogs and cats with suspected inflammatory liver conditions. However, because there is much overlap in the sonographic changes that can occur with different disease processes, histology is still recommended for definitive diagnosis.[34,35]

Dogs and cats can be diagnosed with acute or chronic forms of hepatitis. With all imaging modalities, liver size, margination, and parenchymal changes can be used to assess the liver. In chronic forms of hepatitis, the liver may be small, irregularly marginated, and have a heterogeneous parenchyma (**Fig. 6**). With acute hepatitis, the liver may be of normal size or enlarged and have a normal or abnormal parenchymal appearance. Biliary tract inflammation can manifest as thickening of the gallbladder wall, gallbladder intraluminal contents, and/or dilation of the biliary tract. Changes in hepatic parenchymal contrast enhancement may be identified with CT or MRI. Determining the specific type of acute or chronic hepatitis requires definitive diagnosis with histology.

MR and CT imaging are commonly used in people to diagnose inflammatory conditions in the liver and biliary tract.[9–11,36] A unique MR sequence named MR cholangiography (MRCP) highlights fluid within the biliary tract and pancreatic ducts to diagnose intrahepatic and extrahepatic biliary tract inflammation or obstruction, fluid-filled structures, or inflammation of the pancreas (**Fig. 7**).[9,10,36] In normal dogs, MRCP has been studied and deemed feasible.[37] MR has been used to assess liver, biliary, and pancreatic inflammation in cats.[38,39] The hepatic parenchymal changes were nonspecific; however, biliary tract changes, such as hyperintense intraluminal gallbladder contents/debris, gallbladder wall enhancement, and increased wall thickness were indicators of gallbladder and biliary tract inflammation (**Fig. 8**).[38]

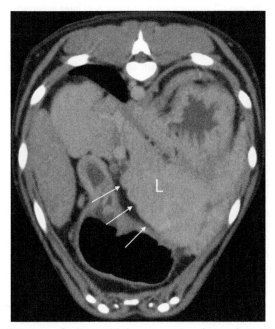

Fig. 6. Transverse CT image of a liver with known canine chronic hepatitis. Delayed phase. Note the irregular liver margins (*arrows*) and poor enhancement of the liver (L).

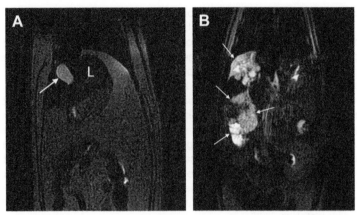

Fig. 7. (*A*) MR MRCP sequence in dorsal imaging plane of a feline liver and gallbladder. Note how the liver (L) and other organs are hypointense and the bile within the gallbladder is hyperintense (*arrow*). Fluid is bright on this sequence for easier evaluation of fluid within the biliary tract and pancreatic ducts. (*B*) Same sequence and plane of the liver and cranial abdomen. The lobulated, hyperintense masses within the liver (*arrows*) are biliary cystadenomas. Because these are predominantly fluid-filled masses, they are hyperintense on this sequence.

Intraluminal calculi in the gallbladder and biliary tract are not common in dogs and cats. However, calculi can be diagnosed by CT and MRI (**Fig. 9**).

In CT imaging, cholangiographic contrast agents are used to highlight the biliary tract.[11,40] CT cholangiography also has been studied in normal dogs and produced high-quality images of the hepatobiliary system.[41] Further studies are needed to determine the utility of MR and CT in diagnosing biliary and liver inflammatory conditions in dogs and cats.

Gallbladder mucoceles are another intraluminal gallbladder disease. These structures represent an abnormal accumulation of mucus that distends the gallbladder and can cause obstruction.[42] Gallbladder mucoceles often have recognizable

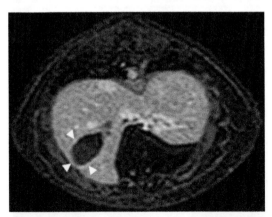

Fig. 8. Transverse MR postcontrast T1-weighted sequence of a feline liver and gallbladder. The gallbladder wall is thickened and mildly contrast enhancing (*arrowheads*). The bile is of mixed intensity, indicating debris within the bile. These changes are consistent with cholangitis and or cholecystitis.

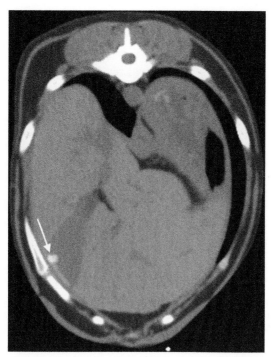

Fig. 9. Transverse precontrast CT image of a canine liver and gallbladder. Note the hyperattenuating, well-defined cholelith (*arrow*) and hyperattenuating amorphous debris in the dependent portion of the gallbladder.

sonographic features and are diagnosed readily with ultrasound.[42,43] There are no studies evaluating gallbladder mucoceles with CT or MRI in veterinary medicine.

Extrahepatic Biliary Obstruction

In dogs and cats, CT and MRI have been used in diagnosis of inflammation of the pancreas and, subsequently, extrahepatic biliary obstruction.[38,44] With both CT and MRI, the extrahepatic portion of the common bile duct can be evaluated for evidence of obstruction and dilation (**Fig. 10**). Secondary to pancreatitis, the surrounding peripancreatic tissues can show evidence of inflammation and be hyperattenuating on CT and T2 hyperintense on MRI.[38,44,45] These changes usually represent regional steatitis or peritonitis (**Fig. 11**). In a study using CT in dogs with acute abdominal signs, "fat-stranding" or increased attenuation of the mesenteric fat due to edema was identified in cases with peritonitis and pancreatitis.[45]

Portal venous thromboses can be diagnosed with CT angiography and MRI.[46] This may be caused by intimal injury and inflammatory mediators associated with pancreatitis or other conditions and has been identified in dogs with pancreatitis.[44]

Liver Fibrosis/Cirrhosis and Portal Hypertension

End-stage liver disease often results in hepatic portal hypertension, which is usually diagnosed with a combination of consistent clinical signs, imaging, or biopsy.[47] Portal hypertension alters blood flow within the portal circulation outside and inside of the liver and can be evaluated with Doppler ultrasound.[47] A recent study using a canine model for imaging liver fibrosis and cirrhosis used CT perfusion to quantitatively

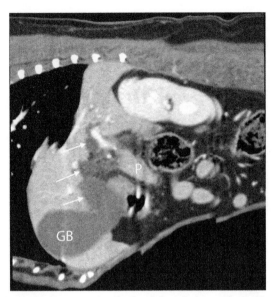

Fig. 10. Sagittal plane CT reconstruction in the delayed phase of a canine liver and dilated biliary tract. The large gallbladder (GB) and dilated common bile duct (*arrows*) are secondary to the inflammation within the pancreas (P).

assess changes in liver blood perfusion.[48] CT perfusion studies demonstrated differences in liver blood flow between normal, fibrotic, and cirrhotic livers.[48] Further studies are needed to determine the reliability of this method for evaluating liver perfusion in fibrotic and cirrhotic livers.

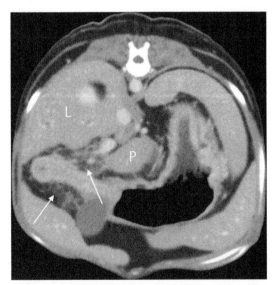

Fig. 11. Transverse angiographic CT image delayed phase of a canine liver (L) and pancreas (P). Note the peripancreatic linear hyperattenuations (*arrows*) due to fluid and inflammation secondary to pancreatitis.

ADVANCED TECHNIQUES IN ULTRASOUND OF THE HEPATOBILIARY SYSTEM
Contrast-Enhanced Ultrasound

Contrast-enhanced ultrasound uses microbubble contrast agents to detect and characterize focal organ lesions. These microbubble contrast agents come in 2 forms: blood pool agents and parenchymal agents.[2,4,49,50] The blood pool agents, such as Sonvue and Definity, remain in the intravascular space. The parenchymal agents, such as Sonazoid, have vascular phases, including arterial and portal phases, and then diffuse into the liver parenchyma where they are phagocytized by Kupffer cells of the reticuloendothelial system.[50] This phagocytosis allows the contrast agent to remain in the liver longer (minutes compared with seconds).

In veterinary medicine, these contrast agents have been studied and have shown to distinguish malignant from benign liver lesions in dogs.[1–4,50] In general, malignant liver lesions, such as metastatic nodules from hemangiosarcoma and primary liver tumors, are hypoechoic to surrounding liver in late vascular phase and parenchymal phases of contrast imaging; whereas benign lesions, such as nodular hyperplasia, are isoechoic to surrounding liver in similar phases.[1–4] In one study, these findings correlated with malignancy with a sensitivity and specificity of 100% and 89%, respectively.[50] However, some benign lesions can demonstrate contrast-enhanced findings of malignancy, so histology or cytology is still recommended for tissue type diagnosis.[50]

Recently, contrast-enhanced ultrasound has been used to assess changes in portal pressure and development of portal hypertension and perfusion changes associated with canine liver fibrosis, noninvasively.[48,51] The blood circulation and tissue perfusion changes associated with liver fibrosis were evaluated with contrast-enhanced ultrasound. In preliminary studies, changes in contrast-enhancement parameters were noted with progressive liver fibrosis.[48,51] This technique might be useful in future evaluation of portal pressure increases and perfusion changes associated with progressive liver fibrosis and development of cirrhosis.

Elastography

This is a technique used to assess the elasticity of tissue and provides information about tissue stiffness (firmness); elastography has been used in people to differentiate benign and malignant lesions, as well as to diagnose hepatic fibrosis.[5,6,52] Strain elastography qualitatively assesses tissue stiffness and can be acquired by manual compression of the tissue with transducer oscillations, which are displayed as an overlying color map based on compressibility of the underlying tissues.[6] Shear elastography allows qualitative and quantitative assessment of the mechanical properties of the tissues by applying a shear wave velocity within the tissues to measure tissue stiffness.[5] Normal shear and strain values and ratios have been established for canine and feline abdominal organs, including the liver, spleen, and kidneys.[5,6,52] With shear wave ultrasound, normal canine liver, spleen, and kidney values were affected by depth of measurement in organ, weight, and gender.[5] Additional veterinary studies are needed to determine feasibility and ability to distinguish normal tissue from abnormal lesions.

SUMMARY

MR, CT, and advanced ultrasound imaging are becoming more common in the diagnosis of hepatobiliary disorders in small animals. With the advent of multislice CT scanners, sedated examinations in veterinary patients are feasible, increasing the utility of this imaging modality. CT and MRI provide additional information for dogs and cats with hepatobiliary diseases due to lack of superimposition of structures, operator dependence, and through intravenous contrast administration. Additionally, contrast-enhanced ultrasound and elastography can provide additional information for patients with hepatic parenchymal diseases. These imaging modalities assist clinicians in a number of ways, by aiding diagnosis, prognostication, and surgical planning.

REFERENCES

1. O'Brien RT. Improved detection of metastatic hepatic hemangiosarcoma nodules with contrast ultrasound in three dogs. Vet Radiol Ultrasound 2007;48(2):146–8.
2. O'Brien RT, Iani M, Matheson J, et al. Contrast harmonic ultrasound of spontaneous liver nodules in 32 dogs. Vet Radiol Ultrasound 2004;45(6):547–53.
3. Ivancic M, Long F, Seiler GS. Contrast harmonic ultrasonography of splenic masses and associated liver nodules in dogs. J Am Vet Med Assoc 2009; 234(1):88–94.
4. Nakamura K, Takagi S, Sasaki N, et al. Contrast-enhanced ultrasonography for characterization of canine focal liver lesions. Vet Radiol Ultrasound 2010;51(1): 79–85.
5. Holdsworth A, Bradley K, Birch S, et al. Elastography of the normal canine liver, spleen and kidneys. Vet Radiol Ultrasound 2014;55(6):620–7.
6. White J, Gay J, Farnsworth R, et al. Ultrasound elastography of the liver, spleen, and kidneys in clinically normal cats. Vet Radiol Ultrasound 2014;55(4):428–34.
7. Remer EM, Baker ME. Imaging of chronic pancreatitis. Radiol Clin North Am 2002;40(6):1229–42, v.
8. Arvanitakis M, Koustiani G, Gantzarou A, et al. Staging of severity and prognosis of acute pancreatitis by computed tomography and magnetic resonance imaging—a comparative study. Dig Liver Dis 2007;39(5):473–82.
9. Palmucci S, Mauro LA, La Scola S, et al. Magnetic resonance cholangiopancreatography and contrast-enhanced magnetic resonance cholangiopancreatography versus endoscopic ultrasonography in the diagnosis of extrahepatic biliary pathology. Radiol Med 2010;115(5):732–46.
10. Maurea S, Caleo O, Mollica C, et al. Comparative diagnostic evaluation with MR cholangiopancreatography, ultrasonography and CT in patients with pancreatobiliary disease. Radiol Med 2009;114(3):390–402.
11. Saad WE, Ginat D. Computed tomography and magnetic resonance cholangiography. Tech Vasc Interv Radiol 2008;11(2):74–89.
12. Jang HJ, Yu H, Kim TK. Imaging of focal liver lesions. Semin Roentgenol 2009; 44(4):266–82.
13. Ichikawa T, Saito K, Yoshioka N, et al. Detection and characterization of focal liver lesions: a Japanese phase III, multicenter comparison between gadoxetic acid disodium-enhanced magnetic resonance imaging and contrast-enhanced computed tomography predominantly in patients with hepatocellular carcinoma and chronic liver disease. Invest Radiol 2010;45(3):133–41.
14. Caceres AV, Zwingenberger AL, Hardam E, et al. Helical computed tomographic angiography of the normal canine pancreas. Vet Radiol Ultrasound 2006;47(3): 270–8.
15. Makara M, Chau J, Hall E, et al. Effects of two contrast injection protocols on feline aortic and hepatic enhancement using dynamic computed tomography. Vet Radiol Ultrasound 2015;56(4):367–73.
16. Strombeck DR. Clinicopathologic features of primary and metastatic neoplastic disease of the liver in dogs. J Am Vet Med Assoc 1978;173(3):267–9.
17. Lawrence HJ, Erb HN, Harvey HJ. Nonlymphomatous hepatobiliary masses in cats: 41 cases (1972 to 1991). Vet Surg 1994;23(5):365–8.

18. Feeney DA, Anderson KL, Ziegler LE, et al. Statistical relevance of ultrasono-graphic criteria in the assessment of diffuse liver disease in dogs and cats. Am J Vet Res 2008;69(2):212–21.
19. Murakami T, Feeney DA, Bahr KL. Analysis of clinical and ultrasonographic data by use of logistic regression models for prediction of malignant versus benign causes of ultrasonographically detected focal liver lesions in dogs. Am J Vet Res 2012;73(6):821–9.
20. Lu MD, Yu XL, Li AH, et al. Comparison of contrast enhanced ultrasound and contrast enhanced CT or MRI in monitoring percutaneous thermal ablation pro-cedure in patients with hepatocellular carcinoma: a multi-center study in China. Ultrasound Med Biol 2007;33(11):1736–49.
21. Jones ID, Lamb CR, Drees R, et al. Associations between dual-phase computed tomography features and histopathologic diagnoses in 52 dogs with hepatic or splenic masses. Vet Radiol Ultrasound 2016;57(2):144–53.
22. Fukushima K, Kanemoto H, Ohno K, et al. CT characteristics of primary hepatic mass lesions in dogs. Vet Radiol Ultrasound 2012;53(3):252–7.
23. Phillips K, Cullen JM, Van Winkle T, et al. CT appearance and vascular character-istics of liver masses in dogs. Proceedings of the American College of Veterinary Radiology, Annual Scientific Meeting. Las Vegas, October 18–21, 2012. 103.
24. Kutara K, Seki M, Ishikawa C, et al. Triple-phase helical computed tomography in dogs with hepatic masses. Vet Radiol Ultrasound 2014;55(1):7–15.
25. Clifford CA, Pretorius ES, Weisse C, et al. Magnetic resonance imaging of focal splenic and hepatic lesions in the dog. J Vet Intern Med 2004;18(3):330–8.
26. Marks AL, Hecht S, Stokes JE, et al. Effects of gadoxetate disodium (Eovist(R)) contrast on magnetic resonance imaging characteristics of the liver in clinically healthy dogs. Vet Radiol Ultrasound 2014;55(3):286–91.
27. Yonetomi D, Kadosawa T, Miyoshi K, et al. Contrast agent Gd-EOB-DTPA (EOB.-Primovist(R)) for low-field magnetic resonance imaging of canine focal liver le-sions. Vet Radiol Ultrasound 2012;53(4):371–80.
28. Louvet A, Duconseille AC. Feasibility for detecting liver metastases in dogs using gadobenate dimeglumine-enhanced magnetic resonance imaging. Vet Radiol Ul-trasound 2015;56(3):286–95.
29. Reimer P, Schneider G, Schima W. Hepatobiliary contrast agents for contrast-enhanced MRI of the liver: properties, clinical development and applications. Eur Radiol 2004;14(4):559–78.
30. Gagne JM, Weiss DJ, Armstrong PJ. Histopathologic evaluation of feline inflam-matory liver disease. Vet Pathol 1996;33(5):521–6.
31. Nakamura M, Chen HM, Momoi Y, et al. Clinical application of computed tomog-raphy for the diagnosis of feline hepatic lipidosis. J Vet Med Sci 2005;67(11):1163–5.
32. Lam R, Niessen SJ, Lamb CR. X-ray attenuation of the liver and kidney in cats considered at varying risk of hepatic lipidosis. Vet Radiol Ultrasound 2014;55(2):141–6.
33. Smallwood JE. Atlas of feline anatomy for veterinarians. In: Hudson L, Hamilton W, editors. Digestive system. Philadelphia: Saunders, W.B; 1993. p. 166–7.
34. Warren-Smith CM, Andrew S, Mantis P, et al. Lack of associations between ultra-sonographic appearance of parenchymal lesions of the canine liver and histolog-ical diagnosis. J Small Anim Pract 2012;53(3):168–73.
35. Kemp SD, Panciera DL, Larson MM, et al. A comparison of hepatic sonographic features and histopathologic diagnosis in canine liver disease: 138 cases. J Vet Intern Med 2013;27(4):806–13.

36. Vitellas KM, Keogan MT, Freed KS. Radiologic manifestations of sclerosing cholangitis with emphasis on MR cholangiopancreatography. Radiographics 2000; 20:959–75.

37. Heo J, Constable P, Naughton J. Dynamic secretin-enhanced magnetic resonance cholangio-pancreatography and pancreatic ultrasonography in normal dogs. Proceedings of the American College of Veterinary Radiology, Annual Scientific Meeting. Las Vegas, October 18–21, 2012. p. 105.

38. Marolf AJ, Kraft SL, Dunphy TR, et al. Magnetic resonance (MR) imaging and MR cholangiopancreatography findings in cats with cholangitis and pancreatitis. J Feline Med Surg 2013;15(4):285–94.

39. Marolf AJ, Stewart JA, Dunphy TR, et al. Hepatic and pancreaticobiliary MRI and MR cholangiopancreatography with and without secretin stimulation in normal cats. Vet Radiol Ultrasound 2011;52(4):415–21.

40. Schindera ST, Nelson RC, Paulson EK, et al. Assessment of the optimal temporal window for intravenous CT cholangiography. Eur Radiol 2007;17(10):2531–7.

41. Miller J, Brinkman-Ferguson EL, Mackin A, et al. Cholangiography using 64 multidetector computed tomography in normal dogs. Proceedings of the American College of Veterinary Radiology, Annual Scientific Meeting; Savannah, GA, October 8–11, 2013. p. 29.

42. Choi J, Kim A, Keh S, et al. Comparison between ultrasonographic and clinical findings in 43 dogs with gallbladder mucoceles. Vet Radiol Ultrasound 2014; 55(2):202–7.

43. Besso JG, Wrigley RH, Gliatto JM, et al. Ultrasonographic appearance and clinical findings in 14 dogs with gallbladder mucocele. Vet Radiol Ultrasound 2000; 41(3):261–71.

44. Adrian AM, Twedt DC, Kraft SL, et al. Computed tomographic angiography under sedation in the diagnosis of suspected canine pancreatitis: a pilot study. J Vet Intern Med 2015;29(1):97–103.

45. Shanaman MM, Schwarz T, Gal A, et al. Comparison between survey radiography, B-mode ultrasonography, contrast-enhanced ultrasonography and contrast-enhanced multi-detector computed tomography findings in dogs with acute abdominal signs. Vet Radiol Ultrasound 2013;54(6):591–604.

46. Scaglione M, Casciani E, Pinto A, et al. Imaging assessment of acute pancreatitis: a review. Semin Ultrasound CT MR 2008;29(5):322–40.

47. Buob S, Johnston AN, Webster CR. Portal hypertension: pathophysiology, diagnosis, and treatment. J Vet Intern Med 2011;25(2):169–86.

48. Liu H, Liu J, Zhang Y, et al. Contrast-enhanced ultrasound and computerized tomography perfusion imaging of a liver fibrosis-early cirrhosis in dogs. J Gastroenterol Hepatol 2016;31(9):1604–10.

49. Ziegler LE, O'Brien RT, Waller KR, et al. Quantitative contrast harmonic ultrasound imaging of normal canine liver. Vet Radiol Ultrasound 2003;44(4):451–4.

50. Kanemoto H, Ohno K, Nakashima K, et al. Characterization of canine focal liver lesions with contrast-enhanced ultrasound using a novel contrast agent-sonazoid. Vet Radiol Ultrasound 2009;50(2):188–94.

51. Zhai L, Qiu LY, Zu Y, et al. Contrast-enhanced ultrasound for quantitative assessment of portal pressure in canine liver fibrosis. World J Gastroenterol 2015; 21(15):4509–16.

52. Jeon S, Lee G, Lee SK, et al. Ultrasonographic elastography of the liver, spleen, kidneys, and prostate in clinically normal beagle dogs. Vet Radiol Ultrasound 2015;56(4):425–31.

Getting the Most Out of Liver Biopsy

Jonathan A. Lidbury, BVMS, PhD

KEYWORDS

- Liver biopsy • Histopathology • Complications • Sampling error
- Interobserver variation • Tru-Cut • Laparoscopy

KEY POINTS

- Liver biopsy often plays an essential role in diagnosing canine and feline hepatobiliary diseases.
- Liver biopsy is generally associated with a low rate of complications but, of these, excess hemorrhage is the most important.
- Despite its value, this technique has several diagnostic limitations, including its invasive nature, sampling error, and suboptimal interobserver agreement associated with histopathologic evaluation.
- The commonly used liver biopsy techniques in dogs and cats are percutaneous needle biopsy, laparoscopic liver biopsy, and surgical liver biopsy. Each has advantages and disadvantages.
- To optimize the value of this procedure it is essential to collect adequately sized biopsy specimens from several liver lobes.

INTRODUCTION

As previously discussed, laboratory testing and diagnostic imaging play an important role in the diagnosis of hepatobiliary disease in dogs and cats (see Yuri A. Lawrence and Jörg M. Steiner's article, "Laboratory Evaluation of the Liver"; and Angela J. Marolf's article, "Diagnostic Imaging of the Hepatobiliary System: An Update," in this issue). In human hepatology it is often possible to use noninvasive or minimally invasive tools to identify the underlying cause of liver disease (eg, serologic diagnosis of hepatitis C).[1] Because of this ability and the availability of validated noninvasive tests for hepatic fibrosis, the necessity for hepatic biopsy is being called into question for many human patients with suspected hepatobiliary disease.[2,3] However, in companion animals a liver biopsy is usually required to definitively diagnose hepatobiliary

Disclosure: The author is affiliated with the Gastrointestinal Laboratory, which offers histopathological evaluation of hepatic biopsies on a fee-for-service basis.
Gastrointestinal Laboratory, Department of Small Animal Clinical Sciences, College of Veterinary Medicine & Biomedical Sciences, Texas A&M University, 4474 TAMU, College Station, TX 77843, USA
E-mail address: jlidbury@cvm.tamu.edu

disease, guide treatment decisions, and provide important prognostic information. Otherwise unobtainable information gained from histopathologic assessment of the liver specimen includes assessment of the structural integrity of the liver tissue, the type and degree of injury, and the patient's response to that injury.[4] Histopathologic assessment also provides the basis for the diagnosis and classification of hepatic tumors.[4] Histopathologic assessment of the liver allows a histomorphologic and sometimes a causal diagnosis to be made. Liver biopsy also allows collection of samples for the quantification of copper, zinc, and/or iron as well as for bacterial and/or fungal culture. However, liver biopsy and histopathologic assessment of hepatic tissue both have important limitations and the success of this diagnostic procedure can be reduced at any stage of the process, including patient preparation, the biopsy procedure, sample processing, histopathologic assessment, and communication between the clinician and pathologist.

This article discusses the indications for liver biopsy, the risks associated with liver biopsy, advantages and disadvantages of different biopsy techniques, and strategies to get as much useful information as possible out of this process (**Box 1**). Fine-needle aspiration and cytologic assessment of the liver are reviewed elsewhere.[5–7]

INDICATIONS FOR LIVER BIOPSY

Every case is different and there are many indications for a liver biopsy. Therefore, it is difficult to make definitive and universal recommendations as to when this procedure is indicated. Although by nature a liver biopsy is invasive and can be costly to perform it is important to remember that a liver biopsy is just a diagnostic tool so, if a clinician thinks that primary liver disease is a possibility, then it is usually indicated. However, when extrahepatic disease is suspected, this should be ruled out before performing a liver biopsy. A liver biopsy is especially valuable for diagnosing hepatic parenchymal disease, such as chronic hepatitis, and biliary tract disease, such as lymphocytic

---

Box 1
Key points to optimize the clinical utility of a liver biopsy

- Before biopsy assess the patient's hemostatic system by performing a platelet count (also check a blood smear), prothrombin time, activated partial thromboplastin time, measurement of fibrinogen concentration, and a buccal mucosal bleeding time.

- Ideally perform laparoscopic or surgical biopsy to optimize sample quality. If performing percutaneous needle biopsy use a 14-gauge needle for dogs and use a 16-gauge needle for small dogs or cats.

- To ensure that representative samples are collected, biopsy several liver lobes. Biopsy specimens of specific lesions should be submitted separately.

- Save samples for aerobic/anaerobic bacterial culture and copper quantification (dogs).

- Collect bile for aerobic/anaerobic bacterial culture and cytologic analysis.

- Consider submitting samples to a pathologist with an interest/expertise in hepatic histopathology.

- Provide the pathologist with a complete but succinct clinical history.

- Staining sections for copper, iron, connective tissue, and lipofuscin can provide additional information.

- Read all parts of the pathology report and ideally talk directly to the pathologist to discuss the findings and make clinical correlations.

cholangitis in cats but is also valuable for diagnosing circulatory and neoplastic disorders.[5] Some of the common reasons to perform a liver biopsy in dogs and cats are presented in **Box 2**.

CONTRAINDICATIONS TO LIVER BIOPSY

The collection of a liver biopsy is contraindicated in patients at high risk for hemorrhage caused by defects of primary or secondary hemostasis (see Cynthia R.L. Webster's article, "Hemostatic Disorders Associated with Hepatobiliary Disease," in this issue). Every patient's situation should be considered individually but suggested contraindications to liver biopsy are presented in **Box 3**. Coagulation times (ie, prothrombin time and activated partial thromboplastin times) are not considered to be reliable predictors of excess hemorrhage postbiopsy because they were not found to be predictive of excess hemorrhage in human patients.[8,9] In a retrospective study of dogs and cats undergoing percutaneous needle biopsy any prolongation of prothrombin time in dogs and activated partial thromboplastin time prolongations greater than 1.5 times the upper limit of the reference interval in cats were found to be risk factors for complications.[10] Hypofibrinogenemia (<50% of the lower limit of the reference interval),[5,11] platelet dysfunction, and severe thrombocytopenia (<80,000/μL)[10] are considered to be contraindications to liver biopsy.

Liver biopsy is also contraindicated in patients that are not stable enough for anesthesia, which is most likely to occur in patients with acute liver failure. In dogs with end-stage chronic hepatitis, acquired portosystemic collateral blood vessels, and ascites it may be too late to successfully intervene and halt the progression of their disease even with biopsy-tailored treatment. Although a liver biopsy is not contraindicated in these

---

Box 2
Common indications for liver biopsy

- Increased serum liver enzyme activities
  - Consider liver biopsy in a dog if:
    - Alanine transaminase (ALT) activity is greater than twice the upper limit of the reference interval for 4 weeks or more
    - Extrahepatic disease is unlikely or ruled out
    - The breed is predisposed to primary hepatic disease (eg, chronic hepatitis)
  - Consider liver biopsy in a cat if:
    - ALT or alkaline phosphatase activity is greater than twice the upper limit of the reference interval for 4 weeks or more
    - Extrahepatic disease (aside from enteritis or pancreatitis) is unlikely or ruled out

- Icterus/hyperbilirubinemia
  - Hemolysis and extrahepatic bile duct obstruction should first be ruled out
  - Icterus/hyperbilirubinemia is persistent and not responding to symptomatic treatment

- Hepatic masses
  - Consider biopsy if fine-needle aspiration does not lead to a diagnosis
  - Avoid needle, laparoscopic, or incisional biopsy if mass is suspected to be a hemangiosarcoma or caused by an infectious agent that could be disseminated

- Hepatic encephalopathy
  - Acquired portosystemic collaterals
    - Consider biopsy of the liver if hepatic disease is suspected and if prehepatic and posthepatic portal hypertension are unlikely or have been ruled out
  - Congenital portosystemic shunts
    - Consider biopsy of the liver if the patient is undergoing surgical shunt attenuation

---

Box 3
Suggested contraindications for liver biopsy

- Platelet count less than 80,000/μL
- Buccal mucosal bleeding time greater than 240 seconds for dogs and greater than 150 seconds for cats
- Prothrombin or activated partial thromboplastin times greater than twice the upper limit of the reference interval
- Plasma fibrinogen concentration less than 50% of the lower limit of the reference interval
- Infectious disease that could be disseminated by biopsy
- Presumed hemangiosarcoma (excisional biopsy may be possible)
- Ascites (relative contraindication; try to treat first)

---

patients and can provide useful information, the clinician should make sure the client has realistic expectations of what can be gained by performing this procedure. Ascites is also a relative contraindication for liver biopsy, because these patients are thought to be at increased risk of hemorrhage.[3] In addition, large-volume ascites can make it technically challenging to perform a percutaneous liver biopsy. Treatment with diuretic agents, such as spironolactone, or therapeutic paracentesis should be performed before biopsy is attempted. Severe obesity could also hinder the successful performance of percutaneous liver biopsy. Patients suspected to have hepatic vascular tumors, such as a hemangiosarcoma, in which bleeding is a major concern or those suspected to have infectious lesions that could be disseminated should also not undergo percutaneous needle or laparoscopic biopsy.

COMPLICATIONS OF LIVER BIOPSY

The risk of morbidity and mortality associated with liver biopsy is fairly low. Although a small amount of bleeding is expected from any biopsy site, excess hemorrhage is a concern. When this does occur it is usually associated with a technical error such as laceration of a larger blood vessel. A retrospective study of 310 dogs and 124 cats undergoing ultrasonography-guided percutaneous hepatic and renal biopsies found that minor bleeding (decrease in packed cell volume of <10% with no treatment needed) occurred in 22% and major bleeding (requiring intravenous fluid therapy or transfusion) occurred in 6% of patients. Bleeding was less likely in patients undergoing hepatic biopsy than renal biopsy. Bleeding was more likely in thrombocytopenic patients and in dogs with a prolonged prothrombin time and cats with a prolonged activated partial thromboplastin time.[10] In a recent study of short-term complications in 106 dogs undergoing laparoscopic liver biopsy, despite 27% of dogs having a coagulopathy before surgery, only 2 dogs required conversion to laparotomy because of splenic laceration. Ninety-five percent of dogs survived to discharge. All the dogs that did not survive to discharge were euthanized because of progression of their hepatic disease and a poor prognosis rather than biopsy-related complications.[12] These findings were similar to those of a previous study that also concluded that laparoscopic liver biopsy is well tolerated and has a low complication rate.[13]

In human patients, other complications of hepatic biopsy that have been reported include pain, bile peritonitis, bile pleuritis, bowel perforation, transient bacteremia, sepsis/abscess formation, pneumothorax, arteriovenous fistula formation, subcutaneous emphysema, or inadvertent biopsy of other organs.[3] Although these complications are also possible in dogs and cats undergoing a liver biopsy they are considered to be uncommon/rare, aside from postbiopsy pain. Importantly, in a case series during biopsy using an automatic Tru-Cut biopsy gun device, 5 out of 26 cats (19%) developed severe shock within 15 minutes of the procedure and could not be resuscitated. The investigators of this series hypothesized that this was caused by intense vagotonia and shock caused by a pressure wave associated with the action of the instrument.[14]

DIAGNOSTIC LIMITATIONS OF LIVER BIOPSY

Despite the unique diagnostic information that liver biopsy can provide, this technique also has diagnostic limitations. First, no matter which biopsy technique is used, a small specimen of this large organ is collected. A standard needle biopsy specimen is estimated to represent only approximately 0.002% of the entire hepatic parenchyma.[3] Many diseases are heterogeneously distributed throughout the hepatic parenchyma, which means that liver biopsy is susceptible to sampling error.[15] In practice, this can mean that the pathologist is presented with tissue that does not represent the lesions that exist in other parts of the liver, possibly leading to misdiagnosis. There can be substantial variation between liver lobes in terms of gross appearance and histologic lesions. In a study of 70 dogs undergoing necropsy, the same diagnosis was made from 6 out of 6 lobes in 39 (56.5%) dogs, 5 out of 6 lobes in 10 (14.5%) dogs, 4 out of 6 lobes in 10 (14.5%) dogs, 3 out of 6 lobes in 7 (10.1%) dogs, and 2 out of 6 lobes in 3 (4.3%) dogs.[16] This finding highlights that it is important to collect biopsy specimens from multiple liver lobes.

Even within an individual liver lobe there can be site-to-site variation. Therefore, bigger specimens are generally more representative. In one study the morphologic diagnosis assigned to needle biopsy specimens (18 gauge) by individual examiners agreed with the morphologic diagnosis assigned to larger wedge biopsy specimens for 56% and 67% of the specimens.[17] In another study of 70 dogs undergoing necropsy, the mean number of portal triads obtained by each sampling method were 2.9 for needle samples (14 gauge), 3.4 for 5-mm laparoscopic cup forceps samples, 12 for 8-mm punch samples, and 30.7 for wedge samples. The diagnoses were in agreement with those from wedge samples in 66% of needle samples, 60% of cup samples, and 69% of punch samples, but these proportions were not significantly different from each other. The investigators concluded that the histopathologic interpretation of a liver biopsy specimen in the dog is unlikely to vary if it contains at least 3 to 12 portal triads.[18] However, these values should be seen as a minimum and it has been recommended that pathologists should be presented with specimens containing at least 11 portal triads.[3] In human hepatology it has been shown that evaluation of samples with fewer portal triads than this results in underestimation of the fibrosis stage.[15]

Sampling error can also affect the analysis of hepatic copper, zinc, and/or iron concentrations. The classic example of this is that, if a regenerative nodule is sampled in a dog with copper-associated chronic hepatitis, the copper concentration can be unrepresentatively low, which could lead to misdiagnosis. In a study in which the livers of 2 dogs with copper-associated chronic hepatitis were repeatedly biopsied during necropsy, the coefficients of variation ranged from 12% to 50%, 4% to 42%, and 6% to 21% for copper, iron, and zinc concentrations, respectively, highlighting site-to-site variations in concentrations of these metals.[19]

Histologic evaluation can be subjective so another disadvantage of liver biopsy is suboptimal interobserver agreement. In one study 3 examiners agreed on the morphologic diagnosis assigned to needle (18 gauge) and wedge biopsy specimens for 44%

and 65% of the specimens, respectively.[17] In another study, currently only represented in abstract form, there was only fair agreement between 6 pathologists who staged hepatic fibrosis for biopsy specimens collected from 50 dogs. However, there was frequently partial agreement between them, which may be acceptable for clinical purposes.[20] This lack of agreement between pathologists is problematic because it can lead to uncertainty for clinicians who have to make decisions based on the histopathologic findings, and this variation could also lead to misdiagnosis.

In addition, because of the high cost of liver biopsy and the risk for complications described earlier, some clients do not consent to their dog or cat undergoing this procedure, which particularly limits how many patients undergo a second liver biopsy to determine disease progression and/or response to therapy.

PATIENT PREPARATION

The patient's general health and hemostatic system should be assessed before the biopsy procedure. This assessment includes collecting a complete history and a physical examination to look for signs of a bleeding diathesis. The platelet count is an essential piece of information and should be confirmed with a blood smear to rule out platelet clumping. This test is usually included as part of a complete blood count. Preexisting anemia is also important to note because this could adversely affect a patient's ability compensate for excessive bleeding. Platelet function should be assessed, admittedly crudely, by performing a buccal mucosal bleeding time. In breeds at increased risk of von Willebrand disease, such as Doberman pinschers, measurement of plasma von Willebrand factor level is also advised. Antithrombotic drugs, such as aspirin or clopidogrel, and anticoagulants, such as heparin, should be discontinued (ideally at least 10 days) before biopsy. Despite the controversy regarding their utility for predicting postbiopsy hemorrhage,[8,10] bleeding times (ie, prothrombin time and activated partial thromboplastin time) are usually measured. Plasma fibrinogen concentrations less than 50% of the lower limit of the reference interval are considered to represent a contraindication to liver biopsy and so should be measured.[5] Vitamin K deficiency can occur in patients with intrahepatic or extrahepatic cholestasis because of decreased absorption of lipid-soluble vitamins from the gastrointestinal tract. Therefore, these patients and also those with a prolonged prothrombin time or activated partial thromboplastin time should be administered 0.5 to 1.5 mg/kg of vitamin K_1 subcutaneously every 12 hours for 3 doses as a precaution and bleeding times may need to be reassessed. Patients with overt coagulopathies may also benefit from transfusion of blood products, such as fresh frozen plasma, before biopsy (see Cynthia R.L. Webster's article, "Hemostatic Disorders Associated with Hepatobiliary Disease," in this issue). High-risk patients should be blood typed and cross-matched before biopsy to save time in case transfusion of packed red blood cells or whole blood is needed.

HEPATIC BIOPSY TECHNIQUES

Detailed descriptions of hepatic biopsy techniques are provided in surgery textbooks. This article focuses on the relative advantages and disadvantages of each technique (Table 1) as well as ways in which to optimize the quality of samples.

Percutaneous Needle Biopsy

Percutaneous needle biopsy of the liver should be performed with ultrasonography guidance. Various types of biopsy needles are available, including aspiration needles, such as the Menghini needle. However, most liver biopsies are currently performed

Table 1			
Disadvantages and advantages of different liver biopsy techniques			
Technique	**Percutaneous Needle Biopsy**	**Laparoscopic Biopsy Using Forceps**	**Surgical Biopsy During Laparotomy**
Invasiveness	Least invasive, can be performed under heavy sedation or light anesthesia	Less invasive than surgical biopsy but general anesthesia is needed	The most invasive; general anesthesia is needed
Adequacy of Specimens	Small, typically 2–4 specimens containing a mean of 2.4 portal triads (18-gauge needle)[18]	Adequate, typically 5–8 specimens containing a mean of 3 portal triads (5-mm forceps)[18]	Large, typically 2–4 specimens containing a mean of 12 portal triads (8-mm punch)[18]
Guidance Method	Ultrasonography	Direct visualization	Direct visualization
Recognition of Hemorrhage	Not possible to observe hemorrhage directly, ultrasonography can be used to detect free abdominal fluid	Hemorrhage can be directly observed	Hemorrhage can be directly observed
Cost and Availability	Relatively cheap; many practices have an ultrasonography unit	More expensive; specialized equipment and training is required	Variable depending on the clinic; no specialized equipment or training are required

using a cutting instrument, such as a Tru-Cut needle. Tru-Cut needles can be semiautomated, in which case the cutting sheath is manually advanced, or automated, in which case this occurs when the device is triggered. Automated devices should be avoided in cats and probably also in small dog because of the risk of vagal events.[14] However, automated devices may collect larger samples of higher quality than manual devices.[21] In most dogs, 14-gauge needles should be used, but in cats and small dogs 16-gauge needles should be used (**Fig. 1**).[5] The samples collected using 18-gauge needles are often small and may be fragmented.[5,17] Specimens should ideally be 2 to 2.5 cm in length.[15] Typically, at least 2 to 3 biopsies are collected from different liver lobes. In one study, 14-gauge needle biopsy specimens contained a mean of 2.9 portal triads.[18]

The advantages of this technique are that it is less invasive than others and in many practices is less costly to perform. These advantages can open up the possibility of repeated biopsy, which is beneficial in some patients; for example, after chelation therapy in a dog with copper-associated chronic hepatitis. It is also possible to acquire tissue from deep within the liver parenchyma, so, if there is a deeper lesion observed on abdominal ultrasonography, percutaneous needle biopsy may be a good option. The main disadvantage of this technique is that the size of the specimens collected is small, which could increase the risk of sampling error and reduce interobserver agreement. In addition, the complication rate of percutaneous biopsy collection seems to be higher than for laparoscopic liver biopsy.[10,12] It is not possible to directly inspect biopsy sites for excess hemorrhage and, if excessive bleeding does occur, there is little that can be done about it other than to provide supportive care or, in rare instances, perform a laparotomy. Usually, excess bleeding occurs because a larger blood vessel has been lacerated. Careful selection of the biopsy sites using ultrasonography, including the use of color flow Doppler, can reduce this risk. Because

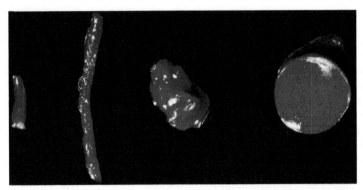

Fig. 1. Four liver specimens collected using different biopsy techniques. From left to right: 18-gauge Tru-Cut biopsy needle, 14-gauge Tru-Cut biopsy needle, 5-mm oval cup laparoscopic biopsy forceps, 8-mm biopsy punch. Note the difference in size between the specimens. (*Courtesy of* Dr Randi Gold, Texas A&M University, College Station, TX.)

of the risk of hemorrhage, typically fewer biopsies are collected than with laparoscopy, which increases the risk of sampling error and suboptimal interobserver agreement. However, percutaneous needle biopsy is the method typically used in human patients and it has diagnostic value in small animals.[3]

Surgical Biopsy

Laparotomy allows liver biopsies to be collected by several techniques, including using a skin punch, ligature, or hemostats. Fairly large biopsies can be collected, which is an important advantage (see **Fig. 1**). For example, using an 8-mm biopsy punch, specimens contained a mean of 12 portal triads.[18] Surgical wedge biopsies should be at least 5 mm and ideally 10 mm deep.[5] In addition, the surface of the liver can be evaluated and specific lesions can be sampled. This method can also allow deeper areas of the parenchyma to be sampled and some lesions can undergo excisional biopsy. The method also allows all of the liver lobes to be biopsied and, when needed, other abdominal organs can also be sampled at the same time. This ability is particularly advantageous in cats, in which hepatobiliary disease often occurs with concurrent pancreatitis and/or intestinal disease.[22] Usually, several liver lobes are sampled and a total of 2 to 4 biopsy specimens are collected. These larger specimens can be subdivided for histologic assessment, copper quantification, and bacterial culture. The biopsy sites can be inspected for excess hemorrhage and, if this occurs, action can be taken to stop it, such as applying direct pressure or Gelfoam. In general, surgical biopsy is considered to have a low rate of serious complications and, in healthy dogs, was associated with minimal hemorrhage.[23] The disadvantage of surgical liver biopsy is that it is the most invasive of the 3 commonly used sampling techniques. It is usually more costly to perform than percutaneous biopsy and in some clinics is more costly than laparoscopic biopsy. However, surgical liver biopsy is fairly simple to accomplish and no specialized equipment or training is required.

Laparoscopic Biopsy

Laparoscopic biopsy allows less invasive collection of multiple biopsies of intermediate size (see **Fig. 1**). In one study, laparoscopic biopsies contained a mean of 3.4 portal triads when 5-mm cup biopsy forceps were used.[18] Typically, 5 to 8 specimens are collected from different liver lobes using direct visualization. In the author's opinion this technique offers a favorable balance between collecting a good number of adequately sized specimens and not being too invasive. It is also possible to biopsy other organs, including the pancreas and small intestine, using modified versions of laparoscopy. Furthermore, excess hemorrhage is easily recognized and direct pressure or Gelfoam can be applied to the affected sites. Typically, the margins of the liver lobes are sampled. Capsular and subcapsular areas of the liver can contain more fibrous tissue than deeper sections and so these biopsies may not be entirely representative (**Fig. 2**).[24] To reduce this effect it is possible to biopsy the surface of liver lobes away from their edges by pushing the biopsy forceps gently into the nonmarginal surface of the liver. This technique seems to be well tolerated. Patients typically recover quickly from this procedure, which is performed under general anesthesia and most patients can go home the same day. The disadvantage of laparoscopic biopsy is that specialized equipment and training are needed. This requirement limits the availability of this technique and also increases the associated cost.

Cholecystocentesis

Because collection of bile for cytologic analysis and bacterial culture is often valuable for the diagnosis of hepatobiliary disease, cholecystocentesis should be performed at the time of liver biopsy whenever possible. Cholecystocentesis can be performed under ultrasonography guidance or by direct visualization during laparotomy or laparoscopy. In either case, as much bile as possible should be removed from the gall bladder to reduce the risk of bile leakage and bile peritonitis. Cholecystocentesis should not be

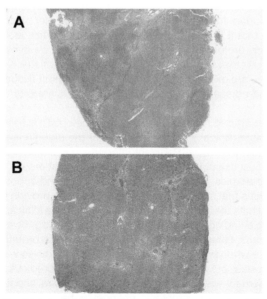

Fig. 2. Representative histologic sections of liver from the margins (*A*) and deeper parenchyma (*B*). Sections prepared from wedge biopsy specimens collected from the same dog during necropsy. (*A*) This sample includes the surface of a liver lobe (*left side*) and shows moderate/marked hepatic fibrosis and lobular collapse. (*B*) Deeper areas of the hepatic parenchyma are included and only mild fibrosis is apparent. (*Courtesy of* Dr John M. Cullen, North Carolina State University, Raleigh, NC.)

attempted in patients with a suspected gall bladder mucocele, compromised gall bladder wall, or complete biliary tract obstruction because the risk of bile peritonitis is significantly increased in these patients.

POSTBIOPSY CARE

Patients should be evaluated carefully during the postbiopsy period. A small amount of hemorrhage from the biopsy sites that can either be visualized directly or observed using abdominal ultrasonography is to be expected. However, it is important to identify greater amounts of bleeding. The patient's demeanor, rectal temperature, pulse rate and quality, respiratory rate and pattern, mucous membrane color, and capillary refill time should be periodically assessed for at least 6 to 12 hours postprocedure. It can also be helpful to check systemic blood pressure and packed cell volume/total solids. However, with acute bleeding, before reequilibration of body fluids can occur, packed cell volume/total solids may not be decreased. In humans, percutaneous liver biopsy is often associated with discomfort,[3] and consequently dogs and cats should be provided with analgesia postprocedure. This analgesia is often accomplished with a full or partial opioid agonist.

SAMPLE HANDLING AND SUBMISSION
Histopathologic Analysis

Several samples from different liver lobes should be promptly placed into 10% neutral buffered formalin and submitted for histopathologic analysis. If there are localized lesions (eg, nodules or liver lobes that appear grossly dissimilar to others) it may be beneficial to submit these in different containers and identify them appropriately. The container should be completely filled with formalin to avoid the specimen being damaged during transit. The tissue should also be placed into sufficient formalin to ensure that it is adequately fixed. The formalin/tissue ratio should be at least 15:1. However, prolonged fixation in formalin should be avoided because this can lead to antigen retrieval problems if immunohistochemistry is to be performed later. Where masses are excised it is good practice to submit tissue from the periphery of the mass and adjacent to it, because their centers are often necrotic and not diagnostic.[5]

When submitting samples for assessment by a pathologist it is essential to provide a succinct but complete clinical synopsis in order for the pathologist to give the most complete interpretation possible. Pertinent information includes the patient's signalment, history, physical examination findings, laboratory test results, diagnostic imaging findings, prior therapies, response to prior therapies, and importantly any clinical suspicion or questions that should be addressed. Failure to provide complete and accurate information limits the ability of the pathologist to make clinical correlations from the histomorphologic findings and could even lead to misdiagnosis.

In a study of humans, differences in the histopathologic interpretation by general pathologists and those who specialize in evaluation of liver biopsies were present in 749 of 1265 (59%) biopsies, of which 505 of 749 (67%) were predicted to affect patient management. Agreement was good in cases with chronic viral hepatitis, fatty liver disease, malignancy, or minimal pathologic changes, whereas diagnostic differences occurred in more than 70% of samples suggestive of biliary disease, autoimmune hepatitis, or vascular/architectural changes.[25] Similar studies have not yet been performed in veterinary medicine. However, there are several veterinary histopathology services that offer assessment of liver tissue by pathologists with a special interest/expertise in hepatic histopathology.

In addition to routine staining of hepatic histologic sections with hematoxylin and eosin (H&E) it is advisable that these sections be stained with a panel of stains, including staining for copper with rhodanine or rubeanic acid, staining for iron (hemosiderin) with Prussian blue, staining for lipofuscin with Schmorl stain, and staining for collagen/connective tissue with Masson trichrome or Sirius red. Histologic stains relevant to the liver are listed in **Table 2**. The practice of only staining for copper granules if hepatic copper accumulation is suspected after evaluation of H&E-stained sections is not advised because it can lead to underdiagnosis of this condition.

Copper Quantification

Although it is possible to reliably quantify copper from paraffin-embedded blocks used to create histologic sections (it is not possible to reliably quantify zinc from them), it is better to collect a liver biopsy specimen especially for copper quantification.[19] Although there is evidence that cats can develop both primary and secondary hepatic copper accumulation, the author currently only collects an extra sample for copper quantification from dogs.[26] When chronic hepatitis is considered a possibility in a canine patient, a sample for copper quantification should be collected and submitted, regardless of the results of histopathologic assessment. The samples should be placed in a metal-free plastic container without formalin, and can be freeze dried before submission. A minimum of 20 to 40 mg of tissue (wet weight) is needed for atomic absorption spectrometry. Typically, this translates to an entire 2-cm long 14-gauge Tru-Cut needle biopsy specimen or a single laparoscopic biopsy sample.[5] The amount of copper is ideally calculated on a dry weight basis because this helps reduce variation between samples. The interpretation of copper quantification should be made in conjunction with the results of copper staining (reviewed in Karen Dirksen and Hille Fieten's article, "Canine Copper-Associated Hepatitis," in this issue). Because typically only 1 biopsy specimen is submitted for quantification of copper

Table 2
Histologic stains used for evaluation of hepatic tissue in small animals

Stain	Comments
Rhodanine/rubeanic acid	Stains copper or copper-binding proteins; used to diagnose hepatic copper accumulation
Prussian blue	Stains iron (hemosiderin); iron coaccumulates with copper and may contribute to oxidative injury
Schmorl stain	Stains lipofuscin, a pigment that is associated with oxidative damage of cell membranes
Masson trichrome	Stains type I collagen fibers; used to assess hepatic fibrosis
Sirius red	Stains type I and III collagen fibers; used to assess hepatic fibrosis
Reticulin	Stains reticulin fibers (type III collagen); used for evaluation of hepatic plates and the reticulin framework of hepatic lobules
Periodic acid-Schiff (with or without diastase)	Stains glycogen when used alone; diastase (amylase) removes glycogen, allowing detection of alpha-antitrypsin globules, basement membranes, debris within macrophages, and/or fungal organisms
Oil red	Stains neutral fat globules; not commonly used because it can only be used for staining frozen sections
Congo red	Stains amyloid; appears bright apple green and birefringent under polarized light

sampling, erroneous results can occur.[19] Biopsies of regenerative nodules should not be sent for copper quantification because they typically contain less copper than the rest of the liver.[19] Discordant copper staining and quantification results are occasionally reported (eg, normal or only mildly increased copper concentrations with abundant copper staining on histologic sections), creating a diagnostic dilemma. A method by which the hepatic copper content can be estimated from rhodanine-stained histologic sections by digital image analysis has been described and may reduce the effect of sampling error because more biopsy specimens can be evaluated.[27]

Bacterial Culture

Hepatic tissue and bile should be submitted for both anaerobic and aerobic bacterial culture. In a study of 248 dogs undergoing liver biopsy the rate of positive culture was higher for bile (30%) than for hepatic tissue (7%).[28] Therefore, cholecystocentesis should be performed whenever possible. Liver samples obtained by surgery or laparoscopy were more likely to yield a positive culture than those obtained by percutaneous needle biopsy.[28] Samples should be collected in a medium and container that preserve both aerobic and anaerobic bacteria. Clinicians should consult a microbiology laboratory to optimize sample handling.

INTERPRETATION OF THE HISTOLOGY REPORT

As previously discussed, histopathologic assessment often plays an essential part in diagnosing hepatobiliary disease in dogs and cats. However, making clinical correlations and decisions based on hepatic histopathologic reports can be challenging for several reasons. First, the histopathologic assessment leads to a histomorphologic diagnosis but does not always provide a causal diagnosis. Clinicians often need to integrate these findings and other clinical information in order to reach a causal diagnosis. In some cases a definitive causal diagnosis cannot be reached despite these integrative efforts. Second, the use of terminology by different pathologists to describe similar changes in the liver is inconsistent. The World Small Animal Veterinary Association formed a Liver Standardization Committee, which published a set of guidelines in 2008 to help resolve this issue.[29] However, not all veterinary pathologists follow these guidelines and alternative terminology is still frequently used. For some lesions, their clinical significance/implications are not currently well defined in the veterinary field. For example, the stage at which liver fibrosis is irreversible is not known in dogs. This uncertainty also extends to the management of certain conditions for which, to date, evidence-based recommendations cannot be made in many instances. For example, some controversy exists about when to treat hepatic copper accumulation with copper chelating agents (see Karen Dirksen and Hille Fieten's article, "Canine Copper-Associated Hepatitis," in this issue).

Because of the first 2 challenges mentioned earlier, it is helpful for clinicians to have some understanding of hepatic histopathology and the terminology used to describe it. A full discussion of hepatic histopathology is beyond the scope of this article but some commonly used terms and their clinical importance are summarized in **Table 3**. Being familiar with the structure of a hepatic lobule and acinus is particularly important because the localization of lesions can be of key importance for the management of the patient. The author highly recommends that clinicians take the time to read the descriptive section of the report as well as the diagnosis and comments sections. It is often possible to glean important clues as to what the pathologist is seeing and thinking from this additional information. The importance of clear and effective

Table 3
Select terminology used to describe histopathologic lesions of the liver

Lesion	Description and Clinical Importance
Periportal	Lesions centered on the portal tracts of the hepatic lobules
Centrilobular	Lesions primarily centered around the central veins of the hepatic lobules
Zone 1 hepatocytes	Hepatocytes closest to the arterial and portal inflow
Zone 2 hepatocytes	Transitional zone between zones 1 and 3
Zone 3 hepatocytes (periacinar)	Hepatocytes nearest the outflow (hepatic venule), exposed to reduced concentrations of oxygen and nutrients
Bridging fibrosis	Fibrosis is said to bridge when fibrous septa connect portal triads to each other (portal-portal bridging fibrosis) or portal triads to central veins (portal-central) This is an important step in the progression of fibrosis and suggests chronicity. However, it is not known what stage of fibrosis is irreversible in dogs
Cirrhosis	There is no universal definition of cirrhosis and some pathologists do not use this term for dogs or cats. In general, there is formation of regenerative nodules surrounded by fibrous septa and vascular disorders
Interface hepatitis (piecemeal necrosis)	Loss and degeneration of hepatocytes at the lobular-portal interface (the limiting plate)
Intrahepatic cholestasis	Interruption of the excretion of bile, characterized by widespread blockage of small biliary ducts
Cholangitis	Inflammation of the large bile ducts This is the preferred term recommended by the WSAVA in cats; cats can have different forms of cholangitis: neutrophilic cholangitis or lymphocytic cholangitis
Cholangiohepatitis	Extension of cholangitis into the adjacent hepatic parenchyma This term is not recommended by the WSAVA as a name for a specific disease or syndrome but is a useful term for describing histopathologic findings

Abbreviation: WSAVA, World Small Animal Veterinary Association Liver Standardization Committee.

Adapted from Cullen JM, Stalker MJ. Liver and biliary system. In: Maxie MG, editor. Jubb, Kennedy & Palmer's pathology of domestic animals, vol. 2. 6th edition. Philadelphia: Saunders Elsevier; 2015.

communication between the clinician and the pathologist cannot be overemphasized. As previously stated, this communication starts with the clinician providing the pathologist with an adequately detailed but succinct history. In human hepatology, clinical conferences are held in which cases are discussed in a multidisciplinary team, including pathologists, hepatologists, and sometimes surgeons, which is thought to have a beneficial effect on patient care.[25] Such clinical conferences may not be practical in veterinary practices where there is no on-site pathologist, but clinicians should speak to a pathologist if the clinical picture does not match the histopathologic assessment, for unusual cases, or if the report does not address their clinical questions.

REFERENCES

1. Strader DB, Wright T, Thomas DL, et al, American Association for the Study of Liver Diseases. Diagnosis, management, and treatment of hepatitis C. Hepatology 2004;39(4):1147–71.

2. Plebani M, Basso D. Non-invasive assessment of chronic liver and gastric diseases. Clin Chim Acta 2007;381(1):39–49.

3. Fox AN, Jeffers LJ, Rajender Reddy K. Liver biopsy and laparoscopy. In: Schiff ER, Maddrey WC, Sorrell MF, editors. Schiff's diseases of the liver. 11th edition. Chichester (United Kingdom): John Wiley; 2012. p. 44–57.

4. Goodman ZD. Hepatic histopathology. In: Schiff ER, Maddrey WC, Sorrell MF, editors. Schiff's diseases of the liver. 11th edition. Chichester (United Kingdom): John Wiley; 2012. p. 152–215.

5. Rothuizen J, Twedt DC. Liver biopsy techniques. Vet Clin North Am Small Anim Pract 2009;39(3):469–80.

6. Bahr KL, Sharkey LC, Murakami T, et al. Accuracy of US-guided FNA of focal liver lesions in dogs: 140 cases (2005-2008). J Am Anim Hosp Assoc 2013;49(3): 190–6.

7. Weiss DJ, Moritz A. Liver cytology. Vet Clin North Am Small Anim Pract 2002; 32(6):1267–91, vi.

8. Ewe K. Bleeding after liver biopsy does not correlate with indices of peripheral coagulation. Dig Dis Sci 1981;26(5):388–93.

9. McVay PA, Toy PT. Lack of increased bleeding after liver biopsy in patients with mild hemostatic abnormalities. Am J Clin Pathol 1990;94(6):747–53.

10. Bigge LA, Brown DJ, Penninck DG. Correlation between coagulation profile findings and bleeding complications after ultrasound-guided biopsies: 434 cases (1993-1996). J Am Anim Hosp Assoc 2001;37(3):228–33.

11. Favier RP. Idiopathic hepatitis and cirrhosis in dogs. Vet Clin North Am Small Anim Pract 2009;39(3):481–8.

12. McDevitt HL, Mayhew PD, Giuffrida MA, et al. Short-term clinical outcome of laparoscopic liver biopsy in dogs: 106 cases (2003-2013). J Am Vet Med Assoc 2016; 248(1):83–90.

13. Petre SL, McClaran JK, Bergman PJ, et al. Safety and efficacy of laparoscopic hepatic biopsy in dogs: 80 cases (2004-2009). J Am Vet Med Assoc 2012; 240(2):181–5.

14. Proot SJ, Rothuizen J. High complication rate of an automatic Tru-Cut biopsy gun device for liver biopsy in cats. J Vet Intern Med 2006;20(6):1327–33.

15. Bedossa P, Dargere D, Paradis V. Sampling variability of liver fibrosis in chronic hepatitis C. Hepatology 2003;38(6):1449–57.

16. Kemp SD, Zimmerman KL, Panciera DL, et al. Histopathologic variation between liver lobes in dogs. J Vet Intern Med 2015;29(1):58–62.

17. Cole TL, Center SA, Flood SN, et al. Diagnostic comparison of needle and wedge biopsy specimens of the liver in dogs and cats. J Am Vet Med Assoc 2002; 220(10):1483–90.

18. Kemp SD, Zimmerman KL, Panciera DL, et al. A comparison of liver sampling techniques in dogs. J Vet Intern Med 2015;29(1):51–7.

19. Johnston AN, Center SA, McDonough SP, et al. Influence of biopsy specimen size, tissue fixation, and assay variation on copper, iron, and zinc concentrations in canine livers. Am J Vet Res 2009;70(12):1502–11.

20. Lidbury JA, Rodrigues Hofmann A, Ivanek R, et al. Interobserver agreement for histological scoring of canine hepatic fibrosis. In: American College of Veterinary Internal Medicine Forum Proceedings 2016. Available at: http://www.vin.com/Members/Proceedings/. Accessed July 12, 2016.

21. Hoppe FE, Hager DA, Poulos PW, et al. A comparison of manual and automatic ultrasound-guided biopsy techniques. Vet Rad 1986;27(4):99–101.

22. Fragkou FC, Adamama-Moraitou KK, Poutahidis T, et al. Prevalence and clinico-pathological features of triaditis in a prospective case series of symptomatic and asymptomatic cats. J Vet Intern Med 2016;30(4):1031–45.
23. Vasanjee SC, Bubenik LJ, Hosgood G, et al. Evaluation of hemorrhage, sample size, and collateral damage for five hepatic biopsy methods in dogs. Vet Surg 2006;35(1):86–93.
24. Petrelli M, Scheuer PJ. Variation in subcapsular liver structure and its significance in the interpretation of wedge biopsies. J Clin Pathol 1967;20(5):743–8.
25. Paterson AL, Allison MED, Brais R, et al. Any value in a specialist review of liver biopsies? Conclusions of a 4-year review. Histopathology 2016;69:315–21.
26. Hurwitz BM, Center SA, Randolph JF, et al. Presumed primary and secondary hepatic copper accumulation in cats. J Am Vet Med Assoc 2014;244(1):68–77.
27. Center SA, McDonough SP, Bogdanovic L. Digital image analysis of rhodanine-stained liver biopsy specimens for calculation of hepatic copper concentrations in dogs. Am J Vet Res 2013;74(12):1474–80.
28. Wagner KA, Hartmann FA, Trepanier LA. Bacterial culture results from liver, gallbladder, or bile in 248 dogs and cats evaluated for hepatobiliary disease: 1998-2003. J Vet Intern Med 2007;21(3):417–24.
29. Cullen JM. Summary of the World Small Animal Veterinary Association Standardization Committee guide to classification of liver disease in dogs and cats. Vet Clin North Am Small Anim Pract 2009;39(3):395–418.

Hepatic Encephalopathy

Adam G. Gow, BVM&S, PhD

KEYWORDS

- Portosystemic shunting • Ammonia • Inflammation • Manganese • Neurotransmitter

KEY POINTS

- Clinicians should be aware that hepatic encephalopathy signs can be subtle and intermittent.
- Ammonia is not the only factor that drives hepatic encephalopathy (HE); there is strong evidence for inflammation also playing a key role. Knowledge of these other factors and precipitants improves management of these cases.
- Dietary protein restriction is no longer the cornerstone of HE management.

   Video content accompanies this article at http://www.vetsmall.theclinics.com.

INTRODUCTION

Hepatic encephalopathy (HE) is most usefully defined in veterinary medicine as neurologic dysfunction caused by hepatic disease and/or portosystemic shunting. This definition allows the diverse consequences of liver disease on the central nervous system (CNS) to be encompassed. Broad categories of hepatic disease resulting in HE have been defined in human medicine and are applicable to veterinary medicine (**Table 1**).[1] In veterinary medicine, although acute hepatopathy occurs not infrequently, as a result of the reserve capacity of the liver, acute liver failure (category A) is a relatively uncommon cause of HE in dogs and cats. Category B is the most common cause of HE seen in veterinary practice because of the high prevalence of congenital portosystemic shunts (CPSS). For companion animals it has been suggested that category C should be widened to encompass all chronic intrinsic liver disease, rather than purely the end-stage of cirrhosis.[2]

CLINICAL SIGNS

The spectrum of clinical signs varies from subtle behavioral abnormalities through to coma. Seizures can occur with HE, although these would be part of a constellation of

---

The author has nothing to disclose.
Hospital for Small Animals, Royal (Dick) School of Veterinary Studies, The University of Edinburgh, Easter Bush, Edinburgh EH25 9RG, Scotland
E-mail address: adam.gow@ed.ac.uk

Vet Clin Small Anim 47 (2017) 585–599
http://dx.doi.org/10.1016/j.cvsm.2016.11.008
0195-5616/17/© 2016 Elsevier Inc. All rights reserved.

Table 1
Category of hepatic disease process resulting in hepatic encephalopathy with suggested veterinary modification

HE Type	Disease Process	Subcategory	Subdivision	Veterinary Modification
A	Acute liver failure			
B	Portosystemic bypass with no intrinsic hepatocellular disease			
C	Cirrhosis and portal hypertension or portosystemic shunts	Episodic	Precipitated Spontaneous Recurrent	Intrinsic hepatocellular disease leading to portal hypertension and portosystemic shunting
		Persistent	Mild Severe	
		Minimal		

clinical signs rather than in isolation. A grading scale for humans has been modified for veterinary patients (**Table 2**, Video 1: Dog exhibiting grade II HE).[3,4] In human medicine, a more subtle grade is recognized; minimal HE where individuals seem neurologically normal but cognitive deficits are revealed during psychometric testing. It has been suggested that the human scale undergo revision, combining minimal and grade I, partly because of the subjectivity in accurately defining grade I.[5,6] These would be combined into "covert HE" and grade II-IV termed "overt HE." It is unlikely, beyond research into veterinary HE, that there is a benefit in detecting minimal HE in our patients. It is likely, however, that detecting grade I suffers from increased subjectivity in veterinary medicine; within the confines of a consultation, decreased mental alertness is a relative term and comorbidities (eg, degenerative joint disease in the dog with chronic hepatitis) may contribute to apathy. Therefore it is possible that grade I animals may be classified as asymptomatic and vice versa. Clinical signs of HE often wax and wane with animals moving between symptomatic and asymptomatic. Chronic HE may be subdefined as persistent or episodic (see **Table 1**). Because clinical signs may be subtle and episodic, clinicians should maintain a high index of suspicion in animals at risk of HE. Unrecognized HE may contribute morbidity, and ultimately mortality because of reduced quality of life. Owners are often surprisingly unaware when their animal is displaying obvious behavioral abnormalities, both in young animals with a CPSS and older animals with acquired shunts. Client education improves management of this condition, particularly of cases with episodic HE.

Table 2
Veterinary modification of West Haven grading scale for hepatic encephalopathy

HE Grade	Clinical Signs
0	Asymptomatic
I	Mild decrease in mobility, apathy, or both
II	Severe apathy, mild ataxia
III	Combination of hypersalivation, severe ataxia, head pressing, blindness, circling
IV	Stupor/coma, seizures

Data from Proot S, Biourge V, Teske E, et al. Soy protein isolate versus meat-based low-protein diet for dogs with congenital portosystemic shunts. J Vet Intern Med 2009;23(4):794–800.

TYPE OF HEPATIC ENCEPHALOPATHY
Acute Hepatic Encephalopathy

This is seen in acute liver failure and is part of a constellation of clinical signs, which are rapid and progressive (see Vincent Thawley's article, "Acute Liver Injury and Failure," in this issue). Animals often have multiple metabolic/biochemical derangements, such as electrolyte, or acid/base status disorders, which contribute to their clinical presentation and their hyperammonemia. HE is severe with animals often presenting in stupor or coma (grade III/IV HE). These patients require intensive management (discussed later) and the prognosis is grave.[7]

Chronic Hepatic Encephalopathy

This is the most common presentation seen in veterinary medicine, caused by congenital or acquired portosystemic shunting. Although HE has been described in cases of chronic liver disease where a shunting vessel has not been identified, this is most likely caused by a lack of testing sensitivity for these vessels because the liver has such a large reserve capacity that chronic intrinsic hepatic failure as a cause of HE in isolation is unlikely.

FACTORS IMPLICATED IN THE PATHOGENESIS OF HEPATIC ENCEPHALOPATHY

Many metabolic abnormalities that can occur as a consequence of liver disease may have an impact on the CNS. It has been more than 100 years since HE was described and its pathogenesis investigated in the dog by Nencki and coworkers[8] using surgically created portosystemic shunts. Their groundbreaking work demonstrated that the liver converted ammonia to urea and delivery of ammonia to the systemic circulation and ultimately the CNS produced neurologic abnormalities.

It is unarguable that ammonia has a central role in HE pathogenesis; however, it has long been recognized in human and veterinary medicine that although in a population of individuals with chronic HE there is correlation between ammonia and HE grade, ammonia concentrations are a poor predictor of HE in the individual.[9,10] In human medicine, HE is a diagnosis of exclusion rather than relying on ammonia measurement.[11] This has led to clinical and experimental investigations to understand what other factors are important in HE pathogenesis and the concept of synergism with ammonia. Many factors have been hypothesized to potentiate HE alongside ammonia, and at present the strongest evidence is for inflammation and manganese (**Fig. 1**).

Ammonia

It is now thought that most ammonia produced in the gastrointestinal tract is as a result of enterocyte conversion of glutamine to glutamate for energy needs, with smaller contributions by urease-producing bacteria, and bacterial protein degradation. Portal blood contains ammonia concentrations, which would be neurotoxic if released directly into the systemic circulation.

Hepatic ammonia detoxification
In healthy animals the liver is the major point of ammonia detoxification. This is achieved by two main mechanisms.[12] Periportal hepatocytes convert ammonia to urea via the urea cycle. Urea is substantially less toxic and is excreted by the kidney. Some urea undergoes enterohepatic recirculation via saliva, bile, or direct diffusion into the gastrointestinal tract where it is degraded by urease bacteria. As blood flows toward the centrilobular vein, there is switching of ammonia detoxification to conversion of glutamate to glutamine, via the enzyme glutamine synthetase, consuming

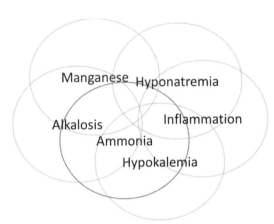

Fig. 1. Representation of factors implicated in hepatic encephalopathy pathogenesis.

ammonia in the process. This transition occurs gradually through the liver lobule such that perivenous hepatocytes mainly use the glutamate/glutamine pathway. Hepatic ammonia detoxification is extremely efficient, thus blood released into the systemic circulation contains low concentrations of ammonia. There is a large reserve capacity and even in the face of severe hepatic insufficiency, ammonia detoxification is often maintained. In portosystemic shunting, dependent on the shunting fraction, variable proportions of the high ammonia concentration blood in the portal vasculature directly reach the systemic circulation.

Renal ammonia metabolism

The kidney plays a crucial role in the defense against hyperammonemia via urea and ammonia excretion. Most ammonia that is excreted in the urine is generated in the kidney.[13] The kidney contains glutaminase with glutamine degradation producing NH_4^+ and HCO_3^-. This mechanism is important in acid/base homeostasis; generated ammonia can either be released into the systemic circulation or excreted in urine. Metabolic acidosis increases urinary ammonia excretion, whereas alkalosis and also hypokalemia increase ammonia production in the kidney, potentiating the development of HE. There is evidence that renal production and urinary excretion of ammonia can increase in hyperammonemic conditions.[14]

Skeletal muscle ammonia metabolism

Skeletal myocytes contain glutamine synthetase and because of the large mass, have significant ability to remove ammonia by conversion to glutamine. This sequestration of ammonia is temporary, however, because glutamine is released into the systemic circulation where glutaminases regenerate ammonia and glutamate.[15] Nonetheless this process can act as an important buffer to ammonia challenges.

Central nervous system ammonia metabolism and hepatic encephalopathy pathogenesis

Astrocytes are the most numerous cell in the brain making up between 25% and 50% of total brain volume. The key to HE pathogenesis is astrocyte dysfunction. These cells contain the enzyme glutamine synthetase and act as a buffer to increasing CNS ammonia concentrations.[16] As a result, glutamate concentrations decrease and glutamine concentrations increase. Glutamate is an excitatory neurotransmitter, whereas glutamine is inhibitory. These neurotransmitters cycle between astrocyte and neurons

(Fig. 2). Glutamine is released from the astrocyte, taken up by neurons, and converted to glutamate by the enzyme glutaminase. Glutamate is released as a neurotransmitter at the synaptic cleft. Astrocytes rapidly reuptake released glutamate. High ammonia concentrations increase extracellular glutamine inhibiting further release from the astrocyte causing increased intracellular concentrations. Ammonia also inhibits key enzymes in the tricarboxylic acid cycle, reducing the astrocytes ability for aerobic respiration, causing a switch to anaerobic respiration and lactate production. Astrocytic mitochondria catabolize glutamine, releasing ammonia, causing oxidative stress and mitochondrial dysfunction.[17] These metabolic effects result in astrocyte swelling. Because astrocytes account for a significant proportion of the brain volume, in acute HE this results in cerebral edema and increased intracranial pressure. Disturbances in control of cerebral blood flow also contribute.[18] This can rapidly lead to herniation, brainstem compression, and death.[17]

In chronic HE, astrocyte swelling is less dramatic but still present, giving rise to Alzheimer type II astrocytes. It is these cases, more commonly seen in veterinary medicine, where the correlation with ammonia concentrations is less pronounced and other factors become more significant.

Inflammation

There is now compelling evidence in human medicine that inflammation is an important potentiator of HE.[19] In support of this, rats with experimentally induced HE have been shown to have restored learning ability after administration of nonsteroidal anti-inflammatory drugs.[20] In dogs with CPSS, C-reactive protein has been shown to be increased in those exhibiting signs of HE and that ammonia and systemic inflammatory response syndrome predict the presence of HE.[10,21] Any process causing a systemic inflammatory response has the potential to precipitate HE. Dogs with CPSS have higher endotoxin concentrations in their portal and peripheral circulations, suggesting that the gastrointestinal tract and microbiome may be an important driver and in support of this, shunt attenuation causes a reduction in circulating inflammatory markers.[22,23]

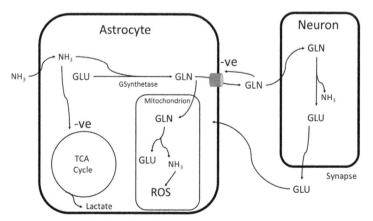

Fig. 2. Representation of ammonia metabolism in astrocyte and neuron. In the face of hyperammonemia, glutamine increases intracellularly, leading to oxidative damage to the mitochondria and ammonia inhibiting the TCA cycle. This disrupts cell metabolism, leading to cell swelling. GLN, glutamine; GLU, glutamate; GSynthetase, glutamine synthetase; ROS, reactive oxygen species.

Proinflammatory cytokines increase cerebral blood flow and compromise the blood brain barrier (BBB), increasing permeability to ammonia. The BBB prevents direct transfer of systemic cytokines into the CNS. However, cytokines can still affect the CNS, possibly through afferent nerves; active transport across the BBB; or via areas lacking the BBB, such as the circumventricular organs.[24] Both inflammatory mediators and ammonia cause microglial activation and neuroinflammation.[19] In humans, it has been demonstrated that inflammation potentiates ammonia in precipitating HE and that systemic inflammation and not ammonia is associated with severe encephalopathy.[9,25]

Ammonia and Innate Immune Dysfunction

In vitro and in vivo studies have shown that neutrophil phagocytic ability is reduced and spontaneous oxidative burst activity increases on exposure to ammonia.[26] Reduced phagocytic ability in the face of hyperammonemia also occurs in canine neutrophils in vitro (Adam G. Gow, unpublished data, 2016). This has important implications in that infection may be more likely in the face of high ammonia concentrations and that increased spontaneous oxidative burst activity, potentiating the inflammatory response syndrome.

Manganese

Manganese (Mn) is an essential trace element with the potential to be neurotoxic, causing psychiatric disturbances and cognitive defects. Most (98%) Mn ingested and absorbed is efficiently removed by the liver and excreted in bile.[27] Portosystemic shunting allows high Mn concentration blood in the splanchnic circulation to reach the systemic circulation. Astrocytes have a high-affinity Mn transport mechanism and concentrations can be 50 times higher than in surrounding cells.[28] This causes oxidative damage and mitochondrial dysfunction; Mn has been shown to produce Alzheimer type II astrocytosis, identical to that of hyperammonemia.[29] In addition, Mn stimulates microglia to release inflammatory cytokines and reactive oxygen species.[30] A direct relationship has been demonstrated between blood Mn, MRI hyperintensity consistent with Mn deposition, and HE severity in humans.[31,32] Dogs with CPSS and chronic liver disease have higher blood Mn compared with control subjects.[33,34] MRI of dogs and cats with CPSS detected CNS lesions consistent with Mn deposition and there is one report of a CPSS dog that had increased CNS Mn concentrations on postmortem examination.[35,36]

Acid/Base and Electrolyte Disturbances

Hyponatremia, hypokalemia, and alkalosis are all recognized as potentiating HE in humans.[37] Hyponatremia potentiates cerebral edema, whereas hypokalemia increases renal ammoniagenesis and reduces renal excretion of ammonia. Although it is likely that they would also potentiate HE in our patients, the evidence for this is lacking and studies to date find no association.[10,38] This may reflect the low prevalence of these abnormalities in our patients, partly because of the differing main etiology of HE (CPSS vs chronic hepatitis) and severity of the disease process; in cases of chronic hepatitis, our patients may be euthanized before these abnormalities occur.[39]

NEUROLOGIC CONSEQUENCE OF ASTROCYTE DYSFUNCTION

In acute HE the major pathologic consequence is cerebral edema and raised intracranial pressure caused by astrocyte swelling. In chronic HE the major consequence of all these factors is neurotransmitter dysregulation. In addition to glutamate/glutamine imbalance, increased "GABAergic tone" has long been recognized in cases of HE. γ-Aminobutyric acid (GABA) is the main inhibitory neurotransmitter, reducing excitability. Initially this increase in tone was hypothesized to be caused by increased GABA synthesis; however, canine studies in dogs with experimentally induced biliary cirrhosis and dogs with experimentally created portocaval shunts found no increase in CNS GABA or GABA receptors.[40] This led to a search for alternative ligands. It is now known that GABA receptors are activated by a group of compounds known as "neurosteroids," which include allopregnanolone and tetrahydrodeoxycorticosterone. These compounds have been shown to be dramatically increased in human patients with HE.[41] Neurosteroids are synthesized in response to activation of a translocator protein in astrocyte mitochondria (formerly known as peripheral-type benzodiazepine receptors). These receptors are increased in humans with cirrhosis. In vitro studies have demonstrated that astrocyte translocator protein is highly upregulated by ammonia and also manganese.[42,43]

DIAGNOSIS OF HEPATIC ENCEPHALOPATHY

Arterial and venous ammonia concentrations are an unreliable marker of HE. A high index of suspicion should be maintained in animals with hepatic disease or those that may have a portosystemic shunt. A high ammonia concentration makes HE likely; however, normal values do not exclude the diagnosis. Careful sample handling for ammonia measurement is important to avoid in vitro increases.[44] Routine clinical pathology allows exclusion of other metabolic causes of neurologic disease and provides support for hepatic disease/insufficiency. The findings from abdominal imaging can provide support for the presence of acquired liver disease and in some cases portosystemic shunting.

TREATMENT OF HEPATIC ENCEPHALOPATHY
Removal of the Underlying Cause

In animals with a CPSS, vessel attenuation often allows a rapid increase in hepatic mass and function.[45] Medical management before shunt attenuation is recommended. Also some cases with CPSS may not be candidates for attenuation because of the client's financial resources, patient comorbidities, or shunt anatomy. Where possible the inciting cause of acute hepatic failure should be addressed; for example, patients with acetaminophen toxicity should undergo gastrointestinal decontamination and replenishment of glutathione, which may help ameliorate ongoing hepatotoxicity.[46]

Assessment and Treatment of Precipitating Factors

Many factors have been implicated in precipitating HE. Cases should be examined for an inflammatory focus/sepsis and their electrolyte and acid/base status should also be assessed. There are many factors implicated in increasing blood ammonia concentrations including dehydration, high-protein meals, gastrointestinal hemorrhage (caused by hemoglobin digestion and also acts as an inflammatory focus), uremia, and constipation. If any are identified then these should be addressed.

Acute Hepatic Encephalopathy Caused by Hepatic Failure

These cases usually have multiple severe comorbidities, most notably coagulopathy and organ dysfunction, all of which require intensive management (see Vincent Thawley's article, "Acute Liver Injury and Failure," in this issue).[7] Cases are often stuporous/comatose, requiring intubation to protect the airway and in some cases mechanical ventilation. Hypoglycemia is common and cases should be monitored for this regularly during hospitalization. Of great concern is cerebral edema as a result of hyperammonemia leading to increased intracranial pressure. To minimize this risk, the patient's head should be raised to a 30° angle and jugular venous drainage should not be compromised (ie, no jugular blood sampling, removal of any collars). Intravenous fluids should be used to maintain a normovolemic state. If cerebral hypertension is suspected, then intravenous mannitol is recommended at a dose of 0.5 to 1 g/kg intravenously given over 20 minutes. This can then be repeated after 4 hours but because of the osmotic diuretic effect, serum/plasma electrolytes should be monitored. Assisted ventilation to maintain a $Paco_2$ between 30 and 40 mm Hg is recommended. Overly aggressive reductions in Pco_2 reduce cerebral perfusion and oxygenation and therefore must be prevented. Ammonia-lowering measures (discussed later) should be instituted. In human medicine, these interventions alongside therapeutic hypothermia, temporary hepatectomy (removing a source of necrosis and inflammation), and ultimately liver transplantation are recommended management strategies.[47] In veterinary medicine, these advanced options are unavailable and as a result of limited treatment options, the prognosis for dogs with fulminant hepatic failure is grave.[7]

Chronic Hepatic Encephalopathy

Any animal with an exacerbation of clinical signs should be thoroughly investigated for precipitating factors (**Fig. 3**). Animals with signs of sepsis require intravenous empiric antibiotic therapy while awaiting culture and sensitivity results. Infection or inflammatory foci should be managed aggressively. Concurrent medications should be reviewed for the potential to cause dehydration, electrolyte disturbances, or hepatotoxicity. Hemorrhage from the upper gastrointestinal tract is often managed with omeprazole and sucralfate alongside other supportive measures. The level of intervention depends on the severity of the clinical signs; grade III/IV animals may require intubation to protect against aspiration (**Fig. 4**).

Intravenous Fluids

Many animals with HE are dehydrated and/or hypovolemic because of obtundation reducing water intake and precipitating causes (eg, diarrhea/gastrointestinal hemorrhage). Restoring euvolemia reduces ammonia concentrations by dilution and improves urinary excretion of ammonia and urea, and prevents ammoniagenesis via urease-producing bacteria in the colon. Diuresis further improves renal excretion. Some clinicians avoid lactate-containing fluids in animals with hepatic failure, because this additive requires hepatic metabolism.

Enemas

Enemas physically remove colonic contents and therefore a source of nitrogen from urease-producing bacteria. Physical removal of hemoglobin from gastrointestinal bleeding prevents bacterial degradation of hemoglobin and ammoniagenesis. Cleansing enemas with warm water or isotonic fluids are used until clear fluid is evacuated. Retention enemas are then used; options include warm water, neomycin, povidone iodine, or nonabsorbable disaccharides (lactulose and lactitol). There are no studies assessing the efficacy of retention enemas in veterinary patients. One human study found that lactulose- and lactitol-containing enemas were more effective than warm water.[48] The author uses one part lactulose to three parts warm water given via a Foley catheter at 10 mL/kg, retained for 30 minutes to 1 hour.

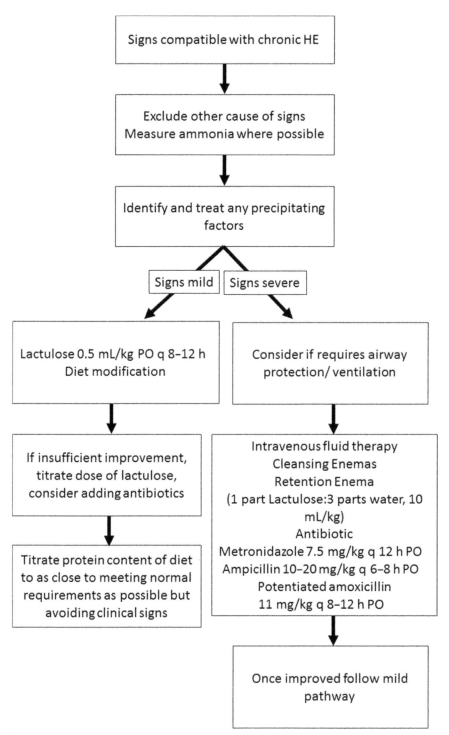

Fig. 3. Suggested approach to patient with signs of hepatic encephalopathy.

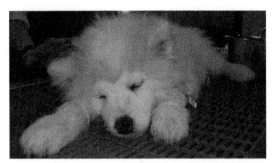

Fig. 4. Samoyed with a congenital portosystemic shunt exhibiting grade III hepatic encephalopathy caused by gastrointestinal hemorrhage. This patient could be roused with stimuli.

Lactulose/Lactitol

These are nonabsorbable disaccharides, which are digested by colonic bacteria to form volatile fatty acids including acetic acid, lactic acid, and butyric acid. Acidification of the colon favors formation of ammonium ions (NH_4^+), which are less able to move through cell membranes, thus forming a colonic ammonia "trap." Lactulose solution in itself is acidic and this may be the reason that lactulose enemas (discussed previously) are effective in improving clinical signs.[49] These volatile fatty acids also act as osmotic laxatives, removing trapped ammonia from the body and nitrogen. Longer term, these products act as probiotics, favoring nonurease bacteria reducing ammonia production from the large intestine. The dose is titrated to produce two to three soft stools per day, starting at a dose of 0.5 mL/kg orally twice daily. Lactitol is a powder and, where available, may be used in animals that do not accept lactulose. Overdose of these agents causes osmotic diarrhea potentially producing hypernatremia and reduced renal excretion of ammonia and urea.

Diet

Although feeding a low-protein diet and thus reducing the potential for ammonia production would seem intuitive, there are potentially deleterious effects to this approach. Failure to feed adequate protein causes tissue catabolism with a reduction in muscle mass, leading to the release of ammonia, reducing the animal's ability to buffer via glutamine synthetase in skeletal muscle. In addition, with acquired shunting caused by portal hypertension, any reduction in serum albumin decreases oncotic pressure, potentiating ascites. Because the bulk of ammoniagenesis is thought to be caused by enterocyte metabolism converting glutamine to glutamate, it is unclear how significant dietary protein is in driving ammonia production. Protein restriction is no longer recommended in humans with HE and dogs with CPSS have identical dietary protein requirements to control animals.[50,51] A highly digestible, high biologic value protein source is recommended but ideally protein content of the diet should be appropriate for the age and growth phase of the animal. The exceptions to this are during the initial stabilization period to control clinical signs or if despite other methods of management clinical signs recur on a standard protein ration. An approximate level of protein restriction of 4 g protein/100 kcal/day would be the starting point on which protein can be titrated upward in the dog. Veterinary commercial canine hepatic diets vary but are generally around this level. Commercial hepatic diets have much to recommend them: restricted in copper to prevent secondary copper accumulation in chronic hepatitis, supplemented with zinc, an antioxidant, required for optimal urea cycle function, and containing protein of high digestibility and biologic value. However commercial hepatic diets are often overly protein restricted for long-term management, especially for young animals. Supplementation with another high-quality protein source, such as cottage cheese or tofu, is required. There is evidence that vegetable protein sources may improve control compared with meat-based diets.[3,52] Because ammoniogenesis in the gastrointestinal tract occurs during digestion, feeding small frequent meals is recommended. Monitoring weight, muscle condition score, and serum albumin is recommended to ensure that calorie and protein requirements are being met for animals on long-term medical management. When in doubt clinicians are advised to consult with a board-certified veterinary nutritionist.

Antibiotics

Antibiotics are used to reduce the numbers of urease-producing bacteria in the gastrointestinal tract. By this rationale, nonabsorbable antibiotics would be a sensible choice. Neomycin was previously recommended; however, some systemic absorption can occur producing renal and ototoxicity.[53] In human medicine, rifaximin-α, a semisynthetic nonabsorbable antibiotic that is effective at treating and preventing HE, is widely used.[54] Pharmacokinetic data are available in the dog that confirms, at least in healthy animals, no systemic uptake.[55] The major hurdle to use of this drug in veterinary medicine is at present the cost.

Because of the previously mentioned problems, systemic antibiotics are often used including metronidazole, ampicillin, and potentiated amoxicillin. Metronidazole undergoes hepatic metabolism therefore a dose reduction to 7.5 mg/kg every 8 to 12 hours is recommended. In view of the increasing concern regarding antibiotic resistance, it is prudent that antibiotics are used short-term or when animals are experiencing an exacerbation. Despite this, there are cases that seem to be clinically improved while on antibiotic treatment.

FUTURE TREATMENT OPTIONS
Increasing Ammonia Metabolism

L-Ornithine L-aspartate is a mixture of two amino acids that are substrates for the urea cycle and also stimulates glutamine production in the liver and skeletal muscle. It is delivered by intravenous infusion and effective in humans with overt HE; however, the effects are short-lived in that on discontinuing the infusion, ammonia concentrations rebound.[56] There is one case series reporting its use in dogs, although no statement can be made as to its efficacy.[57] Like L-ornithine L-aspartate, ornithine phenylacetate increases glutamine synthetase activity; however, glutamine is then bound to phenylacetate, and excreted by the kidney preventing rebound ammonia. This compound is currently undergoing clinical trials in humans.[56] An alternative compound with an identical end-product is glycerol phenylbutyrate, which also seems effective in clinical trials.[58] There is no information on their use in companion animals.

Fecal Microbiome Modulation

The potential benefits of this are reducing urease-producing bacteria, and producing a less proinflammatory microbiome, thus reducing endotoxin and inflammatory cytokine release. Current management with lactulose and vegetable protein may act in this manner. In humans with cirrhosis, intestinal dysbiosis has been demonstrated in humans with HE.[59] There is interest in other prebiotics and probiotics and fecal microbiota transplant to control HE in human medicine.[56,60] It is unknown at present if dysbiosis occurs in companion animals with HE.

Reducing Proinflammatory Cytokines/Inflammation

Because one source of inflammation is the gut microbiome, modulation of this may improve control. An engineered carbon adsorbent (AST-120) given orally is thought to adsorb ammonia, endotoxin, and tumor necrosis factor-α, although an initial study did not demonstrate an improvement in humans with covert HE.[61] Other options are minocycline, which reduces activation of the microglia, and etanercept and infliximab, which neutralize tumor necrosis factor-α, all of which are under investigation to manage HE in human medicine.[30]

SUMMARY

At present, all long-term management strategies to control HE in companion animals are directed toward lowering ammonia concentrations. As a result of intensive research, it is clear that ammonia is not the only factor and that previously held beliefs as to the source of ammonia, and also the mechanisms of action of the current interventions, have changed. Because liver disease and as a consequence HE is increasing in the human population, research into therapeutics is continuing apace. From veterinary research carried out to date, it seems that the pathogenesis of HE in dogs is similar to that in humans and it is hoped that with the necessary validation, advances in human HE management will be transferable to veterinary medicine.

SUPPLEMENTARY DATA

Supplementary video related to this article can be found at http://dx.doi.org/10.1016/j.cvsm.2016.11.008.

REFERENCES

1. Ferenci P, Lockwood A, Mullen K, et al. Hepatic encephalopathy-definition, nomenclature, diagnosis, and quantification: final report of the working party at the 11th World Congresses of Gastroenterology, Vienna, 1998. Hepatology 2002;35(3):716–21.

2. Lidbury JA, Cook AK, Steiner JM. Hepatic encephalopathy in dogs and cats. J Vet Emerg Crit Care 2016;26(4):471–87.

3. Proot S, Biourge V, Teske E, et al. Soy protein isolate versus meat-based low-protein diet for dogs with congenital portosystemic shunts. J Vet Intern Med 2009; 23(4):794–800.

4. Rothuizen J. Important clinical syndromes associated with liver disease. Vet Clin North Am Small Anim Pract 2009;39(3):419–37.

5. Schomerus H, Hamster W. Quality of life in cirrhotics with minimal hepatic encephalopathy. Metab Brain Dis 2001;16(1–2):37–41.

6. Bajaj JS, Cordoba J, Mullen KD, et al. Review article: the design of clinical trials in hepatic encephalopathy. An International Society for Hepatic Encephalopathy and Nitrogen Metabolism (ISHEN) consensus statement. Aliment Pharmacol Ther 2011;33(7):739–47.

7. Lester C, Cooper J, Peters RM, et al. Retrospective evaluation of acute liver failure in dogs (1995-2012): 49 cases. J Vet Emerg Crit Care 2016;26(4):559–67.

8. Nencki M, Pawlow JP, Zaleski J. Ueber den Ammoniakgehalt des Blutes und der Organe und die Harnstoffbildung bei den Säugethieren. Archiv für experimentelle Pathologie und Pharmakologie 1895;37(1):26–51.

9. Shawcross DL, Sharifi Y, Canavan JB, et al. Infection and systemic inflammation, not ammonia, are associated with grade 3/4 hepatic encephalopathy, but not mortality in cirrhosis. J Hepatol 2011;54(4):640–9.
10. Tivers MS, Handel I, Gow AG, et al. Hyperammonemia and systemic inflammatory response syndrome predicts presence of hepatic encephalopathy in dogs with congenital portosystemic shunts. PLoS One 2014;9(1):e82303.
11. Jawaro T, Yang A, Dixit D, et al. Management of hepatic encephalopathy: a primer. Ann Pharmacother 2016;50(7):569–77.
12. Haussinger D, Lamers WH, Moorman AF. Hepatocyte heterogeneity in the metabolism of amino acids and ammonia. Enzyme 1992;46(1–3):72–93.
13. Weiner ID, Verlander JW. Renal ammonia metabolism and transport. Compr Physiol 2013;3(1):201–20.
14. Dejong CH, Deutz NEP, Soeters PB. Metabolic adaptation of the kidney to hyperammonemia during chronic liver insufficiency in the rat. Hepatology 1993;18(4):890–902.
15. Olde Damink SW, Jalan R, Redhead DN, et al. Interorgan ammonia and amino acid metabolism in metabolically stable patients with cirrhosis and a TIPSS. Hepatology 2002;36(5):1163–71.
16. Belanger M, Magistretti PJ. The role of astroglia in neuroprotection. Dialogues Clin Neurosci 2009;11(3):281–95.
17. Scott TR, Kronsten VT, Hughes RD, et al. Pathophysiology of cerebral oedema in acute liver failure. World J Gastroenterol 2013;19(48):9240–55.
18. Jalan R, Olde Damink SW, Deutz NE, et al. Restoration of cerebral blood flow autoregulation and reactivity to carbon dioxide in acute liver failure by moderate hypothermia. Hepatology 2001;34(1):50–4.
19. Aldridge DR, Tranah EJ, Shawcross DL. Pathogenesis of hepatic encephalopathy: role of ammonia and systemic inflammation. J Clin Exp Hepatol 2015;5(Suppl 1):S7–20.
20. Cauli O, Rodrigo R, Piedrafita B, et al. Inflammation and hepatic encephalopathy: ibuprofen restores learning ability in rats with portacaval shunts. Hepatology 2007;46(2):514–9.
21. Gow AG, Marques AI, Yool DA, et al. Dogs with congenital porto-systemic shunting (cPSS) and hepatic encephalopathy have higher serum concentrations of C-reactive protein than asymptomatic dogs with cPSS. Metab Brain Dis 2012;27(2):227–9.
22. Tivers MS, Lipscomb VJ, Smith KC, et al. Lipopolysaccharide and toll-like receptor 4 in dogs with congenital portosystemic shunts. Vet J 2015;206(3):404–13.
23. Tivers MS, Handel I, Gow AG, et al. Attenuation of congenital portosystemic shunt reduces inflammation in dogs. PLoS One 2015;10(2):e0117557.
24. Licinio J, Wong ML. Pathways and mechanisms for cytokine signaling of the central nervous system. J Clin Invest 1997;100(12):2941–7.
25. Shawcross DL, Davies NA, Williams R, et al. Systemic inflammatory response exacerbates the neuropsychological effects of induced hyperammonemia in cirrhosis. Hepatology 2004;40(2):247–54.
26. Shawcross DL, Wright GA, Stadlbauer V, et al. Ammonia impairs neutrophil phagocytic function in liver disease. Hepatology 2008;48(4):1202–12.
27. Davis CD, Zech L, Greger JL. Manganese metabolism in rats: an improved methodology for assessing gut endogenous losses. Proc Soc Exp Biol Med 1993;202(1):103–8.
28. Aschner M, Gannon M, Kimelberg HK. Manganese uptake and efflux in cultured rat astrocytes. J Neurochem 1992;58(2):730–5.

29. Hazell AS, Normandin L, Norenberg MD, et al. Alzheimer type II astrocytic changes following sub-acute exposure to manganese and its prevention by antioxidant treatment. Neurosci Lett 2006;396(3):167–71.

30. Butterworth RF. The liver-brain axis in liver failure: neuroinflammation and encephalopathy. Nat Rev Gastroenterol Hepatol 2013;10(9):522–8.

31. Spahr L, Butterworth RF, Fontaine S, et al. Increased blood manganese in cirrhotic patients: relationship to pallidal magnetic resonance signal hyperintensity and neurological symptoms. Hepatology 1996;24(5):1116–20.

32. Layrargues GP, Rose C, Spahr L, et al. Role of manganese in the pathogenesis of portal-systemic encephalopathy. Metab Brain Dis 1998;13(4):311–7.

33. Gow AG, Marques AI, Yool DA, et al. Whole blood manganese concentrations in dogs with congenital portosystemic shunts. J Vet Intern Med 2010;24(1):90–6.

34. Kilpatrick S, Jacinto A, Foale RD, et al. Whole blood manganese concentrations in dogs with primary hepatitis. J Small Anim Pract 2014;55(5):241–6.

35. Torisu S, Washizu M, Hasegawa D, et al. Measurement of brain trace elements in a dog with a portosystemic shunt: relation between hyperintensity on T1-weighted magnetic resonance images in lentiform nuclei and brain trace elements. J Vet Med Sci 2008;70(12):1391–3.

36. Torisu S, Washizu M, Hasegawa D, et al. Brain magnetic resonance imaging characteristics in dogs and cats with congenital portosystemic shunts. Vet Radiol Ultrasound 2005;46(6):447–51.

37. Frederick RT. Current concepts in the pathophysiology and management of hepatic encephalopathy. Gastroenterol Hepatol 2011;7(4):222–33.

38. Lidbury JA, Ivanek R, Suchodolski JS, et al. Putative precipitating factors for hepatic encephalopathy in dogs: 118 cases (1991-2014). J Am Vet Med Assoc 2015;247(2):176–83.

39. Kilpatrick S, Dreistadt M, Frowde P, et al. Presence of systemic inflammatory response syndrome predicts a poor clinical outcome in dogs with a primary hepatitis. PLoS One 2016;11(1):e0146560.

40. Roy S, Pomier-Layrargues G, Butterworth RF, et al. Hepatic encephalopathy in cirrhotic and portacaval shunted dogs: lack of changes in brain GABA uptake, brain GABA levels, brain glutamic acid decarboxylase activity and brain postsynaptic GABA receptors. Hepatology 1988;8(4):845–9.

41. Butterworth RF. Neurosteroids in hepatic encephalopathy: novel insights and new therapeutic opportunities. J Steroid Biochem Mol Biol 2016;160:94–7.

42. Hazell AS, Desjardins P, Butterworth RF. Chronic exposure of rat primary astrocyte cultures to manganese results in increased binding sites for the 'peripheral-type' benzodiazepine receptor ligand 3H-PK 11195. Neurosci Lett 1999;271(1):5–8.

43. Itzhak Y, Norenberg MD. Ammonia-induced upregulation of peripheral-type benzodiazepine receptors in cultured astrocytes labeled with [3H]PK 11195. Neurosci Lett 1994;177(1–2):35–8.

44. Willard MD, Tvedten H. Small animal clinical diagnosis by laboratory methods. 5th edition. St Louis (MO): Elsevier; 2012.

45. Kummeling A, Vrakking DJ, Rothuizen J, et al. Hepatic volume measurements in dogs with extrahepatic congenital portosystemic shunts before and after surgical attenuation. J Vet Intern Med 2010;24(1):114–9.

46. Bates N, Rawson-Harris P, Edwards N. Common questions in veterinary toxicology. J Small Anim Pract 2015;56(5):298–306.

47. Jalan R. Intracranial hypertension in acute liver failure: pathophysiological basis of rational management. Semin Liver Dis 2003;23(3):271–82.

48. Uribe M, Campollo O, Vargas F, et al. Acidifying enemas (lactitol and lactose) vs. nonacidifying enemas (tap water) to treat acute portal-systemic encephalopathy: a double-blind, randomized clinical trial. Hepatology 1987;7(4):639–43.
49. Elkington SG. Lactulose. Gut 1970;11(12):1043–8.
50. Abdelsayed GG. Diets in encephalopathy. Clin Liver Dis 2015;19(3):497–505.
51. Laflamme DP, Allen SW, Huber TL. Apparent dietary protein requirement of dogs with portosystemic shunt. Am J Vet Res 1993;54(5):719–23.
52. Amodio P, Bemeur C, Butterworth R, et al. The nutritional management of hepatic encephalopathy in patients with cirrhosis: International Society for Hepatic Encephalopathy and Nitrogen Metabolism Consensus. Hepatology 2013;58(1): 325–36.
53. Greenberg LH, Momary H. Audiotoxicity and nephrotoxicity due to orally administered neomycin. J Am Med Assoc 1965;194(7):827–8.
54. Kimer N, Krag A, Moller S, et al. Systematic review with meta-analysis: the effects of rifaximin in hepatic encephalopathy. Aliment Pharmacol Ther 2014;40(2): 123–32.
55. Venturini AP. Pharmacokinetics of L/105, a new rifamycin, in rats and dogs, after oral administration. Chemotherapy 1983;29(1):1–3.
56. Hadjihambi A, Jalan R. Hepatic encephalopathy: new treatments. Clin Liver Dis 2015;5(5):109–11.
57. Ahn JO, Li Q, Lee YH, et al. Hyperammonemic hepatic encephalopathy management through L-ornithin-L-aspartate administration in dogs. J Vet Sci 2015;17(3): 431–3.
58. Rockey DC, Vierling JM, Mantry P, et al. Randomized, double-blind, controlled study of glycerol phenylbutyrate in hepatic encephalopathy. Hepatology 2014; 59(3):1073–83.
59. Rai R, Saraswat VA, Dhiman RK. Gut microbiota: its role in hepatic encephalopathy. J Clin Exp Hepatol 2015;5(Suppl 1):S29–36.
60. Kao D, Roach B, Park H, et al. Fecal microbiota transplantation in the management of hepatic encephalopathy. Hepatology 2016;63(1):339–40.
61. Bajaj JS, Sheikh MY, Chojkier M, et al. Su1685 AST-120 (Spherical Carbon Adsorbent) in covert hepatic encephalopathy: results of the astute trial. Gastroenterology 2013;144(5):S-997.

Hemostatic Disorders Associated with Hepatobiliary Disease

 CrossMark

Cynthia R.L. Webster, DVM

KEYWORDS

- Coagulation • Liver • Portal vein thrombosis • Hyperfibrinolysis • Hemorrhage

KEY POINTS

- Coagulation testing is used diagnostically and prognostically as well as to assess bleeding and thrombotic risk in hepatobiliary disease.
- Both hypocoagulable and hypercoagulable states can exist in hepatobiliary disease.
- Treatment should address perceived bleeding and thrombotic risks and not simply the results of individual coagulation tests.
- Be aware of preexisting conditions and proposed treatments that might shift coagulation balance.
- Best evidence suggests that the minimum bleeding risk assessment should include platelet count, prothrombin time, activated partial thromboplastin time, hematocrit, and fibrinogen.

INTRODUCTION

The liver plays a crucial role in all aspects of coagulation, because most of the factors that regulate procoagulation, anticoagulation, and fibrinolysis are produced and/or cleared by the liver (**Table 1**). The liver is also the site of vitamin K (VK)–dependent activation of factors II, VII, XI, X protein C (PC); and protein S. In health, a balanced homeostasis exists with considerable buffering capacity among the 3 arms of hemostasis. However, with hepatobiliary disease, homeostasis is disrupted and the system is rebalanced with little buffering capacity.[1–3] Thus hypocoagulable, hypercoagulable, and/or hyperfibrinolytic states can emerge, leading to an increased propensity to bleed or clot.

Hemostasis requires the combined activity of vascular, platelet, and plasma factors and is maintained through 3 events: primary hemostasis, secondary hemostasis, and fibrinolysis. For a detailed discussion of hemostasis, the reader is referred to recent

Disclosure: The author has nothing to disclose.
Department of Clinical Sciences, Cummings School of Veterinary Medicine at Tufts University, 200 Westboro Road, North Grafton, MA 01536, USA
E-mail address: Cynthia.Leveille-Webster@tufts.edu

Vet Clin Small Anim 47 (2017) 601–615
http://dx.doi.org/10.1016/j.cvsm.2016.11.009
0195-5616/17/© 2016 Elsevier Inc. All rights reserved.

Table 1
The liver's role in coagulation: coagulation factors synthesized by the liver

Procoagulants	Anticoagulants	Profibrinolysis	Antifibrinolysis
• Fibrinogen	• Protein C	• Factor XIIa	• Plasminogen activator
• Prothrombin	• Protein S	• Plasminogen	inhibitor-1
• Factor V	• Tissue factor		• Alpha-antiplasmin
• Factor VII	pathway inhibitor		• Tissue activatable
• Factor VIII	• Antithrombin		fibrinolysis inhibitor
• Factor IX			
• Factor X			
• Factor XI			
• Factor XII			
• Factor XIII			
• Thrombopoietin			

reviews.[2,4–6] Briefly, primary hemostasis is activated by vascular injury and involves interaction between platelets and the endothelial surface to form an initial platelet plug. Endothelial cell production of von Willebrand factor (vWF) promotes platelet aggregation and activation. Maintenance of platelet number requires thrombopoietin. During secondary hemostasis a cascade of coagulation factors becomes activated, leading to the generation of thrombin. Thrombin cleaves soluble fibrinogen, leading to the formation of an insoluble cross-linked fibrin network that stabilizes the initial platelet plug. Fibrinolysis, the degradation of the fibrin clot, prevents excessive clot formation. Fibrinolysis is initiated by activation of plasminogen to plasmin though the action of tissue plasminogen activator (TPA), which is produced by activated endothelial cells. Plasmin breaks down the fibrin clot into fibrin degradation products, which include D-dimer.

Several regulatory mechanisms modulate normal hemostasis. First, because platelets cannot adhere to normal vascular endothelium, maintenance of vascular integrity prevents inappropriate activation of primary hemostasis. Several pathways regulate thrombin function and thus final clot stabilization. Antithrombin (AT) and tissue factor pathway inhibitor limit thrombin formation by inactivating factor Xa. Thrombin also binds to thrombomodulin on the endothelial cell membrane, which activates the anticoagulant, PC. Activated PC combines with protein S to form a complex that can cleave and inactivate factor Va and factor VIIIa, effectively stopping the generation of thrombin. The fibrinolytic system is kept in check by alpha2-antiplasmin, which inactivates plasmin and tissue plasminogen activator inhibitor (PAI; which inactivates TPA) and tissue activatable fibrinolysis inhibitor (TAFI; acts directly on the fibrin clot).

HOW TO ASSESS COAGULATION?

Table 2 summarizes the clinical tests most commonly used to assess primary and secondary hemostasis and fibrinolysis. Initial assessment of primary hemostasis is by determination of platelet count. Assessment of platelet function is more complicated. In the presence of normal platelet numbers, prolonged buccal mucosal bleeding time (BMBT) is used as a crude indication of qualitative platelet disorders (such as vWF deficiency). However, BMBT can also be prolonged by hypofibrinogenemia and anemia. Light transmission aggregometry and the PFA-100 (platelet function assay) measure platelet response to variety of in vitro agonists (collagen, adenosine diphosphate [ADP]) but are not amenable to routine clinical practice.

Table 2 Clinical tests to assess bleeding and thrombotic risk assessment in dogs and cats with hepatobiliary disease	
Assessment of:	**Coagulation Test**

Primary hemostasis	• Platelet count
	• Platelet function
	  ○ Aggregometry
	  ○ PLA-100
	• vWF activity
	• Buccal mucosal bleeding time
	• Thromboelastography
	  ○ Maximum amplitude, G

Secondary hemostasis	• Procoagulants
	  ○ PT
	  ○ aPTT
	  ○ Fibrinogen
	  ○ Factor levels
	• Anticoagulants
	  ○ Antithrombin activity
	  ○ PC activity
	• Both
	  ○ Thromboelastography
	  ○ R, K, and angle

Fibrinolysis	• D-dimers • Fibrin degradation products • Thromboelastography ○ LY 30
Endothelial function	• vWF • Factor VIII

Abbreviations: aPTT, activated partial thromboplastin time; LY 30, percentage clot lysis 30 minutes after maximum amplitude is reached; PT, prothrombin time.

Prothrombin time (PT), activated partial thromboplastin time (aPTT), and fibrinogen are considered standard tests for assessment of procoagulant status during secondary hemostasis. PT measures initial activation of the coagulation cascade (factors II, V, VII, X) and the final common pathway. Because factor VII is the VK-dependent factor with the shortest half-life, PT is considered an early indicator of VK deficiency. aPTT tests the integrity of the intrinsic and final common pathway of the coagulation cascade and are prolonged with deficiencies of factors XII, XI, IX, and VIII, or with more long-standing VK deficiency. Specialized testing for anticoagulants, such PC or AT, is indicated in some dogs with hepatobiliary disease.

The integrity of the fibrinolytic system is not routinely monitored by conventional coagulation testing. Increased fibrinolytic activity can be inferred from increases in serum concentration of D-dimers and other fibrin degradation products. Assessing the contribution of endothelial dysfunction to hemostasis is also difficult. Most commonly this is suggested by the presence of soluble mediators released by stressed endothelial surfaces, such as vWF and factor VIII.

Thromboelastography (TEG) is a whole-blood assay that evaluates clot formation as a dynamic process, measuring clot time and strength, as well as the kinetics of clot formation.[7,8] As such, TEG analysis gives simultaneous integrated information about primary and secondary hemostasis and fibrinolysis. Thromboelastography variables are measured and integrated to establish whether a hypocoagulable or hypercoagulable state exists. The reaction time (R) is a measure of time for initial fibrin formation and depends on coagulation cascades. The clot formation time (K) is the time from the end of R until the clot reaches 20 mm and depends on coagulation cascades and fibrinogen. The angle is the tangent of the curve made as K is reached and indicates the rapidity of fibrin cross-linking. The maximum amplitude (MA) indicates overall clot firmness. Both angle and MA rely on normal fibrinogen levels and platelet function. The LY 30 is the percentage clot lysis 30 minutes after MA is reached. The G value, a mathematical manipulation of MA, is commonly used to define overall coagulation status. A hypocoagulable TEG has a prolonged K and R, and a decreased angle, MA, and G, whereas a hypercoagulable TEG has a short K and R and an increased angle, MA, and G. Increased LY 30 indicates the presence of a hyperfibrinolytic state.

WHY ASSESS COAGULATION IN LIVER DISEASE?

The goals of coagulation assessment in patients with hepatobiliary disease are 3-fold. First, coagulation testing can provide diagnostic information. In patients with recent onset of liver disease and hyperbilirubinemia, a prolongation in PT more than 1.5 times the upper limit of the reference interval subclassifies acute liver disease (ALD) as acute liver failure (ALF), an important differentiation because it carries a grave prognosis.[9,10] Low PC activity in dogs with congenital portosystemic shunts (CPSS) helps to distinguish this condition from primary hypoplasia of the portal vein.[11] Second, coagulation tests provide prognostic information in acute and chronic hepatopathies in dogs (see **Table 2**).[2,10] In addition, abnormalities in coagulation testing guide therapy in those patients with active bleeding or thrombosis or those at risk for these conditions.

COAGULATION ABNORMALITIES IN DOGS WITH HEPATOBILIARY DISEASE
Acute Liver Disease/Acute Liver Failure

Coagulation abnormalities in dogs with hepatobiliary disease are summarized in **Table 3**. Dogs with ALD often have a mild to moderate thrombocytopenia, prolongations in PT and aPTT, low plasma fibrinogen concentrations, and decreases in AT and PC.[2] As indicated earlier, moderate to marked increases in PT determine when acute injury is severe enough to warrant a designation of ALF.[9,10] On TEG analysis dogs with ALD have variable states of coagulation, with most being hypocoagulable or normocoabulable.[12] Dogs with ALF are more likely hypocoagulable and hyperfibrinolytic. The hypocoagulable state (low MA) is associated with low fibrinogen and PC activity, whereas hyperfibrinolysis (high LY 30) correlates with low PC activity and increased white blood cell count. The hyperfibrinolysis seems to be primary because it is not accompanied by evidence of secondary hyperfibrinolysis, such as increases in D-dimers, red blood cell fragmentation, or end-organ damage from microthrombi. The pathogenesis of this hyperfibrinolytic state is unknown. In people with liver disease it is caused by increased endothelial cell production and decreased hepatic clearance of TPA and PAI, as well as decreased hepatic synthesis of TAFI and antiplasmin.[13] Whether or not this hyperfibrinolytic state leads to an increased tendency to bleed in dogs as it does in humans[13,14] has not been investigated. In a recent retrospective study of ALD in dogs, spontaneous bleeding, particularly from the gastrointestinal tract, did occur,[9] although none of the dogs had TEG analysis to check for hyperfibrinolysis. In the same study, thrombosis of the splanchnic vasculature was also found in several dogs at necropsy, suggesting that, under the right conditions, dogs with ALD can by hypercoagulable as well.

Table 3
Common coagulation abnormalities in dogs with various hepatobiliary diseases

Disease	ALD	Chronic Hepatitis/Cirrhosis	CPSS	Biliary Disease	Neoplasia
Reported coagulation abnormalities	• ↓Platelets (mild-moderate) • ↓PT • ↑aPTT • ↓PC • ↓Antithrombin • Hyperfibrinolytic with ALF	• ↓Platelets (mild-moderate) • ↑PT • ↑PTT • ↓Fibrinogen • Variable tracing on TEG • Hyperfibrinolysis and hypocoagulable with cirrhosis on TEG	• ↓Platelets (mild) • ↓PC • ↓Antithrombin • ↑vWF • ↑Factor VIII • Hypercoagulable on TEG	• ↑Partial thromboplastin time • ↑Fibrinogen • Hypercoagulable on TEG	• ↑Platelets with hepatocellular carcinoma

CHRONIC HEPATITIS/CIRRHOSIS

Several retrospective studies have documented mild to moderate thrombocytopenia in dogs with chronic hepatitis (CH; see **Table 2**).[2,15–18] Thrombocytopenia is more likely in late-stage disease and is correlated with decreased survival in Labrador retrievers with CH.[14,18] The contribution of thrombocytopathia to coagulation disorders in CH is poorly characterized. In an older study, 5 dogs with various liver diseases had decreased platelet aggregation and 3 out of 5 had bleeding tendencies, suggesting that alternations in platelet function may be important clinically.[2]

Multiple veterinary studies have documented prolongations in PT and/or aPTT in dogs with CH.[2,15–19] Decreased fibrinogen level is also a common feature, particularly in late-stage disease. Dogs with cirrhosis but not those with CH had decreases in factor II, V, VII, VIII, IX, X, XI, and XII activity, likely reflecting decreased synthetic capacity.[17] Despite reporting the loss of these procoagulants, no spontaneous bleeding tendencies were reported in these dogs, likely because the loss of procoagulants is balanced by a decrease in the activity of anticoagulants, AT and PC.[2,15–19]

In a recent preliminary report of TEG analysis in dogs with CH, overall coagulation status was variable.[20] Dogs with higher clinical scores, lower fibrinogen levels, and those with complications associated with end-stage disease (portal hypertension) tended to be hypocoagulable. Hyperfibrinolysis also occurred in 23% of dogs. Unlike the hyperfibrinolytic states in ALF, which correlated more with inflammation, in CH hyperfibrinolysis was associated with the severity of injury as assessed by serum transaminase levels.

The risk of spontaneous bleeding or bleeding after provocative procedures in dogs with CH seems to be low. In one study of 80 dogs undergoing laparoscopic biopsy, 22% had prolonged PT or aPTT, and 3 dogs (4%) required perioperative transfusion.[21] Because there was no attempt to correlate hemorrhage with histologic diagnosis, it is unknown whether the dogs with complications had CH. In another study of 94 laparoscopic liver biopsy procedures, 26% of dogs had a prolonged PT or aPTT, but no perioperative blood product support was necessary.[22] The results of histologic analysis were not given in this study but it is likely that at least some dogs had CH. Because neither study objectively measured the amount of intraoperative bleeding, bleeding that did not require intervention could have occurred in some dogs. A single study has assessed bleeding from percutaneous ultrasonography-guided hepatic biopsy.[23] The retrospective study investigated both kidney and liver biopsies in both dogs and cats. Minor bleeding (reduction in packed cell volume >10%) was seen in 18.5% of dogs. The overall major complication rate (defined as requiring intervention) for 310 dogs was 5.9%. Three out of 13 major complications were in dogs undergoing liver biopsies. Data from the article do not permit calculation of the complication rate in just liver biopsies but, because liver biopsies represented about one-half of the procedures, a major complication rate of around 2% can be extrapolated.

Several studies suggest that dogs with CH are also at risk for venous thrombosis, particularly in the splanchnic vasculature. In a retrospective study of dogs with portal vein thrombosis, 42% had hepatic disease (CH, congenital vascular disease, or cancer).[24] The hepatic disease in these dogs was often complicated by other concurrent hypercoagulable conditions such as alterations in blood flow, administration of corticosteroids, pancreatitis, protein-losing nephropathy, or transfusion of blood products that helped to shift the balance to a more hypercoagulable state.

Congenital Portosystemic Shunts

Several studies have examined coagulation parameters in dogs with CPSS.[11,15,25–27] Although dogs with CPSS have lower platelet counts compared with a reference population, few dogs have thrombocytopenia. Their platelet function seems to be normal.[2] Increases in factor VIII and vWF levels occur and may reflect activation of the endothelium. Many dogs have mild prolongations in aPTT and mild decreases in some factors and most have decreases in PC activity.[11,25,26] The low PC activity may simply reflect decreased hepatoportal perfusion and not synthetic failure.[11] Surgical attenuation of the shunt normalizes all of these coagulation parameters.[25]

A recent study of TEG analysis in dogs with CPSS showed that many dogs have mild hypercoagulability (as evaluated by G).[26] G value correlated with platelet count and fibrinogen levels. Dogs with high G values were also more likely to have hepatic encephalopathy and high fibrinogen levels, suggesting that the proinflammatory state of hepatic encephalopathy may contribute to the thrombotic tendency.[26,28] Portal vein thrombosis has been reported as a complication of CPSS,[23] whereas bleeding is rare.[2]

Miscellaneous

Gallbladder mucocele is one of the most common biliary diseases in dogs. Many of these patients undergo surgery, but perioperative bleeding complications are rare. This observation fits with the results of a recent TEG analysis in dogs with extrahepatic bile duct obstruction (including 2 dogs with mucocele) in which all the dogs were hypercoagulable.[29] Many dogs also had high fibrinogen and increased D-dimer levels. Considering the high mortality with biliary surgery in the dog, the role that these hypercoagulable parameters and associated occult thrombosis might play in the reported morbidity and mortality associated with gallbladder mucocele treatment needs further study.

Thrombocytosis has also been reported with hepatocellular carcinoma in dogs.[30] Round cell tumors (lymphoma and malignant histiocytosis), which are an important cause of ALF in dogs, can be associated with thrombocytopenia.[9]

HEMOSTASIS IN CATS WITH LIVER DISEASE

Coagulation abnormalities in cats with hepatobiliary disease are summarized in **Table 4**. Thrombocytopenia is rare in cats with hepatobiliary disease except if there is ALF.[2] Alterations in secondary hemostasis are more common. In 2 studies of cats with hepatic lipidosis, cholangitis, or hepatic neoplasia, the most frequently reported coagulation changes were PT prolongation; reduced factor II, VII, and X activities; and/or increased PIVKA (protein invoked by VK absence), all of which are suggestive of VK deficiency.[31–33] Factor XIII deficiency in also common in cats with cholangitis, lipidosis, and neoplasia.[33] Factor XIII is important in the final stabilization of the fibrin clot. In humans, acquired deficiency is usually not associated with spontaneous bleeding but can result in delayed bleeding after provocative procedures. Similar to dogs, levels of

Table 4
Common coagulation abnormalities in cats with various hepatobiliary diseases

Disease	ALF	Cholangitis	Lipidosis	Neoplasia
Reported coagulation abnormalities	• ↓Platelets • ↑PT • ↑aPTT	• VK deficiency • ↑PT • ↑aPTT • ↓Factor XIII • ↑Fibrinogen	• VK deficiency • ↑PT • ↑aPTT • ↓Factor XIII • ↓Fibrinogen • ↓Factor XIII • ↑D-dimers • ↑Factor V	• ↓Factor XIII

anticoagulants, AT and PC, are also decreased in many cats with liver disease. Decreased fibrinogen levels are common in cats with lipidosis (12 out of 19 patients in one study),[34] whereas hyperfibrinogenemia is more common in cholangitis.[32] Many cats, especially those with inflammatory disease, have increased D-dimer levels caused by secondary fibrinolysis (disseminated intravascular coagulation) or decreased hepatic clearance.

Several studies have reported bleeding tendencies in a small percentage of cats with hepatobiliary disease.[32,34–36] In a study of percutaneous liver and kidney biopsies, major complications occurred in 13% of cats and 60% of these cats had liver biopsies.[23] If it is assumed that half of the biopsies were of the liver, 13% of cats who had a liver biopsy required intervention. Minor hemorrhage (decrease in hematocrit >10%) was seen in 22% of cats. Cats with obstructive jaundice present a unique hemostatic challenge. These cats frequently have significant bleeding associated with surgery and often require blood product support despite a low incidence of prolonged preoperative PT/aPTT.[35,36] Possible explanations for this bleeding tendency include the low sensitivity of PT/aPTT for VK deficiency; the high vascularity of the feline hepatobiliary system; the high incidence of hypotension intraoperatively, which may contribute to the decision to transfuse; and the dilutional coagulopathy that is likely to occur after administration of high volumes of fluids to maintain blood pressure in these patients. In addition, these cats may have undetected factor XIII deficiency or primary hyperfibrinolysis, which would predispose them to delayed bleeding. Studies that closely examine global coagulation status and/or the benefit of prophylactic use of blood products in the perioperative management of cats with obstructive jaundice are urgently needed.

There has been a single study of portal vein thrombosis in cats.[37] All 6 cases over a 5-year period involved hepatobiliary disease (CPSS, cholangitis, or neoplasia).

BLEEDING RISK ASSESSMENT

Bleeding risk assessment is important in the clinical evaluation of dogs and cats with hepatic disease (**Table 5**). The decision as to whether it is safe to perform an invasive procedure (liver biopsy, abdominocentesis, central catheter placement) in a patient with liver disease is complicated. There is no clear consensus as to which coagulation tests should be done and what degree of abnormality represents a risk too severe to perform provocative procedures. A single study in the veterinary literature of liver and kidney biopsies suggests that platelet counts less than 80,000/μL in the dog and cat, any prolongation of PT in the dog, and aPPT prolongation greater than 1.5 times the

Table 5
Coagulation abnormalities identified in dogs and cats with hepatobiliary disease that may predispose to hemorrhage or thrombosis

Hemorrhage	Thrombosis
Thrombocytopenia	Increased vWF activity
Thrombocytopathia	Increased factor VIII
Decreased coagulation factor synthesis	Decreased PC activity
Decreased coagulation factor activation (VK deficiency)	Decreased antithrombin activity
Hypofibrinogenemia	Hyperfibrinogenemia
Hyperfibrinolysis	Portal hypertension/multiple acquired portosystemic shunts

upper limit of the reference interval in cats may be risk factors for complications from percutaneous ultrasonography-guided liver or kidney biopsy.[23] However, the bleeding risk for just liver biopsy was not assessed separately in this study. For laparoscopic liver biopsy, risk factors for major bleeding complications in dogs include platelet count less than 150,000/µL and increased PT.[21]

In human patients with cirrhosis, TEG has been shown to be superior to PT or platelet count in estimating the risk of rebleeding from esophageal varices.[2] In addition, reliance on TEG to determine coagulation status led to the use of fewer blood products in cirrhotics undergoing invasive procedures compared with PT-guided blood product therapy.[38] Furthermore, TEG has a long history of success in guiding blood product transfusion during liver transplant.[14] There is also evidence in dogs with nonhepatic disease that TEG may be able to predict clinical bleeding.[39–42] Similar studies have not been done in dogs with liver disease.

Emerging evidence suggests that plasma fibrinogen concentration is an important determinant of bleeding and thrombotic risk assessment in people with liver disorders.[43] Low fibrinogen levels from synthetic failure or consumption can be associated with bleeding and increased concentrations typically secondary to inflammatory disease and the acute phase response correlate with increased risk of thrombosis.[44] Studies with TEG in dogs with hepatobiliary disease have shown that fibrinogen level correlates positively with G and MA parameters and thus may reflect the state of coagulation.[12,26,29,45] Further investigations evaluating the utility of fibrinogen for the assessment of hemostasis in dogs and cats with hepatobiliary disease are necessary.

THROMBOSIS RISK ASSESSMENT

Prediction of thrombotic tendencies in patients with liver disease is difficult (see **Table 5**). Although studies have shown hypercoagulability in TEG parameters in dogs with various liver diseases,[12,26,28] no studies to date have assessed whether these changes are correlated with thrombosis. Recent studies in dogs with nonhepatic disease have failed to find a correlation between thrombosis and TEG parameters of hypercoagulability; instead, a shortened PT was more predictive.[46,47]

In humans there is evidence that clinically occult microvascular thrombosis occurs in chronic liver disease and contributes to the ongoing disorder in a phenomenon called parenchymal extinction.[48,49] Microthrombi in the hepatic vasculature lead to tissue ischemia, thrombin generation in platelets, and activation of hepatic stellate cells to myofibroblasts that produce large amounts of extracellular matrix. In murine models of hepatotoxicity or cholestasis, inhibition of thrombin, thrombocytopenia, or administration of low-molecular-weight heparin attenuates the development of hepatic fibrosis. These studies suggest that anticoagulant therapy might be beneficial in slowing the progression of hepatic fibrosis.

DISRUPTION OF THE HEMOSTATIC BALANCE IN LIVER DISEASE

Several concurrent conditions or therapeutic interventions can shift the balance of hemostasis in patients with liver disease to predispose to hemorrhage or thrombosis (**Table 6**).

TREATMENT OF COAGULATION DISORDERS

Once a coagulation status is determined, treatment to prevent the complications associated with these alterations in hemostasis can be planned (**Table 7**). Ideally this should be designed to reverse clinically relevant problems (bleeding, thrombosis)

Table 6
Disruption of the coagulation balance in dogs and cats with hepatobiliary disease

Predispose to Hemorrhage	Predispose to Thrombosis
Infection	Pancreatitis
Systemic inflammatory response syndrome	Administration of blood products
	Aggravated portal hypertension
Hypervolemia	Hepatic encephalopathy
Anemia	Corticosteroids
Uremia	Neoplasia
Ascites	Concurrent prothrombotic conditions:
Anesthesia/surgery	PLE, PLN, IMHA, ITP, neoplasia
Acidosis	
Hyperthermia	

Abbreviations: IMHA, immune-mediated hemolytic anemia; ITP, idiopathic thrombocytopenia purpura; PLE, protein-losing enteropathy; PLN, protein-losing nephropathy.

and not to reverse abnormal laboratory parameters, which may or may not provide an accurate assessment of bleeding/thrombotic risk.[2]

In the human literature, multiple studies have shown that attempted correction of prolonged PT and aPTT values or thrombocytopenia with fresh frozen plasma

Table 7
Treatment of coagulation abnormalities in hepatobiliary disease

Condition	Treatment	Side Effects
VK deficiency	VK_1: 0.5 mg/kg SC BID for 3 d then weekly	Anaphylaxis if given IV Prooxidant in excess
Thrombocytopenia	Platelet-rich plasma	Rarely reported
Thrombocytopathia	DDAVP: 1–2 μg/kg SC	None
Prolonged PT or aPTT	Fresh frozen plasma: 5–15 mL/kg IV Whole blood (if there is concurrent anemia)	Prothrombotic Proinflammatory Volume overload Immunologic reactions
Hypofibrinogenemia	Fresh frozen plasma: 5–15 mL/kg IV Cryoprecipitate: 1 unit/10 kg IV	See above Volume overload less likely with cyroprecipitate
Hyperfibrinolysis	Aminocaproic acid: 50–100 mg/kg IV or 15 mg/kg PO q 8 h	GI upset
Evidence of acute thrombosis	Clopidogrel: 2 mg/kg PO q 24 h Low-molecular-weight heparin Dalteparin: 150 units/kg SC q 8 h Enoxaparin: 0.8 mg/kg SC q 8 h Rivaroxaban[a]	Bleeding

Abbreviations: BID, twice a day; DDAVP, desamino-D-arginine vasopressin (arginine vasopressin); GI, gastrointestinal; IV, intravenously; PO, by mouth; q, every; SC, subcutaneously.
[a] Dose not well established in veterinary medicine.

administration or platelet transfusions, respectively, does not always have an effect on the incidence of postprocedural bleeding.[1,3,50] These observations suggest that bleeding tendencies in people with hepatobiliary disease may not be entirely caused by defects in coagulation factors or platelet function, but instead may be secondary to some component of the coagulation cascade that is not affected by replenishment of soluble factors or platelets, such as vascular endothelial dysfunction or hyperfibrinolysis.

Despite the limitations in current coagulation testing and often inadequate response to procoagulant therapy, because of ethical and legal considerations, the practice of prophylactic therapy remains common among human hepatologists.[50] When trends for fresh frozen plasma administration in veterinary medicine are examined, the same seems to be true in veterinary medicine.[51,52] Factors that should be considered in the decision to give prophylactic blood product therapy include a history of a bleeding disorder, the perceived bleeding risk associated with the procedure (aspirate vs biopsy vs surgery), the likelihood that rescue therapy will be successful after the proposed procedure, the cost of the intervention, the ease of managing potential complications, and the side effects of prophylactic treatment. Potential side effects of blood product support include transmission of infectious agents, occurrence of transfusion-related lung injury or other immune-related transfusion reactions, and volume overload.[50–52] Volume overload may be particularly deleterious because there is literature to support the observation that volume overload potentiates portal hypertension, which promotes greater bleeding.

MANAGEMENT OF NONBLEEDING PATIENTS

Despite the inherent limitations of bleeding risk assessment, there are guidelines that can be applied to the management of coagulation status in patients with hepatobiliary disease. Considering the poor sensitivity of the PT and aPTT in detecting VK deficiency, it may be prudent to prophylactically treat all cholestatic (hyperbilirubinemic) patients with VK_1 (see **Table 7**), particularly feline patients. Prompt initiation of VK_1 therapy avoids delays in doing provocative procedures like hepatic biopsy. If thrombocytopathia is suspected, the use of desmopressin may be beneficial.[2]

In patients with prolonged clotting times but no evidence of spontaneous bleeding, and if no provocative procedures are planned, there is no need to administer blood products solely for the sake of improving bleeding times. Even if provocative procedures are necessary there is a growing opinion in human hepatologists that, if there are mild alterations in clotting times, these patients should not receive prophylactic therapy but instead should be provided with rescue therapy, if necessary.[2,48,50] Before performing invasive procedures in these patients, clinicians should be prepared to address any postprocedure hemorrhage by ensuring that patients are blood typed and that blood products are available.

MANAGEMENT OF PATIENTS WITH ACTIVE HEMORRHAGE

Fresh frozen plasma is the first-line treatment modality for spontaneous hemorrhage or iatrogenic bleeding because it supplies the widest range of coagulation factors and is readily available. Given the previously discussed poor correlation of clotting times with bleeding tendency, the author recommends using discontinuation of bleeding as an end point for fresh frozen plasma transfusions and not correction of PT and aPTT. Cryoprecipitate is indicated for hypofibrinogenemia (fibrinogen level <100 mg/dL), and can also be used to supply factor VIII, vWF, and factor XIII. The advantages of cryoprecipitate include a decreased volume of administration and the provision of targeted correction. Platelet transfusions are not typically used in veterinary medicine because of the expense and very short duration of effect.

Antifibrinolytic therapy may be indicated if hyperfibrinolysis is documented with TEG or suspected based on delayed bleeding from mucosal surfaces. The protease inhibitor, aminocaproic acid, which inhibits plasmin, is the most commonly used antifibrinolytic agent. In humans undergoing liver transplant, protease therapy reverses hyperfibrinolysis on TEG, and case series suggest that it is effective in controlling hemorrhage in patients with cirrhosis that are undergoing liver transplant.[13,14] Veterinary studies have shown that aminocaproic acid use is safe in dogs and can decrease postoperative bleeding in greyhounds, but its use in veterinary patients with liver disease and hyperfibrinolysis has not been reported.[53,54]

MANAGING HYPERCOAGULABLE STATES

At this time, the role of treatment of hypercoagulability in liver disease is poorly defined. It is recommended that patients with an acute thrombotic event (most often portal vein thrombosis) be treated with anticoagulation (warfarin or heparin) for at least 6 months.[2] The treatment of chronic thrombosis with anticoagulants is more controversial, because studies show little benefit in thrombus resolution with treatment. A recent study in dogs with portal vein thrombosis suggested that treatment with anticoagulant improved survival.[24] Other treatment options for hypercoagulable states include platelet inhibitors such as clopidogrel or nonsteroidal antiinflammatory drugs (NSAIDs). Because veterinary patients with hepatic disease are already predisposed to gastrointestinal ulceration, NSAIDs are contraindicated because of their ulcerogenic potential. Clopidogrel, which works by inhibiting ADP receptors on the platelet membrane, may be a safer choice in liver disease. Treatment is recommended in patients with current evidence of thrombosis, or high risk of thrombosis based on TEG or underlying disease process. Anticoagulants and platelet inhibitors should be discontinued at least several days (ideally 10 days) before liver biopsy.

Emerging evidence suggests that anticoagulation may be beneficial in patients with cirrhosis.[48,49,55] Small clinical trials in human patients with CH/cirrhosis have shown reduced fibrosis and improved survival in those treated with low-molecular-weight heparin.[49] Although existing data do not support the routine use of anticoagulation as an antifibrotic therapy, it is becoming evident that activity of the coagulation cascade has a profound influence on tissue fibrogenesis.[55]

REFERENCES

1. Lisman T, Porte RJ. Rebalanced hemostasis in patients with liver disease: evidence and clinical consequences. Blood 2010;116:878–85.
2. Kavanagh C, Shaw S, Webster CR. Coagulation in hepatobiliary disease. J Vet Emerg Crit Care (San Antonio) 2011;21:589–604.
3. Northup PG, Caldwell SH. Coagulation in liver disease: a guide for the clinician. Clin Gastroenterol Hepatol 2013;11:1064–74.
4. Brooks MB, Catalfamo JL. Current diagnostic trends in coagulation disorders among dogs and cats. Vet Clin North Am Small Anim Pract 2013;43:1349–72.
5. Smith SA. Antithrombotic therapy. Top Companion Anim Med 2012;27:88–94.
6. McMichael M. New models of hemostasis. Top Companion Anim Med 2012;27: 40–5.
7. McMichael MA, Smith SA. Viscoelastic coagulation testing: technology, applications, and limitations. Vet Clin Pathol 2011;40:140–53.

8. Hanel RM, Chan DL, Conner B, et al. Systematic evaluation of evidence on veterinary viscoelastic testing part 4: definitions and data reporting. J Vet Emerg Crit Care (San Antonio) 2014;24:47–56.

9. Lester C, Cooper J, Peters RM, et al. Retrospective evaluation of acute liver failure in dogs (1995-2012): 49 cases. J Vet Emerg Crit Care (San Antonio) 2016;26:559–67.

10. Weingarten MA, Sande AA. Acute liver failure in dogs and cats. J Vet Emerg Crit Care (San Antonio) 2015;25:455–73.

11. Toulza O, Center SA, Brooks MB, et al. Evaluation of plasma protein C activity for detection of hepatobiliary disease and portosystemic shunting in dogs. J Am Vet Med Assoc 2006;229:1761–71.

12. Kelley D, Lester C, Shaw S, et al. Thromboelastographic evaluation of dogs with acute liver disease. J Vet Intern Med 2015;29:1053–62.

13. Ferro D, Celestini A, Violi F. Hyperfibrinolysis in liver disease. Clin Liver Dis 2009;13:21–31.

14. Mallett SV. Clinical utility of viscoelastic tests of coagulation (TEG/ROTEM) in patients with liver disease and during liver transplantation. Semin Thromb Hemost 2015;41:527–37.

15. Poldervaart JH, Favier RP, Penning LC, et al. Primary hepatitis in dogs: a retrospective review (2002-2006). J Vet Intern Med 2009;23:72–80.

16. Strombeck DR, Miller LM, Harrold D. Effects of corticosteroid treatment on survival time in dogs with chronic hepatitis: 151 cases (1977-1985). J Am Vet Med Assoc 1988;193:1109–13.

17. Prins M, Schellens CJ, van Leeuwen MW, et al. Coagulation disorders in dogs with hepatic disease. Vet J 2010;185:163–8.

18. Shih JL, Keating JH, Freeman LM, et al. Chronic hepatitis in Labrador retrievers: clinical presentation and prognostic. J Vet Intern Med 2007;21:33–9.

19. Favier RP, Poldervaart JH, van den Ingh TS, et al. A retrospective study of oral prednisolone treatment in canine chronic hepatitis. Vet Q 2013;33:113–20.

20. Fry W, Etadali N, Lester C, et al. Thromboelastography in dogs with chronic hepatopathies. J Vet Intern Med 2015;29(4). In press.

21. Petre SL, McClaran JK, Bergman PJ, et al. Safety and efficacy of laparoscopic hepatic biopsy in dogs: 80 cases (2004-2009). J Am Vet Med Assoc 2012;240:181–5.

22. McDevitt HL, Mayhew PD, Guiffride MA, et al. Short-term clinical outcome of laparoscopic liver biopsy in dogs: 106 cases (2003-2013). J Am Vet Med Assoc 2016;248:83–90.

23. Bigge LA, Brown DJ, Penninck DG. Correlation between coagulation profile findings and bleeding complications after ultrasound-guided biopsies: 434 cases (1993-1996). J Am Anim Hosp Assoc 2001;37:228–33.

24. Respess M, O'Toole TE, Taeymans O, et al. Portal vein thrombosis in 33 dogs: 1998-2011. J Vet Intern Med 2012;26:230–7.

25. Kummeling A, Teske E, Rothuizen J, et al. Coagulation profiles in dogs with congenital portosystemic shunts before and after surgical attenuation. J Vet Intern Med 2006;20:1319–26.

26. Kelley D, Lester C, DeLaforcade A, et al. Thromboelastographic evaluation of dogs with congenital portosystemic shunts. J Vet Intern Med 2013;27:1262–7.

27. Niles JD, Williams JM, Cripps PJ. Hemostatic profiles in 39 dogs with congenital portosystemic shunts. Vet Surg 2001;30:97–104.

28. Tivers MS, Handel I, Gow AG, et al. Hyperammonemia and systemic inflammatory response syndrome predicts presence of hepatic encephalopathy in dogs with congenital portosystemic shunts. PLoS One 2014;9(1):e82303.

29. Mayhew PD, Savigny MR, Otto CM, et al. Evaluation of coagulation in dogs with partial or complete extrahepatic biliary tract obstruction by means of thromboelastography. J Am Vet Med Assoc 2013;242:778–85.

30. Liptak JM, Dernell WS, Monnet E, et al. Massive hepatocellular carcinoma in dogs: 48 cases (1992-2002). J Am Vet Med Assoc 2004;225:1225–30.

31. Center SA, Warner K, Corbett J, et al. Proteins invoked by vitamin K absence and clotting times in clinically ill cats. J Vet Intern Med 2000;14:292–7.

32. Lisciandro SC, Hohenhaus A, Brooks M. Coagulation abnormalities in 22 cats with naturally occurring liver disease. J Vet Intern Med 1998;12:71–6.

33. Dircks B, Nolte I, Mischke R. Haemostatic abnormalities in cats with naturally occurring liver diseases. Vet J 2012;193:103–8.

34. Center SA, Crawford MA, Guida L, et al. A retrospective study of 77 cats with severe hepatic lipdosis:1975-90. J Vet Intern Med 1993;7:349–59.

35. Buote NJ, Mitchell SL, Penninck D, et al. Cholecystoenterostomy for treatment of extrahepatic biliary tract obstruction in cats: 22 cases (1994-2003). J Am Vet Med Assoc 2006;228:1376–82.

36. Mayhew PD, Holt DE, McLear RC, et al. Pathogenesis and outcome of extrahepatic biliary obstruction in cats. J Small Anim Pract 2002;43:247–53.

37. Rogers CL, O'Toole TE, Keating JH, et al. Portal vein thrombosis in cats: 6 cases (2001-2006). J Vet Intern Med 2008;22:282–7.

38. De Pietri L, Bianchini M, Montalti R, et al. Thromblelastography-guided blood product use before invasive procedures in cirrhosis with severe coagulopathy. A randomized controlled trial. Hepatology 2016;63:566–73.

39. Wiinberg B, Jensen AL, Rozanski E, et al. Tissue factor activated thromboelastography correlates to clinical signs of bleeding in dogs. Vet J 2009;179:121–9.

40. Bucknoff MC, Hanel RM, Marks SL, et al. Evaluation of thromboelastography for prediction of clinical bleeding in thrombocytopenic dogs after total body irradiation and hematopoietic cell transplantation. Am J Vet Res 2014;75:425–32.

41. Lynch AM, deLaforcade AM, Meola D, et al. Assessment of hemostatic changes in a model of acute hemorrhage in dogs. J Vet Emerg Crit Care (San Antonio) 2016;26:333–43.

42. Vilar-Saavedra P, Stingle N, Iazbik C, et al. Thromboelastographic changes after gonadectomy in retired racing greyhounds. Vet Rec 2011;169:199.

43. Drolz A, Horvatits T, Roedl K, et al. Coagulation parameters and major bleeding in critically ill patients with cirrhosis. Hepatology 2016;64(2):556–68.

44. Zocco MA, Di Stasio E, De Cristofaro R, et al. Thrombotic risk factors in patients with liver cirrhosis: correlation with MELD scoring system and portal vein thrombosis development. J Hepatol 2009;51:682–9.

45. Dengate AL, Morel-Kopp MC, Beatty JA, et al. Differentiation between dogs with thrombosis and normal dogs using the overall hemostasis potential assay. J Vet Emerg Crit Care (San Antonio) 2016;26:446–52.

46. Song J, Drobatz KJ, Silverstein DC. Retrospective evaluation of shortened prothrombin time or activated partial thromboplastin time for the diagnosis of hypercoagulability in dogs: 25 cases (2006-2011). J Vet Emerg Crit Care (San Antonio) 2016;26:398–404.

47. Thawley VJ, Sánchez MD, Drobatz KJ, et al. Retrospective comparison of thromboelastography results to postmortem evidence of thrombosi in critically ill dogs: 39 cases (2005-2010). J Vet Emerg Crit Care (San Antonio) 2016;26:428–36.

48. Kopec AK, Joshi N, Luyendyk JP. Role of hemostatic factors in hepatic injury and disease: animal models de-liver. J Thromb Haemost 2016;14:1337–49.

49. Intagliata NM, Northrup PG. Anticoagulant therapy in patients with cirrhosis. Semin Thromb Hemost 2015;41:514–9.

50. Shah NL, Intagliata NM, Northup PG, et al. Procoagulant therapeutics in liver disease: a critique and clinical rationale. Nat Rev Gastroenterol Hepatol 2014;11:675–82.

51. Snow SJ, Jutkowitz LA, Brown AJ. Trends in plasma transfusion at a veterinary teaching hospital: 308 patients (1996–1998 and 2006–2008). J Vet Emerg Crit Care (San Antonio) 2010;20:441–5.

52. Logan JC, Callan MB, Drew K, et al. Clinical indications for use of fresh frozen plasma in dogs: 74 dogs (October through December 1999). J Am Vet Med Assoc 2001;218:1449–55.

53. Davis M, Bracker K. Retrospective study of 122 dogs that were treated with the antifibrinolytic drug aminocaproic acid: 2010-2012. J Am Anim Hosp Assoc 2016;52:144–8.

54. Marín LM, Iazbik MC, Zaldivar-Lopez S, et al. Epsilon aminocaproic acid for the prevention of delayed postoperative bleeding in retired racing greyhounds undergoing gonadectomy. Vet Surg 2012;41:594–603.

55. Hugenholtz GC, Northrup PG, Porte RJ, et al. Is there a rational for treatment of chronic liver disease with antithrombotic therapy? Blood Rev 2015;29:127–36.

Acute Liver Injury and Failure

Vincent Thawley, VMD

KEYWORDS

- Liver jury • Liver failure • Hepatic encephalopathy • Coagulopathy

KEY POINTS

- Acute liver failure is the result of a rapid loss of functional hepatic mass, such that the synthetic functions of the liver are compromised.
- Treatment of acute liver injury/acute liver failure is largely supportive and directed at ameliorating the complications that arise as a result of severe liver dysfunction.
- Although some patients may make a clinical recovery with intensive care, the prognosis for acute liver failure is generally considered poor.

INTRODUCTION

Acute liver injury (ALI) and acute liver failure (ALF) are clinical syndromes that are frequently life threatening, characterized by a rapid loss of hepatocyte function in a patient without pre-existing liver disease.[1] Numerous definitions for ALF have been proposed in the published literature, most of which involve a combination of an acute onset of clinical signs, the presence of coagulopathy, icterus, and the development of hepatic encephalopathy (HE).[2] In people, ALF is further characterized as hyperacute, acute, or subacute based on the time interval between the development of icterus and the onset of HE, because this seems to have prognostic significance.[3] Similarly, in the veterinary literature, a variety of diagnostic criteria have been used to define ALF. A recently published retrospective case series involving canine patients defined ALF as the acute onset of clinical signs in conjunction with serum hyperbilirubinemia and a prothrombin time (PT) greater than 1.5 times the upper reference range, with or without evidence of HE.[4] In contrast to ALF, ALI is generally thought to involve an acute hepatic insult with sustained hepatic function. This article reviews the pathophysiology and clinical approach to the ALI/ALF patient, with a particular emphasis on the diagnostic evaluation and care in the acute setting.

The author has nothing to disclose.
Emergency and Critical Care Medicine, Department of Clinical Studies, Matthew J. Ryan Veterinary Hospital of the University of Pennsylvania, 3900 Delancey Street, Philadelphia, PA 19104, USA
E-mail address: vthawley@upenn.edu

Vet Clin Small Anim 47 (2017) 617–630
http://dx.doi.org/10.1016/j.cvsm.2016.11.010
vetsmall.theclinics.com

PATHOPHYSIOLOGY

In health, the liver is responsible for a multitude of homeostatic, synthetic, and excretory functions, including protein, carbohydrate, and lipid metabolism; detoxification of metabolites and chemical compounds; immune regulation; fat digestion; albumin production; and storage of vitamins, fats, and glycogen. Hepatic Kupffer cells are tissue macrophages that typically reside in hepatic sinusoids but can migrate into areas of hepatic tissue injury. These cells are highly efficient phagocytes; consequently, the liver is a major site of blood filtration and removal of circulating microbes and microbial antigens.[5]

Histologically, hepatocytes are arranged into 3 zones around the hepatic blood supply. Zone 1 contains hepatocytes that are closest to the arterial or portal inflow; cells in this region are exposed to blood with a higher concentration of oxygen, hormones like insulin and glucagon, and products of nutrient metabolism. Given their proximity to vascular inflow, hepatocytes in zone 1 are susceptible to injury from directly acting toxicants. Zone 2 contains transitional midzone hepatocytes, and zone 3 contains the periacinar hepatocytes, which are closest to the hepatic venule and thus receive a lower concentration of oxygen and nutrients, making them more susceptible to hypoxic injury. In addition, many of the hepatic biotransformation pathways are active in zone 3; thus, hepatocytes in this zone are more susceptible to injury caused by toxic metabolites of the cytochrome P450 systems.[5]

The liver has an extensive reserve system and clinical signs or biochemical manifestations of ALF often are not apparent until there has been loss of more than 70% of the functional hepatic mass.[6] However, in the setting of acute hepatocyte necrosis or hepatic cellular or lipid infiltrates, clinical signs may progress rapidly to those consistent with fulminant liver failure.

CAUSE

ALI/ALF may occur as a result of prolonged ischemia, toxin or toxicant exposure, idiosyncratic or dose-dependent drug reaction, neoplasia, metabolic disorders, and infectious and immune-mediated processes. In humans, ALF is considered relatively uncommon particularly in the developed world.[7] Drug-induced liver failure, most notably a result of accidental or intentional acetaminophen overdose, is a leading cause of human ALF in the United States, whereas there is a higher incidence of viral hepatitis in other parts of the world.[7–11] In a retrospective case series of 49 dogs with ALF, neoplasia was the most common underlying cause (13 of 49 dogs, 27%), followed by presumptive leptospirosis (4/49 dogs, 8%). In one dog, evidence of thrombi within a branch of the hepatic artery and hepatic veins was found on post-mortem examination, thus ischemia-induced ALF was suspected. No definitive cause was identified in 31 dogs, but 15 of these dogs had exposure to potential hepatotoxins.[4] In addition, ALI and ALF have been documented in several reports in the veterinary literature; **Table 1** summarizes the confirmed or suspected causes.[4,12–43] A comprehensive discussion of the various causes of ALI and ALF can be found elsewhere in the literature.[44]

CLINICAL APPROACH TO THE ACUTE LIVER INJURY/ACUTE LIVER FAILURE PATIENT

Quite often the presenting clinical signs in a patient with ALI or ALF can be vague and potentially attributable to numerous disease processes. Common chief complaints include anorexia, lethargy, vomiting, diarrhea with or without hematochezia or melena, weakness or other neurologic signs resulting from HE. Owners may note the presence

Table 1
Reported inciting causes of acute liver injury/acute liver failure in dogs and cats

Toxins	Drugs	Infectious	Other
• Aflatoxins	• Acetaminophen	• Infectious canine	• Ischemia
• Amanita mushrooms	• Oral benzodiazepines	hepatitis	• Hepatic lipidosis
• Blue-green algae	(cats)	• Feline infectious	• Neoplasia
• Cycad palms	• Carprofen	peritonitis	
• Xylitol	• Lomustine	• Leptospirosis	
	• Mitotane	• *Platynosum fastosum*	
	• Phenobarbital	• Salmonellosis	
	• Phenazopyridine	• Toxoplasmosis	
	• Stanazol		
	• Sulfonamides		
	• Zonisamide		

of icteric skin, sclera, or mucous membranes, or appreciate abdominal distention in patients with ascites. Polydipsia and polyuria are occasionally reported.[4] Because clinical signs of liver failure are not apparent until there has been a loss of a critical mass of functional hepatocytes, it is not uncommon for patients to have only a short duration of clinical signs despite evidence to suggest a chronic underlying cause. Given the variability and nonspecific nature of the clinical signs associated with ALI/ALF, definitive diagnosis is typically contingent on integration of data from the history, physical examination, and results of diagnostic testing.

History

In addition to an inquiry as to the nature and progression of clinical signs, additional questions during the medical interview that may help to identify risk factors for ALI/ALF or point toward possible underlying causes include

- Vaccination status and potential exposure to infectious disease
- Travel history, particularly to regions where leptospirosis is endemic
- Potential for exposure to recognized hepatotoxins
- Dietary history, including the introduction of new foods or treats
- Therapeutic drug history, including herbal remedies and nutritional supplements, because many medications have been implicated in the development of ALI/ALF in either a dose-dependent or an idiosyncratic manner

Initial Physical Examination and Stabilization

As with any sick patient, an initial primary survey is conducted at presentation to assess for stability with a particular focus on the respiratory, cardiovascular, and neurologic systems.

Signs of respiratory compromise can include tachypnea, orthopnea, abnormal breathing patterns, abducted elbows and straightening of the head and neck, open-mouth breathing, and in with patients with severe hypoxemia, cyanotic mucous membranes.[45] Causes of respiratory distress in the ALI/ALF patient include pleural effusion resulting from low intravascular oncotic pressure, aspiration pneumonia, atelectasis secondary to recumbency, and, perhaps less commonly, neurogenic pulmonary edema, acute respiratory distress syndrome, pulmonary thromboembolism, or pulmonary hemorrhage. Pulse oximetry or arterial blood gas analysis is useful in assessing the degree of hypoxemia, and early thoracic imaging is indicated to delineate the cause for respiratory compromise. When pleural effusion is suspected, needle thoracocentesis is warranted, because this may be both diagnostic and therapeutic.

Assessment of the cardiovascular system involves evaluation of the mucous membrane color and capillary refill time, heart rate and rhythm, and palpation of the peripheral pulses. Signs of circulatory shock include pale or hyperemic mucous membranes, slow capillary refill time, tachycardia, cool extremities, decreased rectal temperature, and either bounding, reduced, or absent peripheral pulses. In the author's experience, cats in circulatory shock are more commonly bradycardic than tachycardic. Shock in the ALI/ALF patient may be the result of volume loss, for example, from reduced oral intake coupled with vomiting, diarrhea, polyuria, hemorrhage, or ascites, from inappropriate vasodilation secondary to sepsis or systemic inflammation, or a combination of the 2.[46] Frequently patients with ALI are presented in a dehydrated state, but it is imperative to differentiate dehydration from signs of circulatory shock, as the latter requires immediate resuscitation.

Intravenous (IV) fluid resuscitation, aimed at restoring perfusion and improving tissue oxygen delivery, is a cornerstone of therapy for circulatory shock. The shock dose of an isotonic crystalloid solution is 15 to 25 mL/kg (dog) or 10 to 15 mL/kg (cat), given rapidly as a bolus with subsequent patient reassessment and redosing as needed.[47] Isotonic crystalloids containing lactate should be avoided, because patients with liver dysfunction may not be able to effectively metabolize lactate to bicarbonate.[48] For hypoproteinemic patients, a synthetic colloid like hydroxyethyl starch may be administered in aliquots of 3 to 5 mL/kg.[47] It should be noted, however, that administration of hydroxyethyl starch solutions has been associated with the development of impaired coagulation[49] and acute kidney injury.[50] Resuscitation with blood products is generally reserved for patients with evidence of hemorrhagic shock or for those with a documented coagulopathy and active hemorrhage, in which case transfusing plasma may be indicated. Patients with persistent hypotension despite adequate volume resuscitation may require vasopressor administration. The author's preferred vasopressor in this setting is norepinephrine, although there are insufficient data in the published veterinary literature to suggest superiority of any one particular vasopressor.[51] Administration of supraphysiologic dosages of hydrocortisone can be considered for patients in shock with vasopressor-refractory hypotension.[52]

Neurologic impairment in the ALI/ALF patient may be the result of diminished cerebral perfusion secondary to circulatory shock, hypoglycemia and neuroglycopenia, or HE. Signs of HE can include lethargy, behavioral changes, obtundation, head pressing, circling, blindness, tremors, or seizures.[53] Hypoglycemia may cause similar clinical signs and so measurement of whole blood or plasma glucose is indicated. For patients with symptomatic hypoglycemia, a 0.5- to 1-g/kg bolus of dextrose is administered IV followed by supplementation of dextrose to the intravenous fluids. Further discussion of the management of HE is found in later discussion and in Adam G. Gow's article, "Hepatic Encephalopathy," in this issue.

Following the initial patient assessment and once stabilization, as necessary, is underway, a comprehensive physical examination is performed. Common findings include icterus, abdominal pain, cranial organomegaly, and abdominal distention. Patients with a large volume of ascites may have a ballottable abdominal fluid wave. Rectal examination may reveal hematochezia or melena. Occasionally patients may present with fever or clinical signs referable to dysfunction of other organ systems. Assessment of body condition and lean muscle mass may provide information as to the chronicity of the underlying condition. Most physical examination findings, however, are not specific for acute liver dysfunction, and clinical experience suggests that a diagnosis of ALI/ALF can rarely be made on the basis of physical examination alone.

DIAGNOSTIC EVALUATION OF THE ACUTE LIVER INJURY/ACUTE LIVER FAILURE PATIENT

The diagnostic evaluation of a patient with suspected ALI/ALF includes a combination of blood testing, imaging, and potentially obtaining a sample of liver tissue via fine-needle aspiration (FNA) or biopsy. Comprehensive discussions focusing on laboratory evaluation of the liver, coagulation abnormalities, and liver biopsy can be found elsewhere (see Yuri A. Lawrence and Jörg M. Steiner's article, "Laboratory Evaluation of the Liver," and Cynthia R.L. Webster's article, "Hemostatic Disorders Associated with Hepatobiliary Disease," and Jonathan A. Lidbury's article, "Getting the Most Out of Liver Biopsy," in this issue).

Biochemistry Panel

Evaluation of serum hepatobiliary enzyme activities, including alanine aminotransferase (ALT), aspartate aminotransferase (AST), alkaline phosphatase, and gamma-glutamyl transpeptidase, can be used to screen for hepatobiliary disease.[54] ALT is the most liver-specific cytosolic enzyme, and the magnitude of an increase in ALT may provide insight as to the degree of hepatocyte injury. These enzymes are produced inside the hepatocyte, and therefore, serum activities can decrease in end-stage liver failure.[54] Microcystins, produced by blue-green algae, impair hepatic synthesis of ALT, and so activity of this enzyme may be diminished in the face of acute hepatic necrosis due to microcystin toxicity.[12]

Common biochemistry findings in ALF that suggest diminished hepatic synthetic function include decreased serum blood urea nitrogen, hypoglycemia, hypocholesterolemia, and hypoalbuminemia.[55] Hyperbilirubinemia may be prehepatic, hepatic, or posthepatic in origin. In the setting of ALI/ALF, hyperbilirubinemia is often the result of hepatocyte dysfunction and intrahepatic cholestasis leading to impaired uptake, conjugation, and excretion of bilirubin.[55] A concomitant reduction or normalization of hepatic transaminase activity in the face of evidence for hepatic synthetic or excretory dysfunction suggests a significant loss of hepatic functional parenchyma.[54]

Other common serum biochemical abnormalities include hypokalemia, hyperkalemia, hyponatremia, hypernatremia, hyperphosphatemia, hyperammonemia, and elevated creatinine concentration.[4] Hyperammonemia is a common finding in patients with HE, and in both people[56] and dogs,[57] the degree of hyperammonemia is correlated with the severity of HE.

Complete Blood Count

On a complete blood count, microcytic anemia is more commonly documented with chronic liver disease, and regenerative anemia may suggest blood loss. Spontaneous hemorrhage due to coagulopathy is uncommon; however, hepatic disease is a recognized risk factor for gastroduodenal ulceration.[58] Microcytic, hypochromic anemia is suggestive of chronic gastrointestinal blood loss. A leukocytosis or leukopenia may result from systemic inflammation or sepsis. Thrombocytopenia in patients with ALI/ALF can occur as a result of impaired production due to diminished hepatic synthesis of thrombopoietin, splenic sequestration, or consumption following hemorrhage, thrombosis, or disseminated intravascular coagulation.[59]

Urinalysis

Urinalysis with sediment evaluation is warranted in any sick patient and, in the setting of ALI/ALF, bilirubinuria is a common finding. It should be noted that bilirubinuria can be identified in normal dogs because they have the ability to produce and conjugate bilirubin within their renal tubules; however, bilirubinuria is always a pathologic finding in cats.[60] Granular casts can be seen with concurrent acute kidney injury and may occasionally be seen in patients with aflatoxicosis even in the absence of azotemia.[12]

Coagulation Testing

Abnormalities in tests of coagulation are common in ALF, which is not surprising considering that increased PT (or elevated international normalized ratio [INR], which is calculated based on the measured PT) is one of the most commonly cited criterium for diagnosing ALF.[2] Given this, patients with ALF have historically been considered at risk for bleeding complications, although studies in human patients have found that significant spontaneous hemorrhage is rare in ALF patients and, when it occurs is most frequently of gastrointestinal origin as a result of portal hypertension with bleeding varices.[61,62] Indeed, some studies have found an increased risk of thrombotic complications in patients with ALF.[62] Investigation into this paradox has led to the concept of "rebalanced hemostasis," that is, the suggestion that the hemostatic system is balanced between a proclivity toward hemorrhage and a tendency toward thrombosis. This is thought to be the result of decreased hepatic synthesis of procoagulant factors being balanced by decreased synthesis of anticoagulant factors, although the presence of procoagulant platelet microparticles and altered fibrinolytic activity may play a role.[63,64] (Please also see Cynthia R.L. Webster's article, "Hemostatic Disorders Associated with Hepatobiliary Disease," in this issue.)

Recent studies have evaluated the use of thromboelastography (TEG) in ALF as a means of assessing overall hemostasis. Briefly, TEG is a whole blood viscoelastic test of coagulation that provides information on clot kinetics, including the speed of clot formation, clot strength, and rapidity of fibrinolysis. In a study of 51 human patients with ALI or ALF, all of whom had an elevated INR, mean and median TEG parameters were within the normal range for the entire study population, suggesting overall normal hemostasis.[62] In one veterinary study investigating the use of TEG in 21 dogs with either ALI or ALF, TEG was found to be discordant with traditional tests of coagulation 25% of the time, with 4/8 dogs deemed hypocoagulable based on elevated PT, partial thromboplastin time (PTT), or both having normocoagulable TEG results.[63] The authors of this study suggested that conventional tests of coagulation might overestimate a tendency toward hypocoagulability, particularly early in the ALI/ALF disease spectrum.[63] As viscoelastic coagulation assays are not yet widely available, the routine measurement of PT, PTT, platelet count, and fibrinogen is recommended for patients with ALI or ALF; however, the data available call into question the routine use of plasma transfusion to treat an increased PT or PTT without evidence of active hemorrhage or intention to perform an invasive procedure that could cause bleeding.

Diagnostic Imaging

In the emergency setting, cage-side use of ultrasound can be used to quickly detect and facilitate sampling of free abdominal, pleural, or pericardial fluid, particularly in patients that are not cardiovascularly stable.[65] When available, the author recommends the routine use of abdominal- and thoracic-focused assessment with sonography for trauma ultrasound techniques for any patient with evidence of shock, abdominal distention, or abdominal pain.

Abdominal radiographs may show evidence of hepatomegaly or poor organ serosal detail, which may suggest the presence of peritoneal effusion. Thoracic radiography is warranted in any patient with respiratory compromise to evaluate for alveolar infiltrates or pleural effusion as well as in patients with ALI/ALF for whom underlying neoplasia is a concern as a screening test for metastasis.

Complete abdominal ultrasound is likely the imaging modality with the most utility in the ALI/ALF patient, as a means of evaluating the overall size and architecture of the liver as well as to assess for comorbidities like pancreatitis or gastrointestinal ulceration. Dogs with ALF may have variable degrees of hepatomegaly and hepatic echogenicity, with the liver appearing sonographically normal in some cases.[4] In one study, ALF due to hepatic neoplasia was associated with moderate to marked hepatomegaly seen on ultrasound, although some dogs with hepatomegaly had nonneoplastic causes of ALF.[4]

Hepatic Cytology/Histopathology

Liver tissue sampling can enable a definitive histopathologic diagnosis to be made in cases of ALI and ALF; however, in the author's experience, this is rarely performed in the acute setting often due to concern for hemorrhage. FNA of the liver with ultrasound guidance can be considered, because this is relatively noninvasive and is generally thought to be associated with a low risk of hemorrhage; however, in comparison to a biopsy sample, a smaller number of cells are retrieved and the overall architecture of the hepatic parenchyma cannot be evaluated. Despite these limitations, FNA may have utility in the diagnosis of some infiltrative liver diseases, such as hepatic lipidosis or diffuse neoplasia.[4,66] Liver biopsy, performed either percutaneously with ultrasound guidance or via laparoscopy or laparotomy, will provide larger tissue samples but may carry an increased risk of hemorrhage. Before obtaining a biopsy, a coagulation panel including assessment of PT, PTT, and platelet count should be performed. One retrospective study that evaluated the incidence of complications following ultrasound-guided percutaneous organ biopsy found that an increased incidence of postprocedural bleeding was associated with thrombocytopenia (platelet count $<80 \times 10^3/\mu L$) in both dogs and cats, PTT greater than 1.5 times the upper limit of the reference range in cats but not dogs, and PT above the reference range in dogs but not cats.[67] Administration of fresh frozen plasma or fresh whole blood before biopsy may minimize the risk of hemorrhage in patients with mild elevations in PT/PTT. For a more complete discussion of hepatic biopsy techniques, please see Jonathan A. Lidbury's article, "Getting the Most Out of Liver Biopsy," in this issue.

MANAGEMENT OF THE ACUTE LIVER INJURY/ACUTE LIVER FAILURE PATIENT

Clinical management of the ALI/ALF patient is largely supportive in nature because there is not a definitive therapy for most causes of acute liver dysfunction and because liver transplantation is, to the author's knowledge, not yet available for small animal patients. Frequently these patients are critically ill and require aggressive care and intensive monitoring. The discussion that follows details general guidelines on various aspects of care for these patients.

Fluid Therapy

IV fluid therapy is an integral part of the management of the ALI/ALF patient, used to restore and maintain perfusion, to correct dehydration, and to maintain euhydration in patients that are not amenable to oral fluid administration. Balanced electrolyte solutions are used most commonly; however, as stated previously, fluids containing lactate as a buffer should generally be avoided.[48] Although acidifying, 0.9% sodium chloride may be considered for use in patients with HE because this fluid, compared with other isotonic crystalloids, is less likely to decrease osmolality, which might otherwise facilitate movement of water into the brain parenchyma.[48] Careful attention to fluid balance is essential because excessive administration of crystalloid fluids can lead to the development of interstitial edema, pleural effusion, and ascites, particularly in patients with hypoalbuminemia and low colloid osmotic pressure, or in patients with systemic inflammation and increased capillary permeability. Synthetic colloids could be considered for patients with hypoalbuminemia to increase and maintain intravascular colloid osmotic pressure; however, these fluids should be used cautiously in patients at risk for coagulopathy or acute kidney injury.[48]

Blood Products

Transfusion of whole blood or packed red blood cells is indicated in patients symptomatic for moderate or severe anemia; however, it should be noted that ammonia concentration of stored blood increases over time in both canine[68] and feline[69] packed red blood cells, which may be deleterious in a patient with compromised liver function. As previously mentioned, spontaneous hemorrhage appears to be uncommon in patients with ALF; consequently, the author only recommends the use of plasma transfusions in patients with a documented coagulopathy and active hemorrhage or before a planned invasive procedure that will likely cause bleeding.

Treatment for Hepatic Encephalopathy

HE is a common complication of ALF, likely resulting from a combination of hyperammonemia, excitatory neurotoxicity, oxidative stress, altered permeability of the blood-brain barrier, inflammation, and neurosteroid-induced GABA-receptor modulation within the central nervous system.[70] Signs of HE may be precipitated by hypokalemia, which increases renal proximal tubule ammoniagenesis,[71] hyponatremia, which is a risk factor for cerebral edema via reduced extracellular osmolarity,[72] and metabolic alkalosis, which facilitates diffusion of ammonia into the central nervous system.[73] In addition, gastrointestinal hemorrhage[74] and systemic inflammation[75] or infection may increase the risk for HE in the ALF patient. For a comprehensive review of the pathophysiology of HE, please see Adam G. Gow's article, "Hepatic Encephalopathy," in this issue.

HE should be suspected in any patient with evidence of moderate to severe liver dysfunction and concurrent signs of central nervous system depression or hyperexcitability. A blood ammonia level can be measured to document the presence of hyperammonemia, but a normal ammonia level does not rule out HE. Precipitating factors, for example, electrolyte disturbances or hypoglycemia, should be treated as necessary. For patients that develop seizures, the author uses levetiracetam (20–60 mg/kg IV loading dose, then 20 mg/kg IV every 8 hours) in preference to diazepam, because there is some evidence to suggest that increased levels of endogenous benzodiazepine receptor ligands play a role in the pathogenesis of HE.[76]

For emergent stabilization of an encephalopathic crisis, a warm water cleansing enema (10 mL/kg) may be administered to reduce the number of urease-producing bacteria in the lower gastrointestinal tract. Following this, a lactulose retention enema can be administered. Various doses have been reported, including 2 mL/10 kg of lactulose diluted 1:1 in warm water.[77] Lactulose is a nonabsorbable disaccharide that acts as an osmotic laxative and additionally decreases the intraluminal pH of the colon, limiting systemic uptake of ammonia.[78] Metronidazole (7.5 mg/kg IV every 12 hours) is administered to reduce the number of intestinal urease-producing bacteria. Mannitol (0.5–1 g/kg IV over 20 minutes) can be considered when intracranial hypertension due to cerebral edema is suspected. Once the patient becomes stable and tolerant of oral medications, lactulose can be continued at a dose of 1 to 3 mL/10 kg orally every 6 to 8 hours with the dose titrated such that the patient produces soft but not watery feces a few times per day. Oral antibiotic therapy, with, for example, metronidazole, is continued.[77]

Antimicrobial Prophylaxis

In people with ALF, infection, most commonly originating from the respiratory or urinary tracts or bloodstream, is a major cause of death and has been associated with precipitation of HE.[79,80] Prophylactic antimicrobial administration has been shown to reduce the incidence of infection, but there was no demonstrated effect on survival.[81] Current guidelines in the human literature therefore suggest considering antimicrobial prophylaxis only in patients with vasopressor-refractory hypotension, progression of HE, evidence for systemic inflammatory response syndrome, or when surveillance bacterial cultures are positive.[79] When considering prophylactic antimicrobials, empiric therapy should be broad spectrum targeting gram-positive and gram-negative organisms and ideally narrowed based on culture/susceptibility data, when available.

Antacid Therapy

Liver disease is a recognized risk factor for gastroduodenal ulceration, which may ultimately result in bleeding into the gastrointestinal tract.[58] Consequently, antacid therapy is warranted for patients with ALI/ALF. The author prefers to use a proton-pump inhibitor (pantoprazole or omeprazole, 1 mg/kg IV or orally every 12–24 hours) because there is evidence to suggest better gastric acid suppression with this class of antacid as compared with famotidine.[82]

VITAMIN K

Vitamin K deficiency may occur in patients with liver dysfunction as a result of poor oral intake, intrahepatic or extrahepatic cholestasis, or the use of systemic antimicrobials, which disrupts the normal intestinal flora that synthesize vitamin K_2. Vitamin K deficiency may contribute to coagulation dysfunction, because vitamin K is necessary for normal function of clotting factors II, VII, IX, and X.[83] Therefore, empiric administration of vitamin K_1 is recommended at a dose of 1 mg/kg subcutaneously once daily.

Hepatoprotectants

A variety of hepatoprotective medications have been evaluated in the treatment of liver disease, although there is limited information in the published literature to support their efficacy.[84] Silymarin (10–20 mg/kg/day orally, divided every 8 hours),[60] an extract from the seed of the milk thistle plant *Silybum marianum*, may help attenuate hepatic oxidative stress.[85] S-adenosylmethionine (17–22 mg/kg orally every 24 hours)[60] is a substrate that initiates hepatic transmethylation and transsulfuration pathways, thereby playing a role in the stabilization of hepatocyte cell membranes and generation of glutathione, an endogenous antioxidant.[24] Vitamin E (15 IU/kg/d orally) inhibits lipid peroxidation of cell membranes and thus may reduce hepatic oxidative injury.[84]

NUTRITION

Early provision of nutritional support is indicated and, when tolerated, enteral feeding is preferable to parenteral. Milk and vegetable proteins are less likely to potentiate HE compared with animal proteins. Restricted protein diets should only be considered for patients with HE.[60]

The resting energy requirement (RER) should be calculated as kilocalories per day = $70 \times$ body weight $(kg)^{3/4}$. Aim to provide sufficient food, such that a minimum

25% to 50% of the RER is provided on the first day, and slowly increase to 100% of the RER over the next 2 to 3 days, depending on the patient's tolerance. Antiemetics and antacids may improve patient tolerance. Placement of a feeding tube may be considered for patients tolerant of enteral nutrition but not consuming adequate calories voluntarily.

PROGNOSIS

The prognosis for ALI is variable depending on the inciting cause and response to therapy. Unfortunately, once ALF has developed, the prognosis appears to be poor, with one study reporting only 14% survival to discharge.[4]

REFERENCES

1. Lee WM. Acute liver failure. Semin Respir Crit Care Med 2012;33(1):36–45.
2. Wlodzimirow KAK. Systematic review: acute liver failure—one disease, more than 40 definitions. Aliment Pharmacol Ther 2012;35(11):1245–56.
3. O'Grady JG, Schalm SW, Williams R. Acute liver failure: redefining the syndromes. Lancet 1993;342(8866):273–5.
4. Lester C, Cooper J, Peters RM, et al. Retrospective evaluation of acute liver failure in dogs (1995-2012): 49 cases. J Vet Emerg Crit Care (San Antonio) 2016; 26(4):559–67.
5. Maxie MG, editor. Jubb, Kennedy and Palmer's pathology of domestic animals. 6th editon. St Louis (MO): Elsevier; 2016. No. 2.
6. MacKenzie R, Furnival C, O'Keane MA, et al. The effect of hepatic ischaemia on liver function and the restoration of liver mass after 70 per cent partial hepatectomy in the dog. Br J Surg 1975;62(6):431–7.
7. Bernal W, Hyyrylainen A, Gera A, et al. Lessons from look-back in acute liver failure? A single centre experience of 3300 patients. J Hepatol 2013;59(1):74–80.
8. Adukauskiene D, Dockiene I, Naginiene R, et al. Acute liver failure in Lithuania. Medicina (Kaunas, Lithuania) 2008;44(7):536–40.
9. Bower WA, Johns M, Margolis HS, et al. Population-based surveillance for acute liver failure. Am J Gastroenterol 2007;102(11):2459–63.
10. Escorsell A, Mas A, de la Mata M. Acute liver failure in Spain: analysis of 267 cases. Liver Transpl 2007;13(10):1389–95.
11. Ostapowicz G, Fontana RJ, Schiodt FV, et al. Results of a prospective study of acute liver failure at 17 tertiary care centers in the United States. Ann Intern Med 2002;137(12):947–54.
12. Dereszynski DM, Center SA, Randolph JF, et al. Clinical and clinicopathologic features of dogs that consumed foodborne hepatotoxic aflatoxins: 72 cases (2005-2006). J Am Vet Med Assoc 2008;232(9):1329–37.
13. Puschner B, Wegenast C. Mushroom poisoning cases in dogs and cats: diagnosis and treatment of hepatotoxic, neurotoxic, gastroenterotoxic, nephrotoxic, and muscarinic mushrooms. Vet Clin North Am Small Anim Pract 2012;42(2): 375–87, viii.
14. Tokarz D, Poppenga R, Kaae J, et al. Amanitin toxicosis in two cats with acute hepatic and renal failure. Vet Pathol 2012;49(6):1032–5.
15. van der Merwe D, Sebbag L, Nietfeld JC, et al. Investigation of a Microcystis aeruginosa cyanobacterial freshwater harmful algal bloom associated with acute microcystin toxicosis in a dog. J Vet Diagn Invest 2012;24(4):679–87.

16. Simola O, Wiberg M, Jokela J, et al. Pathologic findings and toxin identification in cyanobacterial (Nodularia spumigena) intoxication in a dog. Vet Pathol 2012; 49(5):755–9.

17. Sebbag L, Smee N, van der Merwe D, et al. Liver failure in a dog following suspected ingestion of blue-green algae (Microcystis spp.): a case report and review of the toxin. J Am Anim Hosp Assoc 2013;49(5):342–6.

18. Albretsen JC, Khan SA, Richardson JA. Cycad palm toxicosis in dogs: 60 cases (1987-1997). J Am Vet Med Assoc 1998;213(1):99–101.

19. Ferguson D, Crowe M, McLaughlin L, et al. Survival and prognostic indicators for cycad intoxication in dogs. J Vet Intern Med 2011;25(4):831–7.

20. Dunayer EK, Gwaltney-Brant SM. Acute hepatic failure and coagulopathy associated with xylitol ingestion in eight dogs. J Am Vet Med Assoc 2006;229(7): 1113–7.

21. Schmid RD, Hovda LR. Acute hepatic failure in a dog after xylitol ingestion. J Med Toxicol 2016;12(2):201–5.

22. DuHadway MR, Sharp CR, Meyers KE, et al. Retrospective evaluation of xylitol ingestion in dogs: 192 cases (2007-2012). J Vet Emerg Crit Care (San Antonio) 2015;25(5):646–54.

23. Richardson JA. Management of acetaminophen and ibuprofen toxicoses in dogs and cats. J Vet Emerg Crit Care (San Antonio) 2000;10(4):285–91.

24. Wallace KP, Center SA, Hickford FH, et al. S-adenosyl-L-methionine (SAMe) for the treatment of acetaminophen toxicity in a dog. J Am Anim Hosp Assoc 2002;38(3):246–54.

25. Center SA, Elston TH, Rowland PH, et al. Fulminant hepatic failure associated with oral administration of diazepam in 11 cats. J Am Vet Med Assoc 1996; 209(3):618–25.

26. Park FM. Successful treatment of hepatic failure secondary to diazepam administration in a cat. J Feline Med Surg 2012;14(2):158–60.

27. MacPhail CM, Lappin MR, Meyer DJ, et al. Hepatocellular toxicosis associated with administration of carprofen in 21 dogs. J Am Vet Med Assoc 1998; 212(12):1895–901.

28. Skorupski KA, Hammond GM, Irish AM, et al. Prospective randomized clinical trial assessing the efficacy of Denamarin for prevention of CCNU-induced hepatopathy in tumor-bearing dogs. J Vet Intern Med 2011;25(4):838–45.

29. Webb CB, Twedt DC. Acute hepatopathy associated with mitotane administration in a dog. J Am Anim Hosp Assoc 2006;42(4):298–301.

30. Holahan ML, Littman MP, Hayes CL. Presumptive hepatotoxicity and rhabdomyolysis secondary to phenazopyridine toxicity in a dog. J Vet Emerg Crit Care (San Antonio) 2010;20(3):352–8.

31. Harkin KR, Cowan LA, Andrews GA, et al. Hepatotoxicity of stanozolol in cats. J Am Vet Med Assoc 2000;217(5):681–4.

32. Wong VM, Marche C, Simko E. Infectious canine hepatitis associated with prednisone treatment. Can Vet J 2012;53(11):1219–21.

33. Twedt DC, Diehl KJ, Lappin MR, et al. Association of hepatic necrosis with trimethoprim sulfonamide administration in 4 dogs. J Vet Intern Med 1997; 11(1):20–3.

34. Miller ML, Center SA, Randolph JF, et al. Apparent acute idiosyncratic hepatic necrosis associated with zonisamide administration in a dog. J Vet Intern Med 2011; 25(5):1156–60.

35. Schwartz M, Munana KR, Olby NJ. Possible drug-induced hepatopathy in a dog receiving zonisamide monotherapy for treatment of cryptogenic epilepsy. J Vet Med Sci 2011;73(11):1505–8.
36. Hartmann KK. Feline infectious peritonitis. Vet Clin North Am Small Anim Pract 2005;35(1):39–79.
37. Guerra MA. Leptospirosis. J Am Vet Med Assoc 2009;234(4):472–8, 430.
38. Xavier FG, Morato GS, Righi DA, et al. Cystic liver disease related to high Platynosomum fastosum infection in a domestic cat. J feline Med Surg 2007;9(1):51–5.
39. Giuliano A, Meiring T, Grant AJ, et al. Acute hepatic necrosis caused by salmonella enterica serotype I 4,5,12:-:1,2 in a dog. J Clin Microbiol 2015;53(11): 3674–6.
40. Nagel SS, Williams JH, Schoeman JP. Fatal disseminated toxoplasmosis in an immunocompetent cat. J S Afr Vet Assoc 2013;84(1):E1–6.
41. Center SA, Crawford MA, Guida L, et al. A retrospective study of 77 cats with severe hepatic lipidosis: 1975-1990. J Vet Intern Med 1993;7(6):349–59.
42. Borchers A, Epstein SE, Gindiciosi B, et al. Acute enteral manganese intoxication with hepatic failure due to ingestion of a joint supplement overdose. J Vet Diagn Invest 2014;26(5):658–63.
43. Dayrell-Hart B, Steinberg SA, VanWinkle TJ, et al. Hepatotoxicity of phenobarbital in dogs: 18 cases (1985-1989). J Am Vet Med Assoc 1991;199(8):1060–6.
44. Weingarten MA, Sande AA. Acute liver failure in dogs and cats. J Vet Emerg Crit Care 2015;25(4):455–73.
45. Sigrist NE, Adamik KN, Doherr MG, et al. Evaluation of respiratory parameters at presentation as clinical indicators of the respiratory localization in dogs and cats with respiratory distress. J Vet Emerg Crit Care 2011;21(1):13–23.
46. O'Grady JG. Pathogenesis of acute liver failure. Trop Gastroenterol 1996;17(4): 199–201.
47. Davis H, Jensen T, Johnson A, et al. 2013 AAHA/AAFP fluid therapy guidelines for dogs and cats. J Am Anim Hosp Assoc 2013;49(3):149–59.
48. Silverstein DC, Santoro-Beer K. Daily intravenous fluid therapy. In: Silverstein DC, Hopper K, editors. Small animal critical care medicine. 2nd edition. St Louis (MO): Elsevier/Saunders; 2015. p. 316–21.
49. Adamik KN, Yozova ID, Regenscheit N. Controversies in the use of hydroxyethyl starch solutions in small animal emergency and critical care. J Vet Emerg Crit Care 2015;25(1):20–47.
50. Hayes G, Benedicenti L, Mathews K. Retrospective cohort study on the incidence of acute kidney injury and death following hydroxyethyl starch (HES 10% 250/0.5/ 5:1) administration in dogs (2007-2010). J Vet Emerg Crit Care 2016;26(1):35–40.
51. Silverstein DC, Beer KA. Controversies regarding choice of vasopressor therapy for management of septic shock in animals. J Vet Emerg Crit Care 2015;25(1): 48–54.
52. Peyton JLJL. Critical illness-related corticosteroid insufficiency in a dog with septic shock. J Vet Emerg Crit Care (San Antonio) 2009;19(3):262–8.
53. Lidbury JA, Ivanek R, Suchodolski JS, et al. Putative precipitating factors for hepatic encephalopathy in dogs: 118 cases (1991-2014). J Am Vet Med Assoc 2015;247(2):176–83.
54. Alvarez L, Whittemore J. Liver enzyme elevations in dogs: physiology and pathophysiology. Compend Contin Educ Vet 2009;31(9):408–10, 412–3; [quiz: 414].
55. Chapman SE, Hostutler RA. A laboratory diagnostic approach to hepatobiliary disease in small animals. Vet Clin North Am Small Anim Pract 2013;43(6): 1209–25, v.

56. Ong JP, Aggarwal A, Krieger D, et al. Correlation between ammonia levels and the severity of hepatic encephalopathy. Am J Med 2003;114(3):188–93.

57. Rothuizen J, van den Ingh TS. Arterial and venous ammonia concentrations in the diagnosis of canine hepato-encephalopathy. Res Vet Sci 1982;33(1):17–21.

58. Stanton ME, Bright RM. Gastroduodenal ulceration in dogs. Retrospective study of 43 cases and literature review. J Vet Intern Med 1989;3(4):238–44.

59. Allison MG, Shanholtz CB, Sachdeva A. Hematological issues in liver disease. Crit Care Clin 2016;32(3):385–96.

60. Berent A. Hepatic failure. In: Silverstein DC, Hopper K, editors. Small animal critical care medicine. 2nd edition. St Louis (MO): Elsevier/Saunders; 2015. p. 615–21.

61. Stravitz RT, Ellerbe C, Dukalski V, et al. Spontaneous bleeding complications in acute liver failure (ALF). Hepatology 2013;58(Suppl 4):347A.

62. Stravitz RT, Lisman T, Luketic VA, et al. Minimal effects of acute liver injury/acute liver failure on hemostasis as assessed by thromboelastography. J Hepatol 2012; 56(1):129–36.

63. Kelley D, Lester C, Shaw S, et al. Thromboelastographic evaluation of dogs with acute liver disease. J Vet Intern Med 2015;29(4):1053–62.

64. Lisman T, Stravitz RT. Rebalanced hemostasis in patients with acute liver failure. Semin Thromb Hemost 2015;41(5):468–73.

65. McMurray J, Boysen S, Chalhoub S. Focused assessment with sonography in nontraumatized dogs and cats in the emergency and critical care setting. J Vet Emerg Crit Care (San Antonio) 2016;26(1):64–73.

66. Wang KY, Panciera DL, Al-Rukibat RK, et al. Accuracy of ultrasound-guided fine-needle aspiration of the liver and cytologic findings in dogs and cats: 97 cases (1990-2000). J Am Vet Med Assoc 2004;224(1):75–8.

67. Bigge LA, Brown DJ, Penninck DG. Correlation between coagulation profile findings and bleeding complications after ultrasound-guided biopsies: 434 cases (1993-1996). J Am Anim Hosp Assoc 2001;37(3):228–33.

68. Waddell LS, Holt DE, Hughes D, et al. The effect of storage on ammonia concentration in canine packed red blood cells. J Vet Emerg Crit Care (San Antonio) 2001;11(1):23–6.

69. Cummings KA, Abelson AL, Rozanski EA, et al. The effect of storage on ammonia, cytokine, and chemokine concentrations in feline whole blood. J Vet Emerg Crit Care (San Antonio) 2016;26(5):639–45.

70. Lidbury JA, Cook AK, Steiner JM. Hepatic encephalopathy in dogs and cats. J Vet Emerg Crit Care (San Antonio) 2016;26(4):471–87.

71. Weiner ID, Wingo CS. Hypokalemia–consequences, causes, and correction. J Am Soc Nephrol 1997;8(7):1179–88.

72. Iwasa M, Sugimoto R, Mifuji-Moroka R, et al. Factors contributing to the development of overt encephalopathy in liver cirrhosis patients. Metab Brain Dis 2016; 31(5):1151–6.

73. Taboada J, Dimski DS. Hepatic encephalopathy: clinical signs, pathogenesis, and treatment. Vet Clin North Am Small Anim Pract 1995;25(2):337–55.

74. Olde Damink SW, Dejong CH, Deutz NE, et al. Effects of simulated upper gastrointestinal hemorrhage on ammonia and related amino acids in blood and brain of chronic portacaval-shunted rats. Metab Brain Dis 1997;12(2):121–35.

75. Tivers MS, Handel I, Gow AG, et al. Hyperammonemia and systemic inflammatory response syndrome predicts presence of hepatic encephalopathy in dogs with congenital portosystemic shunts. PLoS One 2014;9(1):e82303.

76. Aronson LR, Gacad RC, Kaminsky-Russ K, et al. Endogenous benzodiazepine activity in the peripheral and portal blood of dogs with congenital portosystemic shunts. Vet Surg 1997;26(3):189–94.

77. Holt D. Hepatic encephalopathy. In: Silverstein DC, Hopper K, editors. Small animal critical care medicine. 2nd edition. St Louis (MO): Elsevier/Saunders; 2015. p. 458–61.

78. Kodali S, McGuire BM. Diagnosis and management of hepatic encephalopathy in fulminant hepatic failure. Clin Liver Dis 2015;19(3):565–76.

79. Stravitz RT, Kramer AH, Davern T, et al. Intensive care of patients with acute liver failure: recommendations of the U.S. Acute Liver Failure Study Group. Crit Care Med 2007;35(11):2498–508.

80. Rolando N, Harvey F, Brahm J, et al. Prospective study of bacterial infection in acute liver failure: an analysis of fifty patients. Hepatology 1990;11(1):49–53.

81. Rolando N, Gimson A, Wade J, et al. Prospective controlled trial of selective parenteral and enteral antimicrobial regimen in fulminant liver failure. Hepatology 1993;17(2):196–201.

82. Tolbert K, Bissett S, King A, et al. Efficacy of oral famotidine and 2 omeprazole formulations for the control of intragastric pH in dogs. J Vet Intern Med 2011; 25(1):47–54.

83. Pereira SP, Rowbotham D, Fitt S, et al. Pharmacokinetics and efficacy of oral versus intravenous mixed-micellar phylloquinone (vitamin K1) in severe acute liver disease. J Hepatol 2005;42(3):365–70.

84. Vandeweerd JM, Cambier C, Gustin P. Nutraceuticals for canine liver disease: assessing the evidence. Vet Clin North Am Small Anim Pract 2013;43(5):1171–9.

85. Filburn CR, Kettenacker R, Griffin DW. Bioavailability of a silybin-phosphatidylcholine complex in dogs. J Vet Pharmacol Ther 2007;30(2):132–8.

Canine Copper-Associated Hepatitis

Karen Dirksen, DVM, PhD, Hille Fieten, DVM, PhD*

KEYWORDS

- Dog • Liver • Bedlington terrier • Labrador retriever • Wilson disease • *ATP7A*
- *ATP7B* • *COMMD1*

KEY POINTS

- Canine copper-associated hepatitis shares similarities with human copper accumulation disorders.
- Copper-associated hepatitis is recognized in several dog breeds and differences exist in causal genes and inheritance patterns between breeds.
- Clinical signs are usually noted late in disease stage when severe liver damage due to hepatic copper accumulation is already present.
- D-Penicillamine (DPA) is the most commonly used chelator to treat hepatic copper accumulation and treatment is most effective in early stages of disease.
- A low-copper/high-zinc diet can help to prevent accumulation or reaccumulation of hepatic copper in dogs with complex forms of copper-associated hepatitis.

INTRODUCTION: PATHOPHYSIOLOGY OF COPPER HOMEOSTASIS AND CELLULAR COPPER METABOLISM

Copper Homeostasis

Copper is an essential trace element necessary for many vital functions in the body. Free copper is toxic, however, due to the potential to create reactive oxygen species. Therefore, copper uptake, distribution, and excretion are tightly regulated.[1] Dietary copper is predominantly absorbed in the small intestine. Copper uptake by the enterocyte is mainly mediated by copper transporter 1 (CTR1), a high-affinity copper transporter. The copper transporter ATPase copper transporting alpha (ATP7A) is located at the basal membrane of the enterocytes and facilitates copper transport into the portal circulation. In the portal blood, copper is predominantly bound to albumin and is delivered to the hepatocellular cytosol via apically located CTR1. The liver is the most important organ in copper metabolism and is responsible for copper storage,

Disclosure Statement: The authors have nothing to disclose.
Department of Clinical Sciences of Companion Animals, Faculty of Veterinary Medicine, Utrecht University, Utrecht, The Netherlands
* Corresponding author. Yalelaan 108, 3584 CM, Utrecht, The Netherlands.
E-mail address: H.Fieten@uu.nl

redistribution to other tissues and organs, and excretion of excess copper via the biliary system. The kidneys excrete a small proportion of excess body copper.

Cellular Copper Metabolism

After copper enters the hepatocytes, it is immediately bound by proteins to prevent oxidative damage (**Fig. 1**). Copper scavengers, including the small proteins metallothionein (MT) and glutathione (GSH), are the first to bind and store copper. Special delivery proteins, the copper chaperones, ensure safe handover of copper to their destination molecules.[2] Cyclooxygenase (COX)17 is the copper chaperone for cytochrome C oxidase (CCO), which resides in the inner mitochondrial membrane. CCO is the terminal enzyme in the mitochondrial respiratory chain and thus plays a crucial role in aerobic energy metabolism. The copper chaperone for superoxide dismutase (CCS) shuttles copper to superoxide dismutase (SOD1), which is an important protein in the defense against oxidative stress. Antioxidant 1 copper chaperone (ATOX1) is the copper chaperone for the copper transporters, ATP7A and ATPase, copper transporting, beta (ATP7B). Both ATPases reside in the trans-Golgi network (TGN) under normal copper conditions. When intracellular copper concentrations are rising, they move away from the TGN to their respective destinations. In the TGN, ATP7B loads 6 copper atoms onto the ferroxidase ceruloplasmin (CP), which is secreted into the circulation.[3] CP is the main copper transport protein in the blood. Under elevated copper conditions, ATP7B traffics to a lysosomal or apical membrane-associated cellular component and facilitates excretion of excess copper into the bile.[4] Previously, the main role of ATP7A was presumed to be copper uptake in the intestines, but recently hepatocellular ATP7A was demonstrated to have an important role in mobilizing and redistributing hepatic copper stores in case of peripheral copper deficiency.[5] The copper metabolism (Murr1) domain containing 1 (COMMD1) protein interacts with the amino

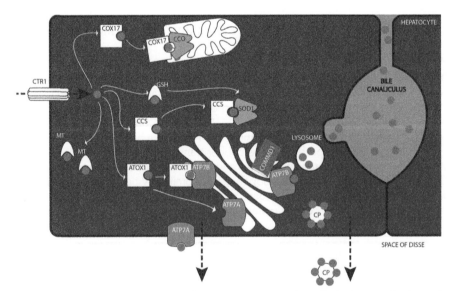

Fig. 1. Hepatocellular copper metabolism. Copper enters the cell via CTR1 and is immediately bound by MTs and/or GSH to prevent oxidative stress. The chaperones COX17, CCS, and ATOX1 transfer copper to their respective destination molecules CCO, SOD1, and ATP7A/ATP7B. ATP7A and ATP7B function in the export of copper to the blood (ATP7A and ATP7B) or to the bile (ATP7B). COMMD1 interacts with both ATPases.

terminus of ATP7B and presumably facilitates biliary excretion of copper. In addition, COMMD1 has a role in the stability and quality control of both ATPases.[6]

COPPER METABOLISM DISORDERS IN HUMANS
Wilson Disease

Wilson disease is an autosomal recessive disorder in humans in which copper accumulates in liver and neuronal tissues. The disease manifests as hepatopathy and/or neurologic or psychiatric symptoms. Wilson disease can result from several mutations in the copper transporter ATP7B. Because of its role in the incorporation of copper into CP, this may lead to low serum CP concentrations, which is one of the diagnostic criteria. Furthermore, urinary copper excretion may be increased in patients with Wilson disease. Conventional treatment consists of lifelong copper chelation with DPA.[7]

Non-Wilsonian Forms of Copper Toxicosis

Other copper storage disorders in humans in which the causative genes have not yet been identified include Indian childhood cirrhosis,[8] endemic Tyrolean infantile cirrhosis,[9] and idiopathic copper toxicosis.[10] In these diseases, a predominant hepatic presentation is observed. A hereditary predisposition in combination with increased (dietary) exposure to copper is thought to be responsible for the observed disease symptoms.

Menkes Disease

Mutations in the copper transporter ATP7A result in X-linked, recessive copper deficiency due to impaired dietary intestinal copper uptake. Patients suffer from severe neurologic impairment and failure to thrive in early childhood, and the disease is often lethal despite parenteral copper supplementation.[11]

HEREDITARY COPPER-ASSOCIATED HEPATITIS IN DOGS
Bedlington Terrier

Historically, the Bedlington terrier was the first dog breed in which canine copper-associated hepatitis was studied extensively and where a causal mutation was identified. The disease is characterized by liver cirrhosis induced by massive, centrolobular copper accumulation (**Fig. 2**A, D). Hepatic copper may be as high as 10,000 mg copper per kg dry weight liver (dwl). The causal mutation is a large deletion in the second exon of the COMMD1 gene, leading to autosomal recessive copper toxicosis.[12] Due to the development of a DNA test, the disease frequency in the Bedlington terrier population has been drastically reduced. Recently, cases of non–COMMD1-related copper toxicosis were observed in Bedlington terriers. Variations in the metal transporter ABCA12 were found to be associated with non-COMMD1 copper toxicosis; however, convincing functional data proving involvement of this gene were lacking.[13]

Labrador Retriever

The Labrador retriever was the second breed in which part of the hereditary background of copper-associated hepatitis was elucidated. In this breed, the disease follows a complex inheritance pattern and genetic as well as dietary factors[14–18] play a role in pathogenesis. A recently performed genome-wide association study showed a significant association of increased hepatic copper concentrations with a mutation in the Wilson disease gene (ATP7B). Concurrent presence of a mutation in the Menkes disease gene (ATP7A) seemed to attenuate hepatic copper accumulation without resulting in a copper-deficient phenotype. Approximately 12% of total heritability can be explained by the 2 identified mutations. Missing heritability may be explained

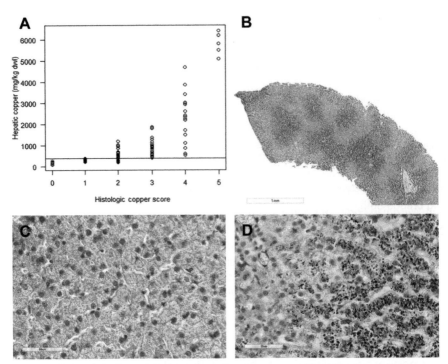

Fig. 2. (*A*) Relation between histologic hepatic copper scores (X axis) and quantitative copper measurements (Y axis) in 109 canine liver samples collected at the Faculty of Veterinary Medicine, Utrecht University, between 2010 and 2016. The horizontal line indicates the cutoff level for normal hepatic copper (400 mg/kg dry weight liver [dwl]). (*B*) Centrolobular copper distribution is clearly visible in a liver biopsy of a *COMMD1*-deficient dog (rubeanic acid stain). (*C*) Copper score 0 (rubeanic acid stain) in a Labrador retriever (quantitative copper concentration 146 mg/kg dwl). (*D*) Copper score 5 (rubeanic acid stain) in a Bedlington terrier (quantitative copper concentration 6540 mg/kg dwl).

by environmental factors or as-yet unidentified genetic mutations. Functional assays in cell lines showed that the *ATP7B* mutation in the conserved arginine resulted in an aberrant retention of the protein in the endoplasmic reticulum in high copper circumstances. The *ATP7A* mutation, located in a conserved phosphorylation site, did not affect trafficking of the protein yet led to a decrease of copper efflux in dermal fibroblasts, indicating a functional impairment of the protein.[19]

Other Breeds

Copper-associated hepatitis with a suspected hereditary background has been described in several other dog breeds including the Dobermann,[20] the West Highland white terrier,[21] and the Dalmatian.[22] Case reports of dogs diagnosed with copper-associated hepatitis include the Skye terrier,[23] Anatolian shepherd,[24] Pembroke Welsh corgi, Cardigan Welsh corgi,[25,26] and the clumber spaniel.[26] More extensive reviews of hepatic copper concentrations in dogs diagnosed with primary hepatitis suggest that there are many more breeds, including crossbreeds, in which copper-associated hepatitis is present.[27,28] The authors think it is unlikely that environmental factors, such as dietary composition, could explain copper accumulation and associated hepatitis in genetically healthy dogs and anticipate that most of the reported breeds have some form of hereditary dysfunction in their copper metabolism. Genetic studies are needed to elucidate the affected genes in these dogs.

DIAGNOSIS
Signalment

The rate of hepatic copper accumulation and development of associated clinical signs depends on genetic predisposition and dietary copper intake and varies between breeds and between individuals within a breed. In Labrador retrievers, the age at which dogs present with clinical signs can range from 2 years old to 12 years old, but most dogs are middle aged (median age of 6 years). Bitches in the postpartum period may be at increased risk for development of clinical signs. A strong female pre-disposition is noted in the Labrador retriever[29] and the Dobermann,[30] whereas in other dog breeds both genders are usually represented equally.

Clinical Signs

The subclinical phase in dogs with inherited copper-associated hepatitis is usually long for 2 reasons. First, hepatic copper accumulation precedes the development of histolog-ic changes in the liver. In Bedlington terriers, it has been shown that copper starts accu-mulating between 6 months and 12 months of age without overt histologic signs of hepatitis.[31] Second, clinical signs only develop when a large portion of liver parenchyma is affected. Because the liver has an enormous reserve capacity, this is usually in the end stage of the disease when chronic hepatitis or cirrhosis becomes overt. Initially, clinical signs are nonspecific and may include anorexia, lethargy, nausea, vomiting, and weight loss. When the disease becomes more progressive, more specific signs pointing toward hepatic failure, such as ascites, hepatic encephalopathy, polyuria/polydipsia, and icterus, can be noticed. Although rare, in the Bedlington terrier an acute hemolytic crisis due to the massive release of copper into the bloodstream has been reported.[32]

Clinical Pathology

The most commonly used biochemical indicators for hepatocellular injury are alanine aminotransferase (ALT) and alkaline phosphatase (ALP).[33] In the subclinical stage of copper accumulation, however, extensive hepatocellular injury is not necessarily pre-sent. The sensitivities of ALP for detection of acute hepatitis, chronic hepatitis, and nonspecific reactive hepatitis in a group of 191 clinically healthy Labrador retrievers that were admitted to the Faculty of Veterinary Medicine, Utrecht University, between 2003 and 2015, were all below 35%. For ALT, sensitivities for the detection of acute hepatitis, chronic hepatitis, and nonspecific reactive hepatitis were 45%, 71%, and 5%, respectively. This group of dogs included 131 Labrador retrievers with hepatic copper accumulation (Fieten and Dirksen, unpublished data, 2016). In affected Bed-lington terriers, hepatocellular injury became visible between 12 and 18 months of age, whereas an increase in ALT and ALP was only detected at 24 months and 18 months of age, respectively.[31] Both observations underline that ALT and ALP are not useful for screening for subclinical copper-associated hepatitis. In a more advanced stage of the disease, an increase of ALT and ALP can be noticed, and a slight decrease in albumin concentration may be observed as well, although concen-trations still may be within the reference range.[22,29,34] Other laboratory indicators include an increase in bile acids, ammonia, bilirubin, prothrombin time, and activated partial thromboplastin time and a decrease in fibrinogen and packed cell volume.[29,34] Serum/plasma ALT and ALP activity as well as bile acid concentration are useful pa-rameters for detecting liver disease but neither is specific for copper-associated liver disease. In dogs, serum copper concentrations do not correlate with hepatic copper concentrations. Decreased CP is a diagnostic hallmark for human Wilson disease. It would be interesting to investigate serum CP concentrations in Labrador retrievers with copper-associated hepatitis due to *ATP7B* mutations.

Fanconi Syndrome

Comparable to observations in humans with Wilson disease, Fanconi syndrome has been recognized in dogs with copper-associated hepatitis.[26,35,36] In these dogs, proximal tubular dysfunction was present due to copper accumulation in the proximal tubular epithelium. Dogs presented with low urinary specific gravity, proteinuria, and normoglycemic glucosuria. The observed abnormalities were reversed by DPA chelation therapy.

Cytology

Fine-needle aspiration and cytology of hepatocytes stained with a specific copper stain (ie, rubeanic acid) may be used as a noninvasive way to get an indication of the presence of copper in individual hepatocytes.[20,37] Limitations of this technique are the impossibility of evaluating zonal copper distribution, degree of hepatocellular injury, and the determination of the exact amount of copper (needed for determination of treatment duration). Further studies into the negative predictive value are necessary, because copper distribution in the liver lobules is zonal and theoretically a negative sample could be obtained from a dog affected with copper-associated hepatitis.

Liver Histopathology

Histologic distribution of copper

A histologic biopsy remains the gold standard for diagnosing copper-associated hepatitis. Samples can be obtained via laparotomy, via laparoscopy or, percutaneously with a needle (14–16 gauge) using ultrasound guidance. Because copper is not visible on routine hematoxylin-eosin stains, additional staining for copper (rubeanic acid[38] or rhodanine[39]) is necessary for the diagnosis. In cases of primary copper-associated hepatitis, copper typically starts to accumulate in the centrolobular regions of the hepatic lobule (zone 3; **Fig. 2**B).[28,29,40] Copper-loaded hepatocytes trigger the emergence of an inflammatory infiltrate, which can be mononuclear or mixed. Because excess copper is excreted into bile, an increase of hepatic copper, especially in the periportal areas of the liver lobules, could be anticipated in dogs with cholestatic diseases. In many cases of cholestatic liver disease, however, no periportal copper accumulation is detectable and the interpretation of rare cases with periportal copper accumulation is not totally clear.[41] In end-stage liver disease, where severe cirrhosis, massive necrosis, and lobular collapse are present, it may be difficult to distinguish the different zones of the liver lobule. Furthermore, in an advanced stage of the disease necrotic hepatocytes have released their copper burden, and newly formed hepatocytes, which arise during the regeneration process, do initially not contain copper,[21,42] neither does scar tissue, further diluting total copper content in the transition to end-stage disease. Mainly because of these unevenly distributed histologic changes, results of both the histologic examination (distribution and scoring) and quantitative copper determination always have to be considered in hepatic copper assessment.

Histologic scoring of copper

A semiquantitative grading system to determine hepatic copper content can be applied on copper-stained sections of liver tissue (see **Fig. 2**A).[40] Scoring is based on zonal location and number of hepatocytes and macrophages containing copper granules. In a grading scale of 0 to 5, copper scores of 2 or higher are considered abnormal (see **Fig. 2**A, C, D). However, each semiquantitative score includes a wide range of quantitative copper concentrations, with overlap between scores (see **Fig. 2**A).

Quantitative copper determination

Hepatic copper concentrations can also be assessed quantitatively by the irradiation of small pieces of liver and the measurement of the induced copper radioactivity.[43] Therefore, an additional biopsy specimen of at least 5 mg is needed, which is freeze dried before analysis to determine dry weight copper. Other methods for quantification are spectrophotometric methods, including atomic absorption spectrometry or inductively coupled plasma emission spectrometry. Normal hepatic copper concentrations in dogs are considered below 400 mg/kg dwl.[44] In dogs affected with copper-associated hepatitis, hepatic copper concentrations are usually above 800 mg/kg dwl but can reach 10,000 mg/kg dwl. In this respect, dogs are markedly different from humans where normal copper concentrations lie in the range of 50 mg/kg dwl, and patients with Wilson disease usually have hepatic copper concentrations in the range of 500 mg/kg dwl.

Digital estimation of copper concentrations

Digital microscopic scanning of copper-stained liver sections has shown to be more accurate than qualitative copper scoring but still allows assessment of zonal histologic lesions.[45] This technique can be applied for histologic slides of liver biopsies where no additional sample for copper quantification is available.

Biomarkers

Because currently the only way to diagnose and monitor copper-associated hepatitis is by (repeated) histologic assessment of liver biopsies, the development of a noninvasive biomarker for copper status from samples of blood or urine is warranted. Such a biomarker could help identify at risk dogs to prevent clinical illness by institution of early treatment and to prevent breeding of affected individuals. Moreover, it would be easier to monitor copper concentrations during treatment using a serum or urine biomarker. The urinary copper/zinc ratio was significantly associated with hepatic copper concentration in Labrador retrievers, but the diagnostic value was limited due to overlap between normal and affected dogs.[46] Copper/zinc SOD1 and its chaperone (CCS) have both been studied as biomarkers in humans and animals with copper deficiency and overload. Erythrocyte CCS and CCS/SOD1 ratio was significantly decreased in a pilot study in Labrador retrievers with copper-associated hepatitis, suggesting promise for future clinical use. Other biomarkers under investigation include microRNAs, which are small noncoding RNAs that regulate gene expression.[47] The hepatocyte-derived microRNA-122 was significantly increased in Labrador retrievers with high hepatic copper concentrations compared with Labrador retrievers with normal copper concentrations, both without histological abnormalities, likely reflecting early copper-induced hepatocellular damage.[48] MicroRNA-122 is not copper-specific and new copper-specific microRNAs should be identified.

TREATMENT
General Recommendations

The goal of treatment in dogs with copper toxicosis is to create a negative copper balance. This can be achieved by restricting copper intake and by increasing urinary copper excretion using copper chelators (**Table 1**). Because treatment has the best outcome early in the disease when hepatocellular injury is limited, it is important that treatment is initiated as soon as possible and ideally in the subclinical phase.

Table 1
Medication for copper-associated hepatitis

Drug	Dose	Adverse Effects	Remarks
DPA	10–15 mg/kg po bid, separate from meals	Anorexia, vomiting, and possibly immune-mediated reactions	Most commonly used Possibly immunomodulatory and antifibrotic properties Prediction model for treatment duration available for Labrador retrievers
Trientene (2,2,2-tetramine)	15 mg/kg po bid	None reported in dogs	
2,3,2-Tetramine	15 mg/kg po bid	None reported in dogs	Not commercially available
Ammonium TTM	Unknown	Anorexia, vomiting	High risk of severe copper deficiency resulting in bone marrow depression
Zinc salts • Zinc acetate • Zinc gluconate • Zinc sulfate	5–10 mg/kg elemental zinc po bid	Generally well tolerated, but gastrointestinal side effects may occur	Should not be the sole therapy in clinical cases Slow onset of action Monitoring of plasma zinc concentrations necessary

Increased hepatic copper concentrations may induce oxidative stress and in this way contribute to progression of hepatocellular injury. It is currently unknown at exactly what concentration of copper this process starts and when chelation therapy should be initiated. For dogs, usually a hepatic copper level of greater than 400 mg/kg dwl is considered increased, which is already high, for example, compared with normal hepatic copper levels in humans (50 mg/kg dwl). In general, clinically ill dogs or dogs with overt hepatocellular injury and increased hepatic copper levels should be treated with a copper chelator and treatment should ideally be monitored by follow-up liver biopsies.

In dogs without clinical signs, with normal hepatic enzymes and moderately increased hepatic copper levels (ie, 400–600 mg/kg dwl), changing to a low-copper/high-zinc diet may be sufficient in normalization of hepatic copper levels. Individual variation in response to diet was noted, however, and continuing copper accumulation may occur despite feeding a low-copper/high-zinc diet.[16] Because it is currently not possible to predict response to diet in individual dogs, a second biopsy is always necessary 6 months after initial diagnosis and dietary change.

D-Penicillamine

DPA is a highly soluble degradation product of penicillin that is excreted by the kidneys. It binds 1 copper atom at its sulfhydryl group and facilitates excretion of copper into the urine.[49] DPA is one of the most potent copper chelators and is also able to form lower avidity complexes with other metals like zinc and iron.[50,51] Besides chelating properties, DPA may have additional favorable immunomodulatory and antifibrotic activities.[52,53] It has been shown to be effective in the treatment of canine copper-associated hepatitis and is the most commonly used chelator.[29,54–56] The recommended dose for use in dogs is 10 mg/kg to 15 mg/kg orally twice daily. To increase bioavailability and to maximize plasma concentrations, DPA should not be given with food.[57] Side effects in dogs are usually limited to gastrointestinal signs, such as anorexia and vomiting.[55,57] Gastrointestinal side effects are easily manageable by temporarily decreasing the dose or by giving antiemetics an hour prior to DPA administration.[55,57]

In humans, DPA may induce immunologic side effects, but these have not been regularly reported in dogs. The authors and editor are aware of 2 cases in which immunologic effects were presumed related to DPA administration. A 4-year-old, female neutered English springer spaniel developed severe protein-losing glomerulonephropathy, resulting in hypoalbuminemia and ascites approximately 4 months after initiation of DPA therapy. Proteinuria and hypoalbuminemia resolved completely within 2 weeks after cessation of DPA. Furthermore, a West Highland white terrier presented with severe dermatologic lesions shortly after starting DPA, which quickly and completely resolved after DPA cessation. Although in both cases a causal link remains difficult to prove, there was a suspicion of DPA-related immunologic side effects.

Recently a model has been published that can be used as a guideline for the calculation of necessary duration of DPA treatment depending on hepatic copper concentrations in Labrador retrievers (**Box 1**).[55] Most likely, this model can also be used for other dog breeds with complex forms of copper-associated liver disease and copper concentrations in a similar range. Treatment should be continued until normal hepatic copper concentrations are achieved.

Continuous DPA therapy may lead to copper and zinc deficiency due to enhanced urinary excretion of these metals.[46,55] Despite 1 case-report of an affected Bedlington terrier developing DPA-induced copper deficiency,[58] affected Bedlington terriers usually need lifelong continuous chelation therapy. In many of these dogs, normalization of hepatic copper concentrations does not occur despite therapy,[54] but progression of disease is precluded. In other dog breeds, lifelong therapy is not recommended. An intermittent treatment regime with recheck biopsies every 1 to 2 years prevents copper (re-) accumulation and concurrently avoids copper and zinc deficiencies.

Trientene (2,2,2-Tetramine)

Trientine is a tetramine chelator that was originally introduced for humans who developed adverse reactions to DPA. Like DPA, trientene is an effective promoter of urinary copper excretion although it may act through a different pool of body copper.[59] In humans, fewer side effects are reported than for DPA,[60] whereas in dogs no side effects have been reported.[61] Studies in dogs, however, are limited. The recommended dose in dogs is 15 mg/kg twice daily. At the time of writing, the cost of trientine in the United States prohibits its use for veterinary patients.

Box 1
Formula to calculate necessary treatment duration with D-penicillamine in Labrador retrievers

$$CuQ_1 = -81.5 + 0.99 \times CuQ_0 + 51.0 \times T - 3.92 \times T^2 - 0.16 \times CuQ_0 \times T + 0.92 \times 10^{-2} \times CuQ_0 \times T^2$$

Abbreviations: CuQ_0, quantitative copper at start of treatment; CuQ_1, quantitative copper at certain period of treatment; T, treatment duration.

2,3,2-Tetramine

2,3,2- Tetramine is another tetramine chelator but was reported to produce a 4-fold to 9-fold greater urinary copper excretion than trientene.[61] 2,3,2-Tetramine therapy was studied in 5 Bedlington terriers with copper toxicosis.[62] After 200 days of treatment, hepatic copper concentrations decreased 55%, without the development of adverse reactions. Besides this study, few data are available and 2,3,2-tetramine is not commercially available.

Ammonium Tetrathiomolybdate

Ammonium tetrathiomolybdate (TTM) is a strong copper chelator that forms a tripartite complex with copper and protein in the intestines, plasma, and liver tissue. It decreases MT-bound hepatic copper by excretion of copper TTM complexes into the bile and blood.[63,64] Due to its extensive decoppering effects, it has antiangiogenic properties, which also make it a candidate for cancer treatment in humans and dogs.[65,66] To date, TTM has not been used for the treatment of copper-associated hepatitis in dogs. One study, conducted in healthy dogs, showed that TTM administration (1 mg/kg) resulted in a significant increase in serum copper concentration, underlining possible potential as a future therapeutic agent.[67]

Zinc

The oral administration of zinc salts (zinc acetate, zinc gluconate, and zinc sulphate) interferes with copper uptake in the enterocytes. Zinc oxide has a limited bioavailability. Increased intestinal zinc concentrations are believed to induce up-regulation of intestinal MT, which has a high affinity for copper. With high levels of copper bound to MT, less copper is available for serosal transfer and passage into the portal circulation is blocked.[68,69] Presumably, zinc may also attenuate the toxicity of copper by inducing MT up-regulation in hepatocytes.[70] In human copper storage diseases, long-term effectivity is similar to that of DPA, but zinc is generally tolerated better.[71,72] Zinc acetate, zinc gluconate, and zinc sulfate have all been used in dogs with copper toxicosis.[14,73,74] Acetate and gluconate salts may be better tolerated than sulfate, but individual differences in response exist. Normal plasma zinc concentrations range from 90 µg/dL to 120 µg/dL. To suppress gastrointestinal copper uptake, a minimal plasma zinc concentration of 200 µg/dL is needed.[73] The recommended dose to achieve a plasma concentration between 200 µg/dL and 300 µg/dL is 5 to 10 mg/kg elemental zinc twice daily or 200 mg of elemental zinc per day, in divided doses. To be effective, zinc salts should not be given with any food. Plasma zinc concentrations exceeding 1000 µg/dL may result in hemolysis. Therefore, plasma zinc concentrations should be monitored during treatment. Because a minimum of 3 months of administration is required to obtain a therapeutic response, zinc therapy is not recommended as the sole treatment in clinical cases. Those cases require more aggressive therapy with copper chelators.

Dietary Management

Dietary intake has a significant impact on hepatic copper accumulation[15,18] and an adjusted diet (low copper and high zinc) may be valuable in the management of dogs with copper-associated hepatitis. A low-copper/high-zinc diet may be beneficial to prevent or postpone reaccumulation of copper in dogs that were initially treated with a copper chelator.[14,17] Another role for dietary management could be in subclinical dogs with moderate copper accumulation. In 1 study, hepatic copper concentrations could be normalized with dietary intervention alone in approximately 50% of subclinical Labrador retrievers with increased hepatic copper.[16] Some individuals, however, continued to accumulate copper, even when fed a low-copper/high-zinc diet. Individual variation in response to diet may be influenced by hereditary factors.[19] Because variation in response to low-copper/high-zinc diets occurs, hepatic copper concentrations should be evaluated by repeat biopsy with copper staining and quantification.

REFERENCES

1. Kim BE, Nevitt T, Thiele DJ. Mechanisms for copper acquisition, distribution and regulation. Nat Chem Biol 2008;4(3):176–85.
2. Palumaa P. Copper chaperones. The concept of conformational control in the metabolism of copper. FEBS Lett 2013;587(13):1902–10.
3. Yanagimoto C, Harada M, Kumemura H, et al. Copper incorporation into ceruloplasmin is regulated by Niemann–Pick C1 protein. Hepatol Res 2011;41(5):484–91.
4. Polishchuk EV, Concilli M, Iacobacci S, et al. Wilson disease protein ATP7B utilizes lysosomal exocytosis to maintain copper homeostasis. Dev Cell 2014;29(6):686–700.
5. Kim B, Turski ML, Nose Y, et al. Cardiac copper deficiency activates a systemic signaling mechanism that communicates with the copper acquisition and storage organs. Cell Metab 2010;11(5):353–63.
6. Materia S, Cater MA, Klomp LW, et al. Clusterin and COMMD1 independently regulate degradation of the mammalian copper ATPases ATP7A and ATP7B. J Biol Chem 2012;287(4):2485–99.
7. Roberts EA, Schilsky ML. Diagnosis and treatment of Wilson's disease: an update. Hepatology 2008;47(6):2089–111.
8. Tanner MS. Role of copper in Indian childhood cirrhosis. Am J Clin Nutr 1998;67(5 Suppl):1074S–81S.
9. Müller T, Feichtinger H, Berger H, et al. Endemic Tyrolean infantile cirrhosis: an ecogenetic disorder. Lancet 1996;347(9005):877–80.
10. Scheinberg IH, Sternlieb I. Wilson disease and idiopathic copper toxicosis. Am J Clin Nutr 1996;63(5):842S–5S.
11. Kaler SG. ATP7A-related copper transport diseases-emerging concepts and future trends. Nat Rev Neurol 2011;7(1):15–29.
12. van De Sluis B, Rothuizen J, Pearson PL, et al. Identification of a new copper metabolism gene by positional cloning in a purebred dog population. Hum Mol Genet 2002;11(2):165–73.
13. Haywood S, Boursnell M, Loughran MJ, et al. Copper toxicosis in non-COMMD1 bedlington terriers is associated with metal transport gene ABCA12. J Trace Elem Med Biol 2016;35:83–9.
14. Hoffmann G, Jones PG, Biourge V, et al. Dietary management of hepatic copper accumulation in labrador retrievers. J Vet Intern Med 2009;23(5):957–63.
15. Fieten H, Hooijer-Nouwens B, Biourge V, et al. Association of dietary copper and zinc levels with hepatic copper and zinc concentration in Labrador retrievers. J Vet Intern Med 2012;26(6):1274–80.
16. Fieten H, Biourge VC, Watson AL, et al. Dietary management of Labrador retrievers with subclinical hepatic copper accumulation. J Vet Intern Med 2015;29(3):822–7.
17. Fieten H, Biourge VC, Watson AL, et al. Nutritional management of inherited copper-associated hepatitis in the Labrador retriever. Vet J 2014;199(3):429–33.

18. Johnston AN, Center SA, McDonough SP, et al. Hepatic copper concentrations in labrador retrievers with and without chronic hepatitis: 72 cases (1980–2010). J Am Vet Med Assoc 2013;242(3):372–80.

19. Fieten H, Gill Y, Martin AJ, et al. The Menkes and Wilson disease genes counteract in copper toxicosis in labrador retrievers: a new canine model for copper-metabolism disorders. Dis Model Mech 2016;9(1):25–38.

20. Mandigers PJ, van den Ingh TS, Bode P, et al. Association between liver copper concentration and subclinical hepatitis in Doberman pinschers. J Vet Intern Med 2004;18(5):647–50.

21. Thornburg LP, Rottinghaus G, Dennis G, et al. The relationship between hepatic copper content and morphologic changes in the liver of west highland white terriers. Vet Pathol 1996;33(6):656–61.

22. Webb CB, Twedt DC, Meyer DJ. Copper-associated liver disease in dalmatians: a review of 10 dogs (1998-2001). J Vet Intern Med 2002;16(6):665–8.

23. Haywood S, Rutgers HC, Christian MK. Hepatitis and copper accumulation in skye terriers. Vet Pathol 1988;25(6):408–14.

24. Bosje JT, van den Ingh TS, Fennema A, et al. Copper-induced hepatitis in an anatolian shepherd dog. Vet Rec 2003;152(3):84–5.

25. Rifkin J, Miller MD. Copper-associated hepatitis in a pembroke welsh corgi. Can Vet J 2014;55(6):573–6.

26. Appleman E, Cianciolo R, Mosenco A, et al. Transient acquired fanconi syndrome associated with copper storage hepatopathy in 3 dogs. J Vet Intern Med 2008; 22(4):1038–42.

27. Poldervaart JH, Favier RP, Penning LC, et al. Primary hepatitis in dogs: a retrospective review (2002-2006). J Vet Intern Med 2009;23(1):72–80.

28. Thornburg LP, Rottinghaus G, McGowan M, et al. Hepatic copper concentrations in purebred and mixed-breed dogs. Vet Pathol 1990;27(2):81–8.

29. Hoffmann G, van den Ingh TS, Bode P, et al. Copper-associated chronic hepatitis in labrador retrievers. J Vet Intern Med 2006;20(4):856–61.

30. Speeti M, Eriksson J, Saari S, et al. Lesions of subclinical doberman hepatitis. Vet Pathol 1998;35(5):361–9.

31. Favier RP, Spee B, Schotanus BA, et al. COMMD1-deficient dogs accumulate copper in hepatocytes and provide a good model for chronic hepatitis and fibrosis. PLoS One 2012;7(8):e42158.

32. Watson A, Middleton D, Ilkiw J. Copper storage disease with intravascular haemolysis in a bedlington terrier. Aust Vet J 1983;60(10):305–7.

33. Center SA. Interpretation of liver enzymes. Vet Clin North Am Small Anim Pract 2007;37:297–333.

34. Smedley R, Mullaney T, Rumbeiha W. Copper-associated hepatitis in Labrador retrievers. Vet Pathol 2009;46(3):484–90.

35. Hill T, Breitschwerdt E, Cecere T, et al. Concurrent hepatic copper toxicosis and fanconi's syndrome in a dog. J Vet Intern Med 2008;22(1):219–22.

36. Langlois D, Smedley R, Schall W, et al. Acquired proximal renal tubular dysfunction in 9 labrador retrievers with Copper-Associated hepatitis (2006–2012). J Vet Intern Med 2013;27(3):491–9.

37. Teske E, Brinkhuis BG, Bode P, et al. Cytological detection of copper for the diagnosis of inherited copper toxicosis in Bedlington terriers. Vet Rec 1992;131(2):30–2.

38. Uzman LL. Histochemical localization of copper with rubeanic acid. Lab Invest 1956;5(3):299–305.

39. Johnson GF, Gilbertson SR, Goldfischer S, et al. Cytochemical detection of inherited copper toxicosis of Bedlington terriers. Vet Pathol 1984;21(1):57–60.

40. Van den Ingh TS, Van Winkle TJ, Cullen JM, et al. Morphological classification of parenchymal disorders of the canine and feline liver. In: WSAVA Standardization Group, editor. WSAVA standards for clinical and histological diagnosis of canine and feline liver diseases. 1st edition. Philadelphia: Saunders Elsevier; 2006. p. 85–101. Updated webversion (January 2016). Available at: http://www.vet visuals.com/home-society-of-comparative-hepatology/sch.

41. Spee B, Arends B, van den Ingh TS, et al. Copper metabolism and oxidative stress in chronic inflammatory and cholestatic liver diseases in dogs. J Vet Intern Med 2006;20(5):1085–92.

42. Thornburg LP. A perspective on copper and liver disease in the dog. J Vet Diagn Invest 2000;12(2):101–10.

43. Bode P. Instrumental neutron activation analysis in a routine way. J Trace Microprobe Tech 1990;8(1–2):139–54.

44. Puls R. Mineral levels in animal health: diagnostic data. 2nd edition. Clearbrook, Canada: Sherpa International; 1994.

45. Center SA, McDonough SP, Bogdanovic L. Digital image analysis of rhodanine-stained liver biopsy specimens for calculation of hepatic copper concentrations in dogs. Am J Vet Res 2013;74(12):1474–80.

46. Fieten H, Hugen S, van den Ingh TS, et al. Urinary excretion of copper, zinc and iron with and without D-penicillamine administration in relation to hepatic copper concentration in dogs. Vet J 2013;197(2):468–73.

47. Krol J, Loedige I, Filipowicz W. The widespread regulation of microRNA biogenesis, function and decay. Nat Rev Genet 2010;11(9):597–610.

48. Dirksen K, Verzijl T, van den Ingh TS, et al. Hepatocyte-derived microRNAs as sensitive serum biomarkers of hepatocellular injury in Labrador retrievers. Vet J 2016;211:75–81.

49. Walshe J. Penicillamine, a new oral therapy for Wilson's disease. Am J Med 1956; 21(4):487–95.

50. Kuchinskas EJ, Rosen Y. Metal chelates of DL-penicillamine. Arch Biochem Biophys 1962;97(2):370–2.

51. Lenz G, Martell A. Metal chelates of some sulfur-containing amino acids. Biochemistry 1964;3(6):745–50.

52. Lipsky PE, Ziff M. The effect of D-penicillamine on mitogen-induced human lymphocyte proliferation: synergistic inhibition by D-penicillamine and copper salts. J Immunol 1978;120(3):1006–13.

53. Siegel RC. Collagen cross-linking. effect of D-penicillamine on cross-linking in vitro. J Biol Chem 1977;252(1):254–9.

54. Favier RP, Spee B, Fieten H, et al. Aberrant expression of copper associated genes after copper accumulation in COMMD1-deficient dogs. J Trace Elem Med Biol 2015;29:347–53.

55. Fieten H, Dirksen K, van den Ingh TS, et al. D-penicillamine treatment of copper-associated hepatitis in Labrador retrievers. Vet J 2013;196(3):522–7.

56. Mandigers PJ, van den Ingh TS, Bode P, et al. Improvement in liver pathology after 4 months of D-penicillamine in 5 Doberman pinschers with subclinical hepatitis. J Vet Intern Med 2005;19(1):40–3.

57. Langlois D, Lehner A, Buchweitz J, et al. Pharmacokinetics and relative bioavailability of d-Penicillamine in fasted and nonfasted dogs. J Vet Intern Med 2013; 27(5):1071–6.

58. Seguin MA, Bunch SE. Iatrogenic copper deficiency associated with long-term copper chelation for treatment of copper storage disease in a Bedlington terrier. J Am Vet Med Assoc 2001;218(10):1593–7, 1580.

59. Sarkar B, Sass-Kortsak A, Clarke R, et al. A comparative study of in vitro and in vivo interaction of D-penicillamine and triethylenetetramine with copper. Proc R Soc Med 1977;70(Suppl 3):13–8.
60. Walshe J. Treatment of Wilson's disease with trientine (triethylene tetramine) dihydrochloride. Lancet 1982;319(8273):643–7.
61. Allen KG, Twedt DC, Hunsaker HA. Tetramine cupruretic agents: a comparison in dogs. Am J Vet Res 1987;48(1):28–30.
62. Twedt DC, Hunsaker HA, Allen KG. Use of 2,3,2-tetramine as a hepatic copper chelating agent for treatment of copper hepatotoxicosis in Bedlington terriers. J Am Vet Med Assoc 1988;192(1):52–6.
63. Gooneratne S, Christensen D. Effect of chelating agents on the excretion of copper, zinc and iron in the bile and urine of sheep. Vet J 1997;153(2):171–8.
64. Komatsu Y, Sadakata I, Ogra Y, et al. Excretion of copper complexed with thiomolybdate into the bile and blood in LEC rats. Chem Biol Interact 2000;124(3):217–31.
65. Brewer GJ, Merajver SD. Cancer therapy with tetrathiomolybdate: antiangiogenesis by lowering body copper–a review. Integr Cancer Ther 2002;1(4):327–37.
66. Kent MS, Madewell BR, Dank G, et al. An anticopper antiangiogenic approach for advanced cancer in spontaneously occurring tumors using tetrathiomolybdate: a pilot study in a canine animal model. J Trace Elem Exp Med 2004;17(1):9–20.
67. Chan CM, Langlois DK, Buchweitz JP, et al. Pharmacologic evaluation of ammonium tetrathiomolybdate after intravenous and oral administration to healthy dogs. Am J Vet Res 2015;76(5):445–53.
68. Fischer PW, Giroux A, L'Abbe MR. Effects of zinc on mucosal copper binding and on the kinetics of copper Absorption. J Nutr 1983;113:462–9.
69. Cousins RJ. Absorption, transport, and hepatic metabolism of copper and zinc: special reference to metallothionein and ceruloplasmin. Physiol Rev 1985;65(2):238–309.
70. Schilsky ML, Blank RR, Czaja MJ, et al. Hepatocellular copper toxicity and its attenuation by zinc. J Clin Invest 1989;84(5):1562–8.
71. Czlonkowska A, Gajda J, Rodo M. Effects of long-term treatment in Wilson's disease with D-penicillamine and zinc sulphate. J Neurol 1996;243(3):269–73.
72. Brewer GJ, Dick RD, Johnson VD, et al. Treatment of wilson's disease with zinc: XV long-term follow-up studies. J Lab Clin Med 1998;132(4):264–78.
73. Brewer GJ, Dick RD, Schall W, et al. Use of zinc acetate to treat copper toxicosis in dogs. J Am Vet Med Assoc 1992;201(4):564–8.
74. Hoogenraad T, Rothuizen J. Compliance in Wilson's disease and in copper toxicosis of Bedlington terriers. Lancet 1986;328(8499):170.

Canine Idiopathic Chronic Hepatitis

Nick Bexfield, BVetMed, PhD, DSAM, FRSB, AFHEA, MRCVS

KEYWORDS

- Idiopathic • Hepatitis • Canine • Diagnosis • Management • Prognosis

KEY POINTS

- Canine idiopathic hepatitis is common, categorized histologically by hepatocellular apoptosis or necrosis, a variable mononuclear or mixed inflammatory cell infiltrate, regeneration and fibrosis.
- Clinical signs are vague and nonspecific, but there are known breed, age, and gender predispositions.
- Results of clinical pathology are nonspecific, but usually include increases in liver enzymes and function impairment; a liver biopsy is required for diagnosis.
- Management involves the use of an antiinflammatory dose of glucocorticoids and other supportive and symptomatic therapies, including ursodeoxycholic acid, antioxidants, diuretics, and diet.
- The prognosis is variable, but there are known prognostic indicators, especially the presence of portal hypertension.

INTRODUCTION

Historically, the term canine chronic hepatitis (CH) has been defined poorly and used to describe a variety of inflammatory liver diseases. However, the World Small Animal Veterinary Association's (WSAVA) Liver Standardization Group have produced standardized criteria for the histologic diagnosis of canine liver diseases, including CH. They define CH by the presence of hepatocellular apoptosis or necrosis (**Fig. 1**), a variable mononuclear or mixed inflammatory cell infiltrate (**Fig. 2**), regeneration (**Fig. 3**), and fibrosis (**Fig. 4**).[1] However, it is clear there are variations in histologic appearance between breeds.[2,3]

Hepatic copper accumulation is an important cause of canine CH (see Karen Dirksen and Hille Fieten's article, "Canine Copper-Associated Hepatitis," in this issue). However, for many cases where copper accumulation has been ruled out, the cause of CH remains unknown despite the patient undergoing a complete diagnostic

The author has nothing to disclose.
School of Veterinary Medicine and Science, University of Nottingham, Sutton Bonington Campus, School Road, Leicestershire LE12 5RD, UK
E-mail address: nick.bexfield@nottingham.ac.uk

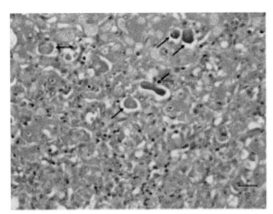

Fig. 1. Photomicrograph of liver tissue from a Labrador retriever with idiopathic chronic hepatitis demonstrating several apoptotic hepatocytes within the hepatic parenchyma (*arrows*; stain, hematoxylin and eosin; original magnification, ×200).

workup. These dogs are said to have idiopathic CH. This article reviews the current theories regarding the etiopathogenesis of canine CH other than copper accumulation, as well as the clinical features, diagnostic findings, and management of idiopathic CH.

PATHOPHYSIOLOGY

The development of fibrosis is the key pathologic change that leads to the development of chronic liver disease, including canine idiopathic CH.[4] The hepatic stellate cell, also known as the Ito cell or lipocyte, is central in the development of fibrosis in humans and rats,[4–7] and evidence also suggests its involvement in the pathogenesis of hepatic fibrosis in dogs.[8] Canine hepatic stellate cells reside in the space of Disse, between the sinusoidal endothelial cells and the hepatocytes.[9] In normal human and rat liver, they are the major storage site of vitamin A, and also synthesize extracellular matrix components, matrix metalloproteinases, cytokines, and growth factors.[4,5]

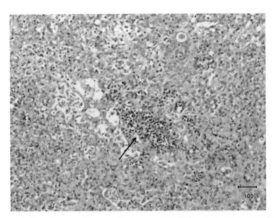

Fig. 2. Photomicrograph of liver tissue from an English springer spaniel with idiopathic chronic hepatitis (same case as **Fig. 1**) demonstrating a foci of inflammatory cells in the hepatic parenchyma (*arrow*). Stain, hematoxylin and eosin; original magnification, ×100.

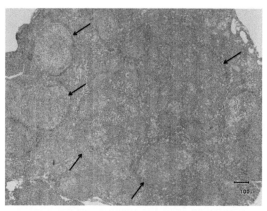

Fig. 3. Low-power photomicrograph of liver tissue from an English springer spaniel with idiopathic chronic hepatitis demonstrating disruption to the normal architecture by regenerative nodules (*arrows*; stain, hematoxylin and eosin; original magnification, ×40).

Although their function in canine liver has not been studied extensively, they likely possess similar roles. In human chronic liver injury, they are stimulated to transform into collagen-secreting, activated stellate cells, which express smooth muscle-specific α-actin, and secrete high-density matrix and collagen into the space of Disse.[7] In most cases of human and experimental animal chronic liver disease, the simulation of stellate cells is believed to be indirect via the release of cytokines from inflammatory cells, although some substances act on them directly to stimulate fibrosis.[4] For instance, activated Kupffer cells in the human liver secrete transforming growth factor-β1, the most potent fibrogenic factor, as well as other cytokines such as platelet-derived growth factor.[4,7] Inflammatory mediators released from neutrophils, lymphocytes, platelets, and necrotic hepatocytes have also been implicated in the pathogenesis of hepatic fibrosis in humans,[7] but their contribution to the development of fibrosis in canine liver disease has not been investigated. Damage to cells and mitochondrial membranes by bile acids in cholestatic liver disease also plays a role in

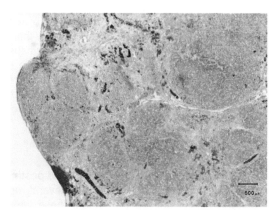

Fig. 4. Low-power photomicrograph of liver tissue from a Doberman pinscher with idiopathic chronic hepatitis demonstrating marked fibrosis (*light green staining*). Masson's trichrome (original magnification, ×40).

producing oxidant damage and stimulating cytokine release.[10] The formation of fibrous tissue within the liver leads to the development of intrahepatic portal hypertension by altering sinusoidal tone and blood flow.[5] The development of portal hypertension results in many of the complications of chronic liver disease, such as ascites and gastrointestinal ulceration.

ETIOLOGY

Although there are several known causes of canine CH, the majority of dogs have idiopathic disease.[3,11,12] A limited number of infectious causes are documented, and include canine adenovirus type I[13] and *Leptospira* spp.[14,15] Although initially postulated as a canine hepatitis causing virus, the recently identified canine homology of human hepatitis C virus, canine hepacivirus,[16] does not seem to be involved in the etiology of canine CH in the United Kingdom[17] or the Netherlands.[18] Although bacteria, especially those originating from the gastrointestinal tract, are known to cause canine cholangitis/cholangiohepatitis,[19,20] their role in the etiology of CH is unknown. Toxins and drug reactions usually cause acute, necrotizing hepatitis,[21] but some agents such as phenobarbitone can cause CH.[22] Defects in copper metabolism leading to the development of CH have been described in several breeds of dog. These include true "copper storage" disease, where the primary initiating event is a build up of copper leading to secondary hepatic damage, and "copper-associated" disease, in which copper accumulates secondary to an underlying liver disease including CH. Copper storage disease was first described in the Bedlington terrier more than 3 decades ago,[23] and since then has been reported in the Dalmatian,[24] Doberman pinscher,[25] and Labrador retriever.[26] Further details on the role of copper in the etiology of CH can be found in Karen Dirksen and Hille Fieten's article, "Canine Copper-Associated Hepatitis," and Penny Watson's article, "Canine Breed-Specific Hepatopathies," in this issue. To date, no data exist to demonstrate convincingly the presence of an underlying autoimmune etiology canine CH. Low concentrations of antinuclear antibodies were present in some dogs with CH, and the occasional dog had high circulating concentrations of antibodies to liver membrane proteins.[27] In another study, 10 of 21 dogs with CH had antibodies to anti–liver membrane protein.[28] More recently, autoantibodies against liver proteins were found in the sera of Doberman pinschers with CH before the onset of clinical signs.[29] Using an indirect immunofluorescence assay on cryostat sections of mouse liver, small numbers of Dobermans with CH had evidence of antinuclear antibodies,[30] and immunoglobulin G autoantibodies against histones.[31] However, the question that remains from all these studies is whether these autoantibodies are the primary cause of the disease, or a secondary phenomenon. Finally, the association of certain susceptibility and resistance major histocompatibility complex class II haplotypes in the Doberman pinschers,[32] and English springer spaniels[33] clearly indicates a role of the immune system in disease development, but does not necessarily point to an autoimmune etiology.

SIGNALMENT

Canine CH is common in the United Kingdom with a reported postmortem prevalence of 12% in a first opinion practice setting.[34] There are several reports of apparent breed, age, and gender predispositions, although these vary depending on geographic location and also the time the study was performed. Moreover, not all dogs in these studies necessarily had idiopathic CH, because comprehensive work to eliminate known causes was not always performed. An early study performed

approximately 2 decades ago on a Swedish population of dogs, and before the estab-
lishment of the WSAVA criteria for the histologic diagnosis of CH, demonstrated that
the American and English cocker spaniel, West Highland white terrier, Labrador
retriever, Doberman pinscher, and Scottish terrier had an increased risk for CH.[35] In
this study, there was a male predisposition in English and American cocker spaniels,
which were a mean of 5 years old, and female predisposition in Labrador retrievers,
which were a mean of 6.9 years old at presentation. A more recent study performed
in the UK assessed for breed predilections to CH by comparing the signalment of
551 cases to that of a large control population.[12] From a total of 61 breeds, the American cocker spaniel, Cairn terrier, Dalmatian, Doberman pinscher, English cocker
spaniel, English springer spaniel, Great Dane, Labrador retriever, and Samoyed
were found to be at increased risk for developing CH (**Table 1**). In this study, the median age for all breeds with CH was 8 years (range, 7 months to 16 years), and the female to male ratio was 1.5:1. In Japan, a predilection of female Labrador retrievers and
Doberman pinschers for CH was reported, and the median age of dogs was 8 years
and 7 months.[36] The mean age of 43 dogs with idiopathic CH in 1 retrospective study
was 7.7 years (range, 0.4–14.2), although there were no data on apparent breed or
gender predispositions.[3] For further details of breed, age, and gender predispositions
to canine idiopathic CH, please see Penny Watson's article, "Canine Breed-Specific
Hepatopathies," in this issue.

HISTORY AND PHYSICAL EXAMINATION FINDINGS

The liver has tremendous functional and structural reserve, and a significant loss of
normal hepatic mass can occur with minimal or no clinical signs.[37] The liver also
has a remarkable capacity to regenerate after injury, providing that the damage is
not too severe or ongoing,[38] and overt liver failure does not develop until at least
70% to 80% of functional capacity is lost.[39] Historical signs in dogs with idiopathic
CH vary and are usually nonspecific and insidious in onset. The more frequently reported include inappetence, lethargy, weight loss, vomiting, and diarrhea.[39,40] Some
dogs with idiopathic CH can be asymptomatic, or alternatively may present with signs
of "acute" disease.[2] The duration of clinical signs also varies, and in 43 dogs with

Table 1			
Age and gender data for breeds with an increased risk for developing canine CH			
Breed	Odds Ratio (95% Confidence Interval)	Median Age at Diagnosis (Range)	Gender
American cocker spaniel	21.6 (9.7–47.9)	5 y 6 mo (2 y to 11 y 3 mo)	1 F, 5 M
Cairn terrier	3.6 (1.9–6.9)	10 y 2 mo (7 y to 13 y 5 mo)	4 F, 5 M
Dalmatian	4.1 (2.2–7.7)	4 y 7 mo (3 y to 12 y)	9 F, 1 M
Doberman pinscher	11.5 (7.6–17.3)	5 y 4 mo (2 y 6 mo to 10 y)	16 F, 8 M
English cocker spaniel	2.4 (1.8–3.2)	8 y 9 mo (1 y 3 mo to 14 y)	34 F, 19 M
English springer spaniel	5.3 (4.2–6.7)	5 y (1 y 2 mo to 11 y)	60 F, 20 M
Great Dane	4.0 (1.9–8.9)	6 y 2 mo (1 y 2 mo to 7 y 11 mo)	3 F, 3 M
Labrador retriever	2.0 (1.6–2.5)	8 y 3 mo (2 y 8 mo to 13 y)	63 F, 32 M
Samoyed	12.6 (5.3–29.9)	10 y (3 y 1 mo to 11 y)	2 F, 3 M

Odds ratios are given based on 2008 control data.
Abbreviations: F, female; M, male.

idiopathic CH, were present for a median of 4.3 weeks before presentation (range, 0.5–14.0).[3] In a study of 101 dogs with both acute hepatitis and CH, the most commonly identified signs were lethargy (n = 56), anorexia (n = 56), vomiting (n = 48), polyuria and polydipsia (n = 27), weight loss (n = 28), and diarrhea (n = 23).[3] In 68 English springer spaniels with idiopathic CH, clinical signs at presentation included lethargy (n = 63), decreased appetite (n = 58), vomiting (n = 34), weight loss (n = 31), diarrhea (n = 21), and polydipsia (n = 21).[2] In 16 Labrador retrievers with CH, signs included vomiting (n = 9), lethargy (n = 8), weight loss (n = 6), decreased appetite (n = 5), diarrhea (n = 2), and polyuria/polydipsia (n = 2).[41]

Physical examination findings are also very variable and likely depend on the duration and severity of disease. Physical examination findings in 101 dogs with both acute and CH included jaundice (n = 24), abdominal distention (n = 21), signs of hepatic encephalopathy (HE; n = 22), hepatomegaly (n = 17), and abdominal pain (n = 8).[3] Physical examination in 68 English springer spaniels with idiopathic CH revealed icterus (n = 37), hyperthermia (n = 24), poor body condition (n = 23), ascites (n = 17), and abdominal pain (n = 9).[2] A range of concurrent diseases, including those of the endocrine, renal, cardiovascular, musculoskeletal, dermatologic, and neurologic systems, are also sometimes documented in dogs with idiopathic CH.[2,3]

CLINICAL PATHOLOGY
Serum Biochemistry

Clinical pathology is the next step in investigating the dog with suspected idiopathic CH. Findings usually include elevations of liver enzyme activities, especially hepatocellular enzymes released as a result of liver cell damage, namely alanine aminotransferase (ALT) and aspartate aminotransferase. In addition, the markers of cholestasis, alkaline phosphatase (ALP) and gamma-glutamyl transferase are invariably elevated. There is a wide variation in absolute values of the various clinical pathology tests, and very occasionally a dog with advanced idiopathic CH may have liver enzyme activity within the reference interval. In addition to increases in liver enzyme activities, owing to the development of fibrosis, liver function in dogs with idiopathic CH is progressively compromised. Markers of reduced liver function include decreased serum albumin, urea, glucose, and coagulation factors, whereas serum bile acids, ammonia, and bilirubin may increase. Of course, none of these tests are specific for canine idiopathic CH, and thus should always be interpreted in the light of other clinical and clinicopathologic findings.

In a variety of breeds of dog with idiopathic CH serum, serum ALP activity was increased in 32 of 33 (mean, 660 U/L) and ALT in 16 of 17 (mean, 403 U/L).[3] Albumin was decreased in 14 of 24 (mean, 26.0 g/L), and glucose in 2 of 8 (mean, 4.9 mmol/L). In 32 of 35 dogs, bile acids were increased (mean, 75.7 μmol/L), whereas resting ammonia was increased in 1 of 7 dogs (mean, 33.9 μmol/L). In 68 English springer spaniels with idiopathic CH, serum ALT and ALP activities were increased in all dogs with median values of 690 and 821 U/L, respectively.[2] Serum aspartate aminotransferase and gamma-glutamyl transferase activities were increased in 75% and 63% of cases with median values of 361 and 26 U/L, respectively. In 76% of cases, resting bile acids were increased with a median of 87 μmol/L, and bilirubin was increased in 69% of cases with a median of 77 μmol/L. Albumin and urea were reduced in 38% and 22% of cases, respectively. In 24 Labrador retrievers with CH, all dogs had increases in serum activity of 1 or more hepatobiliary enzymes, with increased ALP (n = 21), ALT (n = 20), aspartate aminotransferase (n = 20), and gamma-glutamyl transferase (n = 9).[41] Hyperbilirubinemia and hypoalbuminemia were present in 45% and 21% of dogs, respectively, preprandial or postprandial serum bile acid concentrations were increased in 2 of 4 cases, and 1 of 6 dogs tested had hyperammonemia.[41]

Hematology

Nonspecific qualitative and quantitative abnormalities in erythrocytes may be present in dogs with idiopathic CH, in combination with alterations in white cell counts and platelet numbers. Alterations to red cell morphology may also include the presence of acanthocytes and codocytes. Dogs with idiopathic CH may have a neutrophilic leukocytosis, owing to stress or an inflammatory response, and thrombocytopenia may develop owing to platelet sequestration or increased destruction.

In 21 dogs with idiopathic CH, the hematocrit was decreased in 11, with a mean of 0.40 L/L and thrombocytopenia was identified in 4/10, with a mean platelet count of 212 $\times$ 10^9/L.[3] Eleven of 24 dogs had evidence of a leukocytosis (mean, 14.8 $\times$ 10^9/L) with segmented neutrophils present in 10 of 24 dogs. The median white blood cell count was 16.1 $\times$ 10^9/L in 68 English springer spaniels with idiopathic CH, and 77% of cases had an increased white blood cell count.[2] Results of hematology from 24 Labrador retrievers with CH included an increased white blood cell count (n = 9), lymphopenia (n = 7), neutropenia (n = 2), left shift (n = 2), and monocytosis (n = 2).[41] The median hematocrit was 46%, and 7 dogs were anemic (median, 31%; range, 23%–35%). Four dogs had thrombocytopenia (median, 128 $\times$ 10^3/mL; range, 67–177 $\times$ 10^3/mL), and 1 dog had thrombocytosis.

Urinalysis

Nonspecific abnormalities may also be present in the urine of dogs with idiopathic CH, including reduced specific gravity as a result of polyuria and polydipsia, bilirubinuria, and increased urobilinogen. Urate crystals are occasionally seen. A paucity of data exists on the results of urinalysis in dogs with idiopathic CH, but in 14 Labrador retrievers with CH of a variety of causes, bilirubinuria was identified in 7 dogs, transient glucosuria without hyperglycemia in 3, and proteinuria in 2.[41]

Hemostasis

The canine liver plays an important role in maintaining hemostasis, and the resulting decreased function in idiopathic CH may result in abnormalities of coagulation (see Cynthia R.L. Webster's article, "Hemostatic Disorders Associated with Hepatobiliary Disease," in this issue). Hepatocytes not only produce fibrinogen, prothrombin, and the majority of the coagulation factors, but are also responsible for the activation of the vitamin K-dependent factors and protein C.[42] It is, therefore, essential to assess coagulation before a liver biopsy. In humans with chronic hepatocellular disease, levels of vitamin K-dependent clotting factors, particularly factor VII and protein C, may decrease.[43] However, increased activation may also occur in patients with liver diseases and a consumptive coagulopathy, leading to disseminated intravascular coagulation, has been reported in human patients with end stage liver disease.[43]

In 1 study of dogs with CH of various causes, although both mean prothrombin time and activated partial thromboplastin time were above upper reference values, only partial thromboplastin time was prolonged significantly in dogs with CH and cirrhosis.[44] The mean activities of factors II, V, VII, VIII, IX, X, XI, and XI activities, and protein C were lower in dogs with CH and cirrhosis compared with dogs with CH alone.[44] The mean D-dimer concentrations were not increased significantly in dogs with CH or CH and cirrhosis.[44] In 34 dogs with idiopathic CH, an increased prothrombin time (mean, 10.1 seconds) was identified in 14 dogs, an increased partial thromboplastin time (mean, 17.1 seconds) in 12, and reduced fibrinogen concentration in 8 (mean, 2.5 g/L).[3] Prothrombin time and activated partial thromboplastin time were measured in 49 English springer spaniels with idiopathic CH and were increased in 24% and 21%, respectively.[2] Seven of 21 Labrador retrievers with CH had prolonged partial thromboplastin time and 9 dogs had prolonged prothrombin time.[41]

DIAGNOSTIC IMAGING

Diagnostic imaging, including abdominal radiography and ultrasound imaging, is an important part of the investigation of a dog with suspected idiopathic CH, and is performed typically in combination with clinical pathology. Abdominal radiography can be used to assess liver size, position, and shape, and to check for the presence of other abdominal pathology.[45] As a general rule, liver size is decreased in dogs with chronic diseases, such as idiopathic CH. Splenomegaly may also be present in dogs with CH and portal hypertension. Abdominal radiography in dogs with idiopathic CH and ascites secondary to portal hypertension or hypoalbuminemia is generally unhelpful because the fluid obscures abdominal detail. However, radiographic evaluation is poorly sensitive and specific for the diagnosis of idiopathic CH; the liver may seem to be normal radiographically, even when severely diseased. Few studies report the radiographic findings in dogs with idiopathic CH, although among 33 English springer spaniels, 27 had reduced liver size and 16 had splenomegaly.[2]

Ultrasound imaging is an established method for examining the canine liver, and it enable an assessment of its size, shape, echogenicity, and echotexture, as a means of detecting lesions affecting the hepatic parenchyma. However, ultrasound imaging is generally considered unsuitable as a sole method for diagnosis because of the large overlap in the ultrasonographic appearance between different hepatic diseases, including CH.[46,47] In a recent study, a marked variability in ultrasonographic appearance of lesions was observed for all diagnoses, including hepatitis, and no associations between ultrasonographic appearance and diagnosis were found.[46] The sensitivity for the diagnosis of hepatitis of all causes in this latter study was 48%, with 10% of dogs having multifocal hypoechoic parenchymal lesions, and 10% showing diffuse parenchymal heterogenicity. Cirrhosis, the end stage of idiopathic CH, may be associated with a small, irregularly marginated liver; extensive hepatic fibrosis usually results in diffusely increased hepatic echogenicity, often with hypoechoic regeneration nodules scattered throughout the parenchyma and bulging from the hepatic margins.[48] Portal hypertension is a common sequel to hepatic fibrosis, resulting in ascites and the development of acquired portosystemic shunts, which are occasionally visible on ultrasonographic examination.

In 67 dogs with idiopathic and copper-associated CH, 15 had no identifiable ultrasonographic abnormalities, and hepatic size was assessed as normal (n = 26), small (n = 26), or enlarged (n = 8).[3] Hepatic structure was found to be normal in 27, irregular in 31, and 11 had increased echogenicity. Nodular processes were observed in 16 dogs, and ascites was present in 18. On ultrasonographic examination of 68 English springer spaniels with CH, the liver seemed to be small in 49 dogs and normal in size in the remainder.[2] Changes in hepatic parenchymal echogenicity were present in 62 dogs and included hypoechogenicity (n = 12), hyperechogenicity (n = 10), or a combination of hypoechogenicity and hyperechogenicity (n = 40) when compared with the echogenicity of the spleen. Six dogs had a normal appearance to the liver on ultrasound imaging.

HISTOPATHOLOGY

It is not possible to make a definitive diagnose of idiopathic CH from results of signalment, history, physical examination, clinical pathology, or diagnostic imaging. In some cases, a tentative diagnosis can be made, but the gold standard for diagnosis is the histopathologic evaluation of liver tissue. This enables subjective descriptors of severity of inflammation and a subjective assessment about the amount of fibrosis; these factors may be used prognostically and therapeutically. Histopathology is important to rule out significant copper accumulation as a cause of CH. Liver histology will also give vital information to help establish the most appropriate therapy; without a biopsy, therapy of idiopathic CH will be at best nonspecific and at worst counterproductive.

Many methods are available for collection of liver tissue, and the method used will depend on clinician preference, availability of equipment, technical skill, cost, and the clinical stability of the patient (see Jonathan A. Lidbury's article, "Getting the Most Out of Liver Biopsy," in this issue). Cytologic evaluation of liver aspirates is of limited diagnostic accuracy in the diagnosis of idiopathic CH, and is therefore not recommended.[49,50] This relates to both the importance of liver architecture in the categorization of the diagnosis, and the chances of missing inflammatory cells where there are areas of fibrosis or if the distribution is nonuniform. In 1 study, inflammatory disease was accurately identified cytologically in only 5 of 20 dogs.[50] The only real absolute contraindication for liver biopsy is severe coagulopathy (see Jonathan A. Lidbury's article, "Getting the Most Out of Liver Biopsy," in this issue).

Histopathologic evaluation should be carried out in accordance with criteria produced by the WSAVA Liver Standardization Group.[1] The standard histochemical stain used in the assessment of liver tissue is hematoxylin and eosin, but consideration should be given to the use of additional stains for specific features such as Masson's trichrome (connective tissue), Perls' Prussian blue (ferritin), Fouchet's (bile pigments), and periodic acid-Schiff (polysaccharides). In addition, to rule out primary copper accumulation as a cause of CH, specific histochemical stains for copper, such as rubeanic acid or rhodanine, should be used, especially in at-risk breeds. An objective grading and scoring system for CH, akin to those used in human medicine,[51,52] would enable better characterization of the canine disease to improve studies into the etiology, response to treatment, and prognosis. Although bacteria do not seem to be a significant cause of CH, before a diagnosis of the idiopathic disease is made, culture of bile or liver tissues could be performed. Although not undertaken routinely, fluorescent in situ hybridization could also be considered for the identification of intrahepatic bacteria causing CH.[53]

Findings on histopathologic examination depend on the duration and severity of disease. The inflammatory cell infiltrate in dogs with CH has been poorly characterized, primarily owing to a lack of canine-specific reagents. In 1 study, high numbers of CD3[+] lymphocytes were found in liver tissue of dogs with CH,[8] although the etiology of these cases was not clear. These cells were apposed closely to degenerated hepatocytes and a positive correlation between necrosis and the number of portal and lobular CD3[+] lymphocytes was noted. The hepatic T-lymphocyte phenotype has also been characterized in a dog with CH before and after treatment.[54] Before treatment, numerous CD3[+] lymphocytes were present in the liver, and the ratio of CD4[+]/CD8[+] was high, and after treatment, CD3[+] lymphocyte infiltration was reduced along with the ratio of CD4[+]/CD8[+] cells. In English springer spaniels with idiopathic CH, the predominant inflammatory cell type was the lymphocyte, with all dogs having lesser number of plasma cells.[2] Forty-five of 68 dogs also had a neutrophilic inflammatory cell infiltrate, but there were always fewer neutrophils than lymphocytes. The inflammatory cell infiltrate was present both in the portal areas and throughout the hepatic parenchyma. In this latter study, all dogs had evidence of increased fibrous connective tissue on reticulin staining and 38 dogs had bridging fibrosis and of these 22 had cirrhosis. Cases with bridging fibrosis had combinations of portal–portal (n = 30), portal–central (n = 24), and central–central (n = 18) fibrosis. In 24 Labrador retrievers with CH of various causes, all dogs had mild-to-moderate infiltrates of lymphocytes or macrophages, which were most prominent in the portal areas.[41] Thirteen dogs also had a neutrophilic component, and 21 had degenerative hepatocellular changes. Twenty-one dogs had evidence of increased fibrous tissue on hematoxylin and eosin staining, and on examination of Masson's trichome stained sections, 6 dogs had bridging fibrosis, and 4 had cirrhosis. In 43 dogs with idiopathic CH, cirrhosis was observed in 23, including macronodular cirrhosis in 7.[3]

MANAGEMENT

Because the etiology of idiopathic CH is currently not understood, specific therapies are not possible. Nonspecific therapies seem to, however, make a significant difference to the quality of life and probably also the survival time of affected dogs. Hepatocytes have a remarkable capacity for regeneration, which means that early diagnosis and therapy has the potential to reverse disease mechanisms. A key aim of therapy in canine idiopathic CH is to inhibit fibrosis, which, if left to progress, will ultimately lead to functional impairment. Therapy aimed at addressing clinical signs of liver disease, including ascites, gastrointestinal ulceration, and HE is also an important part of therapy of the dog with idiopathic CH. In addition, careful dietary management is very important. Unfortunately, there is a paucity of controlled studies on clinical efficacy and pharmacokinetics of the commonly used drugs in canine idiopathic CH. As a result, many of our current management strategies are either derived from human hepatology, from veterinary clinical experience, or originate from low-quality veterinary clinical studies and anecdotal reports.

Glucocorticoids

Glucocorticoids have antiinflammatory, immune-modulating, and antifibrotic properties.[55] They have a potent indirect antifibrotic action via reducing prostaglandin and leukotriene production from inflammatory cells, and a weak direct antifibrotic action by inhibiting messenger RNA and enzymes. However, glucocorticoids are not without adverse effects, and these can be very severe and potentially life threatening in some dogs with idiopathic CH. Adverse effects include increased protein catabolism, fluid retention, gastrointestinal ulceration, and an increased risk of infection. Glucocorticoids should be used cautiously in dogs with bridging fibrosis or cirrhosis, because these changes can be associated with portal hypertension, ascites, and/or gastrointestinal ulceration.

There have been limited studies evaluating the use of glucocorticoids in dogs with idiopathic CH. In an early study, prednisolone was used in 151 dogs with CH at a dose of 2.2 mg/kg per day orally for 7 to 14 days, and resulted in a significantly increased survival time when compared with untreated dogs.[56] Moreover, complete remission occurred in some dogs with no relapse. However, this study was retrospective and uncontrolled, and it is unknown how many of the dogs would fit the criteria for idiopathic CH according to current WSAVA criteria. In a more recent study, 36 dogs with idiopathic CH were treated with prednisolone at a dose of 1 mg/kg per day orally for at least 6 weeks, and at follow-up 11 dogs were in complete remission, 8 dogs had recurrent clinical signs, and 17 dogs had residual disease.[57] The use of glucocorticoids has also been reported in retrospective studies of dogs with idiopathic CH, although as it is likely that varying doses were used, and most dogs received other medications, it is difficult to draw conclusions on their efficacy.[2,3,41] It seems that clinicians are being selective in the cases they treat with glucocorticoids; for instance, in a retrospective study of 43 dogs with idiopathic CH, prednisone was not used in 12 dogs owing to the presence of only mild inflammation on histology.[3]

The results of these studies, therefore, do support the use of glucocorticoids in dogs with CH. In this author's opinion, glucocorticoids are indicated in the therapy of idiopathic CH when there is biopsy evidence of ongoing inflammation and this is associated with mild to moderate fibrosis. The glucocorticoid most commonly used is prednisolone rather than prednisone, because the latter drug needs to be metabolized into prednisolone by the liver. The ideal dose remains unknown, but because there is currently no evidence for an immune-mediated etiology for canine CH, an immunosuppressive dose does not seem to be warranted. Moreover, this dose is likely to be associated with more severe adverse effects. The author currently uses an antiinflammatory dose of 1 mg/kg per day orally. The duration, or method of dose reduction in dogs with idiopathic CH, is also not known. In human patients, glucocorticoids are continued for at least 6 months beyond remission, and in some cases life-long treatment is given. It is often difficult to assess remission in dogs, particularly because glucocorticoids induce hepatic enzymes and so confuse attempts to follow the disease clinicopathologically. Repeat liver biopsy can be very useful, although they are infrequently performed in our canine patients. The duration of therapy, therefore, remains empirical and some animals remain on life-long therapy. In this situation, the aim is to use a low alternate day dose. There are few data to recommend the use of alternative immune-modulating drugs, such as azathioprine and cyclosporine, in canine idiopathic CH.

Antifibrotics

As detailed, progressive fibrosis in idiopathic CH ultimately leads to decreased function and many of the clinical consequences of advanced liver disease. As yet, there are no widely available therapies to inhibit the action of inflammatory cytokines, such as transforming growth factor-β, on hepatic stellate cells, the main stimulus for fibrous tissue formation. The primary way to inhibit fibrosis is to treat the underlying disease mechanism, which is why antiinflammatory drugs are usually indicated in the management of canine idiopathic CH. In addition to the antifibrotic action of glucocorticoids, other drugs have been reported to have weak direct or indirect antifibrotic actions, including zinc and vitamin E.

Colchicine is a more specific antifibrotic; it is an alkaloid that binds to β-tubulin, thus inhibiting self-assembly and polymerization of microtubules and interfering with several cellular functions.[58] In addition, colchicine modulates the production of chemokines and prostanoids, inhibits neutrophil and endothelial cell adhesion molecules, and eventually decreases neutrophil degranulation, chemotaxis, and phagocytosis, thus reducing the initiation and amplification of inflammation.[59] Although historically it has been used as a hepatic antifibrotic in human medicine, in more recent large clinical studies it seems not to be effective, and so the hunt still goes on for efficacious antifibrotics.[60] There is limited evidence of its use in dogs,[61,62] and only anecdotal reports of its use in the management of idiopathic CH. Adverse effects, including bone marrow suppression, neurologic signs, anorexia, and diarrhea, are seen relatively commonly. As such, this author does not use colchicine in the management of idiopathic CH.

Ursodeoxycholic Acid

Ursodeoxycholic acid (UDCA) is a natural hydrophilic bile acid present in the biliary system, but is also synthesized and manufactured commercially. UDCA is nontoxic to the liver, whereas the less hydrophilic bile acids such as lithocolic acid can be highly toxic. Bile acids exert their toxicity by inducing apoptosis of hepatocytes, and disrupting the mitochondrial electron transport chain leading to the formation of free radicals and oxidative damage to cells. UDCA exerts its beneficial effects in the liver by preventing cells from entering apoptosis and preventing mitochondrial damage, likely by displacing toxic hydrophobic bile acids.[63-65] UDCA is also a cholerectic; that is, it stimulates bile flow. In addition, it has also been shown to have immunomodulatory actions by reducing immunoglobulin and interleukin production, and the expression of major histocompatibility complex-1 on hepatocytes. Studies show an additional antioxidant activity of UDCA owing to increased production of glutathione (GSH).

Although UDCA seems to be used very widely in veterinary practice, few data exist on its efficacy in dogs. There is a single case report of a dog with severe cholestasis secondary to suspected idiopathic CH whose sole treatment was UDCA.[66] In this dog, serum activities of liver enzymes and concentrations of cholesterol and total bilirubin all decreased over the course of 7 months of treatment. Concomitant with this improvement, the composition of the serum bile acids changed from the hydrophobic, toxic, endogenous bile acids to the less toxic hydrophilic bile acids. Although there are also several retrospective studies of dogs with idiopathic CH in which UDCA was used, dogs typically received multiple therapies, making it difficult to determine the specific effect of UDCA. At a dose of 15 mg/kg per day by mouth, UDCA seems to be safe, with no adverse effects reported in the literature. Because most dogs with idiopathic CH have bile stasis, and thus would likely benefit from UDCA, this author uses it in all cases.

Antibiotics

Because bacteria are not involved in the etiology of dogs with idiopathic CH, antibiotics are not warranted in general. However, owing to the compromised reticuloendothelial cell function in chronic liver disease,[67] bacterial infections may be a secondary complication of idiopathic CH. The mainstay of antibiotic use in dogs with idiopathic CH is in the management of HE, which arises with the development of portal hypertension and acquired shunts (see Adam G. Gow's article, "Hepatic Encephalopathy," in this issue). In the author's experience, clinical HE is relatively uncommon, even in dogs with advanced liver disease. If there are signs of HE, oral antibiotics to suppress bacterial populations that produce gut-derived encephalopathic toxins are warranted, and these are usually used with lactulose for a synergistic effect.[68] Suitable antibiotics effective against anaerobic organisms include amoxicillin, metronidazole, and neomycin. Metronidazole and amoxicillin have an added advantage over neomycin in that they are absorbed systemically and so may protect against bacteremia.

Antioxidants

Oxidative stress and damage to cells by reactive oxygen species is an important disease mechanism. Free radicals take up electrons from neighboring molecules, which results in oxidative damage to proteins, lipids, and DNA. In liver disease, oxidant stress is increased owing to the effects of inflammation, reduced blood flow, and mitochondrial damage by refluxed bile acids. Normal cellular protective mechanisms against oxidative damage include GSH. Most of the evidence for antioxidants is in acute liver injury, especially that owing to hepatotoxins.[69] Oxidative stress is, however, likely to be 1 factor in the pathogenesis of idiopathic CH, suggesting that antioxidants may have a role in the management of this disease.

Antioxidants include vitamin C, vitamin E, silymarin (silibinin or milk thistle extract), and S-adenosyl-L-methionine (SAMe). Vitamins C and E are normally synthesized by dogs, and it is not known whether deficiencies occur in canine idiopathic CH and therefore if supplementation is beneficial. Silymarin seems to be a strong free radical scavenger, increasing the normal cellular defense mechanisms against oxidative damage. In experimental laboratory animal studies, it has been shown to protect against toxin-induced liver damage, such as that owing to acetaminophen.[70] When given intravenously, its beneficial effects have also been reported in experimental amanita mushroom toxicity in dogs.[71] SAMe is present in hepatocytes and is a precursor for cysteine, one of the amino acids of GSH. SAMe is, therefore, important in the defense against oxygen free radicals. SAMe is produced from methionine, which is activated by SAMe synthase in hepatocytes. In liver disease, it is therefore possible that the production of SAMe and GSH may be reduced, although levels of GSH in canine liver disease vary.[72] Administration of exogenous SAMe could, therefore, restore levels of GSH in hepatocytes. SAMe is also a critical enzyme in many biochemical reactions including the transmethylation, transsulfuration, and aminopropylation pathways, and so is a key metabolite that regulates hepatocyte growth, death, and differentiation.[73] It is widely available as a nutraceutical for dogs, often combined with other antioxidants including silymarin. SAMe in combination with silymarin has been shown to mitigate the apparent prooxidant influences of prednisolone[74] and minimize the increase in liver enzymes in dogs receiving lomustine.[75] There are no controlled studies reporting the effects of SAMe supplementation in canine idiopathic CH, and there is limited evidence for the efficacy of SAMe in human chronic liver disease.[76] Having said that, owing to the potential for oxidative stress and damage, and the fact that adverse effects at therapeutic dosages have not been reported, this author sometimes uses combinations of SAMe and silymarin in canine idiopathic CH.

Diuretics

Dogs with idiopathic CH and ascites formation may require diuretic therapy. Ascites is usually owing to portal hypertension, although in some animals hypoalbuminemia may contribute to the pathogenesis.[77] Portal hypertension results from an increased intrahepatic resistance combined with increased portal blood flow. Increased intrahepatic resistance results from fibrous tissue, sinusoidal endothelial dysfunction leading to impaired intrahepatic sinusoidal relaxation, and intrahepatic vascular shunts. Fluid is then driven into the interstitial space, and when the capacity of the regional lymphatics is overwhelmed, ascites develops. The development of ascites is worsened by the splanchnic vasodilation that accompanies portal hypertension. The subsequent reduction in systemic arterial blood pressure owing to pooling of fluid in the abdomen activates the renin–angiotensin–aldosterone system. Activation of the renin–angiotensin–aldosterone system then leads to further fluid retention and more ascites. Spironolactone, an aldosterone antagonist, is therefore the drug of choice in ascitic dogs with idiopathic CH owing to portal hypertension, usually at an initial dose of 2 mg/kg orally per day. Spironolactone can have a relatively slow onset of activity in humans, taking up to 14 days to causes diuresis; this may also occur in dogs with idiopathic CH. In cases that are refractory to spironolactone, or when a more rapid resolution of ascites is required, furosemide (1–2 mg/kg orally every 12 hours) can also be used. However, therapy with furosemide has been shown to precipitate more complications in humans with ascites, especially electrolyte disturbances, such as hypokalemia.

Dietary Management

Appropriate dietary management is as important as drug therapy in the dog with idiopathic CH. Each case is individual and the diet should be adjusted accordingly, so clinicians should resist the temptation to think that "one diet fits all." No studies have been performed in dogs with idiopathic CH to assess energy needs, or dietary composition, and recommendations are usually derived empirically from studies in humans, with most work having been done in patients with end-stage liver disease complicated by HE.[78] It is this author's experience that many dogs with idiopathic CH are fed diets with inappropriate and excessive protein restriction, which may inhibit hepatic regeneration and result in protein–calorie malnutrition. Negative protein and energy balance in human patients with chronic liver disease has also been linked with abnormal immune responses, sepsis, and mortality.[79] If energy and protein metabolism of dogs with advanced liver disease are similar to those in humans, these patients actually have increased protein requirements, possibly 2- or 3-fold maintenance values.[80] **Table 2**

Table 2 Summary of the dietary recommendations for canine idiopathic CH	
Palatability and frequency	As dogs with idiopathic CH may be inappetent, feed a palatable diet several times per day. Frequent feeding maximizes energy intake and helps to reduce the development of hepatic encephalopathy
Protein	As detailed, protein restriction should be avoided in dogs with idiopathic CH, and only done if necessary to control signs of hepatic encephalopathy. Excessive protein restriction may result in protein:calorie malnutrition and the breakdown of highly ammoniaogenic endogenous proteins. Feed highly digestible, high quality protein such as that from vegetable or casein sources. Regularly assess weight, muscle mass and blood albumin.
Carbohydrates	Dogs with idiopathic CH may have impaired carbohydrate metabolism, so a diet containing highly digestible, complex carbohydrates should be fed.
Fat	Normal amounts of fat should be fed, although fat can be restricted if steatorrhea develops.
Fiber	Fermentable fiber is helpful in dogs with hepatic encephalopathy because it acidifies the colon and traps ammonia. It also increases nitrogen incorporation into bacteria and reduces bacterial ammonia production. Nonfermentable fiber is helpful in preventing constipation, a predisposing factor for hepatic encephalopathy.
Zinc	Zinc is essential to large numbers of metalloenzymes involved in a range of biochemical processes. Zinc is also involved in membrane stability and has free radical and antioxidant effects. Zinc metabolism may become disrupted in patients with liver disease. Zinc deficiency occurs in human CH and may occur in dogs with idiopathic CH, and so supplementation may be required.
Fat-soluble vitamins	These include vitamins A, D, E, and K. Malabsorption of fat-soluble vitamins can occur with disruption to the enterohepatic circulation of bile acids. As detailed, vitamin E is an antioxidant and can be supplemented in dogs with idiopathic CH. Vitamin K supplementation may be necessary if coagulation times are prolonged, especially proceeding biopsy. Vitamins A and D should not probably be supplemented because excess vitamin A can cause hepatic damage and excess vitamin D may result in hypercalcemia.
Water-soluble vitamins	Thiamine (vitamin B_1) is an essential coenzyme in carbohydrate metabolism and deficiency can results in hepatic encephalopathy-like signs. Supplementation with vitamin C is not recommended.

Abbreviation: CH, chronic hepatitis.

summarizes some of the important considerations in the dietary management of canine idiopathic CH.

PROGNOSIS

The prognosis for idiopathic CH is highly variable, and likely depends on multiple factors, especially the stage of disease. The estimated median survival time of 43 dogs with idiopathic CH was 18.3 months, with a range of zero to 49 months.[3] In Labrador retrievers with CH, the median survival was 12.5 months (range, 1 day to 88 months),[41] whereas in English springer spaniels it was 6.3 months (range, 1 day to 40.3 months).[2] The presence of advanced fibrosis and cirrhosis are strongly associated with a reduced survival time in humans with CH, and the presence of bridging fibrosis was a predictor of shorter survival time in dogs with CH of varying causes.[56] Another important prognostic indictor in dogs with CH seems to be the presence of ascites; the time from onset of clinical signs to death was 2 months, compared with 33 months for dogs without ascites.[81] A range of clinical pathology parameters have also been associated with a shorter survival time in dogs with CH, including prolonged prothrombin time, prolonged partial thromboplastin time, thrombocytopenia, hypoalbuminemia, hyperbilirubinuria, and hyperglobulinemia. However, caution should be used when interpreting these data in the individual dog with idiopathic CH, because prognosis depends on multiple variables.

REFERENCES

1. Van den Ingh TSGAM, Van Winkle TJ, Cullen JM, et al. Morphological classification of parenchymal disorders of the canine and feline liver: 2 hepatocellular death, hepatitis and cirrhosis. In: Rothuizen J, Bunch SE, Charles JA, et al, editors. WSAVA Standards for clinical and histological diagnosis of canine and feline liver disease. 1st edition. Philadelphia: Saunders Elsevier; 2006. p. 85–102.
2. Bexfield NH, Andres-Abdo C, Scase TJ, et al. Chronic hepatitis in the English springer spaniel: clinical presentation, histological description and outcome. Vet Rec 2011;169:415.
3. Poldervaart JH, Favier RP, Penning LC, et al. Primary hepatitis in dogs: a retrospective review (2002-2006). J Vet Intern Med 2009;23:72–80.
4. Friedman SL. Seminars in medicine of the Beth Israel Hospital, Boston. The cellular basis of hepatic fibrosis. Mechanisms and treatment strategies. N Engl J Med 1993;328:1828–35.
5. Reynaert H, Thompson MG, Thomas T, et al. Hepatic stellate cells: role in microcirculation and pathophysiology of portal hypertension. Gut 2002;50:571–81.
6. Benyon RC, Iredale JP. Is liver fibrosis reversible? Gut 2000;46:443–6.
7. Bataller R, Brenner DA. Hepatic stellate cells as a target for the treatment of liver fibrosis. Semin Liver Dis 2001;21:437–51.
8. Boisclair J, Dore M, Beauchamp G, et al. Characterization of the inflammatory infiltrate in canine chronic hepatitis. Vet Pathol 2001;38:628–35.
9. Ijzer J, Roskams T, Molenbeek RF, et al. Morphological characterisation of portal myofibroblasts and hepatic stellate cells in the normal dog liver. Comp Hepatol 2006;5:7.
10. Ljubuncic P, Tanne Z, Bomzon A. Evidence of a systemic phenomenon for oxidative stress in cholestatic liver disease. Gut 2000;47:710–6.
11. Watson PJ. Chronic hepatitis in dogs: a review of current understanding of the aetiology, progression, and treatment. Vet J 2004;167:228–41.

12. Bexfield NH, Buxton RJ, Vicek TJ, et al. Breed, age and gender distribution of dogs with chronic hepatitis in the United Kingdom. Vet J 2012;193(1):124–8.

13. Gocke DJ, Morris TQ, Bradley SE. Chronic hepatitis in the dog: the role of immune factors. J Am Vet Med Assoc 1970;156:1700–5.

14. Bishop L, Strandberg JD, Adams RJ, et al. Chronic active hepatitis in dogs associated with leptospires. Am J Vet Res 1979;40:839–44.

15. Adamus C, Buggin-Daubie M, Izembart A, et al. Chronic hepatitis associated with leptospiral infection in vaccinated beagles. J Comp Pathol 1997;117:311–28.

16. Kapoor A, Simmonds P, Gerold G, et al. Characterization of a canine homolog of hepatitis C virus. Proc Natl Acad Sci U S A 2011;108:11608–13.

17. Bexfield NH, Watson PJ, Heaney J, et al. Canine hepacivirus is not associated with chronic liver disease in dogs. J Viral Hepat 2014;21:223–8.

18. van der Laan LJ, de Ruiter PE, van Gils IM, et al. Canine hepacivirus and idiopathic hepatitis in dogs from a Dutch cohort. J Viral Hepat 2014;21:894–6.

19. O'Neill EJ, Day MJ, Hall EJ, et al. Bacterial cholangitis/cholangiohepatitis with or without concurrent cholecystitis in four dogs. J Small Anim Pract 2006;47:325–35.

20. Tamborini A, Jahns H, McAllister H, et al. Bacterial Cholangitis, Cholecystitis, or both in Dogs. J Vet Intern Med 2016;30(4):1046–55.

21. Twedt DC, Diehl KJ, Lappin MR, et al. Association of hepatic necrosis with trimethoprim sulfonamide administration in 4 dogs. J Vet Intern Med 1997;11:20–3.

22. Bunch SE, Castleman WL, Hornbuckle WE, et al. Hepatic cirrhosis associated with long-term anticonvulsant drug therapy in dogs. J Am Vet Med Assoc 1982;181:357–62.

23. Sternlieb I, Twedt DC, Johnson GF, et al. Inherited copper toxicity of the liver in Bedlington terriers. Proc R Soc Med 1977;70(Suppl 3):8–9.

24. Webb CB, Twedt DC, Meyer DJ. Copper-associated liver disease in Dalmatians: a review of 10 dogs (1998-2001). J Vet Intern Med 2002;16:665–8.

25. Mandigers PJ, van den Ingh TS, Bode P, et al. Association between liver copper concentration and subclinical hepatitis in Doberman Pinschers. J Vet Intern Med 2004;18:647–50.

26. Hoffmann G, van den Ingh TS, Bode P, et al. Copper-associated chronic hepatitis in Labrador Retrievers. J Vet Intern Med 2006;20:856–61.

27. Andersson M, Sevelius E. Circulating autoantibodies in dogs with chronic liver disease. J Small Anim Pract 1992;33:389–94.

28. Weiss DJ, Armstrong PJ, Mruthyunjaya A. Anti-liver membrane protein antibodies in dogs with chronic hepatitis. J Vet Intern Med 1995;9:267–71.

29. Dyggve H, Jarva H, Spillmann T, et al. Autoantibodies in Doberman hepatitis. Toulouse (France): ECVIM-CA Congress; 2010.

30. Dyggve H, Meri S, Spillmann T, et al. Anti-nuclear antibodies in Doberman hepatitis. Seville (Spain): ECVIM-CA Congress; 2011.

31. Dyggve H, Meri S, Spillmann T, et al. Anti-histone antibodies in Doberman hepatitis. Maastricht (Netherlands): ECVIM-CA Congress; 2012.

32. Dyggve H, Kennedy LJ, Meri S, et al. Association of Doberman hepatitis to canine major histocompatibility complex II. Tissue Antigens 2011;77:30–5.

33. Bexfield NH, Watson PJ, Aguirre-Hernandez J, et al. DLA class II alleles and haplotypes are associated with risk for and protection from chronic hepatitis in the English Springer spaniel. PLoS One 2012;7:e42584.

34. Watson PJ, Roulois AJ, Scase TJ, et al. Prevalence of hepatic lesions at postmortem examination in dogs and association with pancreatitis. J Small Anim Prac 2010;51:566–72.

35. Andersson M, Sevelius E. Breed, sex and age distribution in dogs with chronic liver disease: a demographic study. J Small Anim Pract 1991;32:1–5.

36. Hirose N, Uchida K, Kanemoto H, et al. A retrospective histopathological survey on canine and feline liver diseases at the University of Tokyo between 2006 and 2012. J Vet Med Sci 2014;76:1015–20.

37. Center SA. Pathophysiology of liver disease: normal and abnormal function. In: Guilford WG, Center SA, Strombeck DR, et al, editors. Strombeck's small animal gastroenterology. 3rd edition. Philadelphia: W.B. Saunders Company; 1996. p. 553–632.

38. Szawlowski AW, Saint-Aubert B, Gouttebel MC, et al. Experimental model of extended repeated partial hepatectomy in the dog. Eur Surg Res 1987;19: 375–80.

39. Watson PJ. Hepatobiliary diseases in the dog. In: Nelson RW, Couto CG, editors. Small animal internal medicine. 5th edition. St Louis (MO): Mosby Elsevier; 2014. p. 559–87.

40. Webster CRL. History, clinical signs, and physical findings in hepatobiliary disease. In: Ettinger SJ, Feldman EC, editors. Textbook of veterinary internal medicine. 7th edition. St Louis (MO): Saunders Elsevier; 2010. p. 1612–26.

41. Shih JL, Keating JH, Freeman LM, et al. Chronic hepatitis in Labrador Retrievers: clinical presentation and prognostic factors. J Vet Intern Med 2007;21:33–9.

42. Prater MR. Acquired coagulopathy II: liver disease. In: Feldman BF, Zinkl JG, Jain NC, editors. Schalm's veterinary hematology. 5th edition. Philadelphia: Williams and Wilkins; 2000. p. 560–4.

43. Mammen EF. Coagulation abnormalities in liver disease. Hematol Oncol Clin North Am 1992;6:1247–57.

44. Prins M, Schellens CJ, van Leeuwen MW, et al. Coagulation disorders in dogs with hepatic disease. Vet J 2010;185:163–8.

45. Schwarz T. The liver and gallbladder. In: O'Brien RT, Barr F, editors. BSAVA manual of canine and feline abdominal imaging. Gloucester (England): BSAVA Publications; 2009. p. 144–56.

46. Warren-Smith CM, Andrew S, Mantis P, et al. Lack of associations between ultrasonographic appearance of parenchymal lesions of the canine liver and histological diagnosis. J Small Anim Pract 2012;53:168–73.

47. Feeney DA, Anderson KL, Ziegler LE, et al. Statistical relevance of ultrasonographic criteria in the assessment of diffuse liver disease in dogs and cats. Am J Vet Res 2008;69:212–21.

48. D'Anjou M. Liver. In: D'Anjou M, Pennick D, editors. Atlas of small animal ultrasonography. 1st edition. Iowa: Blackwell Publishing; 2008. p. 217–62.

49. Cole TL, Center SA, Flood SN, et al. Diagnostic comparison of needle and wedge biopsy specimens of the liver in dogs and cats. J Am Vet Med Assoc 2002;220: 1483–90.

50. Wang KY, Panciera DL, Al-Rukibat RK, et al. Accuracy of ultrasound-guided fine-needle aspiration of the liver and cytologic findings in dogs and cats: 97 cases (1990-2000). J Am Vet Med Assoc 2004;224:75–8.

51. Knodell RG, Ishak KG, Black WC, et al. Formulation and application of a numerical scoring system for assessing histological activity in asymptomatic chronic active hepatitis. Hepatology 1981;1:431–5.

52. Ishak K, Baptista A, Bianchi L, et al. Histological grading and staging of chronic hepatitis. J Hepatol 1995;22:696–9.

53. Recordati C, Gualdi V, Craven M, et al. Spatial distribution of Helicobacter spp. in the gastrointestinal tract of dogs. Helicobacter 2009;14:180–91.

54. Sakai M, Otani I, Ishigaki K, et al. Phenotypic analysis of hepatic T lymphocytes in a dog with chronic hepatitis. J Vet Med Sci 2006;68:1219–21.

55. Rhen T, Cidlowski JA. Antiinflammatory action of glucocorticoids–new mechanisms for old drugs. N Engl J Med 2005;353:1711–23.

56. Strombeck DR, Miller LM, Harrold D. Effects of corticosteroid treatment on survival time in dogs with chronic hepatitis: 151 cases (1977-1985). J Am Vet Med Assoc 1988;193:1109–13.

57. Favier RP, Poldervaart JH, Van den Ingh TS, et al. A retrospective study of oral prednisolone treatment in canine chronic hepatitis. Vet Q 2013;33:113–20.

58. Cocco G, Chu DC, Pandolfi S. Colchicine in clinical medicine. A guide for internists. Eur J Intern Med 2010;21:503–8.

59. Lange U, Schumann C, Schmidt KL. Current aspects of colchicine therapy – classical indications and new therapeutic uses. Eur J Med Res 2001;6:150–60.

60. Friedman SL. Evolving challenges in hepatic fibrosis. Nat Rev Gastroenterol Hepatol 2010;7:425–36.

61. Rutgers HC, Haywood S, Kelly DF. Idiopathic hepatic fibrosis in 15 dogs. Vet Rec 1993;133:115–8.

62. Hill PB, Auxilia ST, Munro E, et al. Resolution of skin lesions and long-term survival in a dog with superficial necrolytic dermatitis and liver cirrhosis. J Small Anim Pract 2000;41:519–23.

63. Guldutuna S, Zimmer G, Imhof M, et al. Molecular aspects of membrane stabilization by ursodeoxycholate. Gastroenterology 1993;104:1736–44.

64. Rodrigues CM, Fan G, Ma X, et al. A novel role for ursodeoxycholic acid in inhibiting apoptosis by modulating mitochondrial membrane perturbation. J Clin Invest 1998;101:2790–9.

65. Yanaura S, Ishikawa S. Choleretic properties of ursodeoxycholic acid and chenodeoxycholic acid in dogs. Jpn J Pharmacol 1978;28:383–9.

66. Meyer DJ, Thompson MB, Senior DF. Use of ursodeoxycholic acids in a dog with chronic hepatitis: effects on serum hepatic tests and endogenous bile acid composition. J Vet Intern Med 1997;11:195–7.

67. Noda T, Mimura H, Orita K. Assessment of Kupffer cell function in rats with chronic liver injury caused by CCl4. Hepatogastroenterology 1990;37:319–23.

68. Bexfield N. Ascites and hepatic encephalopathy therapy for liver disease. In: Bonagura JD, Twedt DC, editors. Kirk's current veterinary therapy XV. St Louis (MO): Elsevier Saunders; 2014. p. 591–4.

69. Song Z, McClain CJ, Chen T. S-Adenosylmethionine protects against acetaminophen-induced hepatotoxicity in mice. Pharmacology 2004;71:199–208.

70. Muriel P, Garciapina T, Perez-Alvarez V, et al. Silymarin protects against paracetamol-induced lipid peroxidation and liver damage. J Appl Toxicol 1992;12:439–42.

71. Vogel G, Tuchweber B, Trost W, et al. Protection by silibinin against Amanita phalloides intoxication in beagles. Toxicol Appl Pharmacol 1984;73:355–62.

72. Center SA, Warner KL, Erb HN. Liver glutathione concentrations in dogs and cats with naturally occurring liver disease. Am J Vet Res 2002;63:1187–97.

73. Mato JM, Lu SC. Role of S-adenosyl-L-methionine in liver health and injury. Hepatology 2007;45:1306–12.

74. Center SA, Warner KL, McCabe J, et al. Evaluation of the influence of S-adenosylmethionine on systemic and hepatic effects of prednisolone in dogs. Am J Vet Res 2005;66:330–41.

75. Skorupski KA, Hammond GM, Irish AM, et al. Prospective randomized clinical trial assessing the efficacy of Denamarin for prevention of CCNU-induced hepatopathy in tumor-bearing dogs. J Vet Intern Med 2011;25:838–45.
76. Guo T, Chang L, Xiao Y, et al. S-adenosyl-L-methionine for the treatment of chronic liver disease: a systematic review and meta-analysis. PLoS One 2015; 10:e0122124.
77. Buob S, Johnston AN, Webster CR. Portal hypertension: pathophysiology, diagnosis, and treatment. J Vet Intern Med 2011;25:169–86.
78. Center SA. Nutritional support for dogs and cats with hepatobiliary disease. J Nutr 1998;128:2733S–46S.
79. O'Keefe SJ, El-Zayadi AR, Carraher TE, et al. Malnutrition and immuno-incompetence in patients with liver disease. Lancet 1980;2:615–7.
80. Elwyn DH. Protein metabolism and requirements in the critically ill patient. Crit Care Clin 1987;3:57–69.
81. Raffan E, McCallum A, Scase TJ, et al. Ascites is a negative prognostic indicator in chronic hepatitis in dogs. J Vet Intern Med 2009;23:63–6.

Canine Breed-Specific Hepatopathies

Penny Watson, MA, VetMD, CertVR, DSAM, FRCVS

KEYWORDS

- Inherited • Congenital • Ductal plate • Portosystemic shunt • Chronic hepatitis
- Vacuolar hepatopathy

KEY POINTS

- Many canine liver diseases have reported breed predispositions, but the genetic cause is usually poorly understood.
- Most canine liver diseases are likely to be polygenic in inheritance and represent an interaction of genes and environment.
- Congenital portosystemic shunts and abnormalities of development of intrahepatic portal veins and ductal plates are likely inherited and probably underrecognized.
- Idiopathic chronic hepatitis in dogs shows strong breed relationships suggesting genetic causes in several breeds, but the reasons for this will vary between breeds.
- Vacuolar hepatopathies and gallbladder mucoceles have also been demonstrated to have some breed relationships.

INTRODUCTION

Liver diseases, congenital and acquired and acute and chronic, are commonly recognized in a wide variety of pedigree dog breeds and crossbreeds. There are well-documented breed predispositions to many liver diseases, demonstrating an inherited tendency. In many cases, these are true breed predilections, but in some cases the claims have not been substantiated by comparison with a reference population (either a biased hospital reference population or less biased Kennel Club or insurance company data). It is important to do this before claiming increased breed prevalence because it is all too easy for false data to become established fact once they are published. Recent increased understanding of disease causes in humans and dogs shows that many inherited diseases represent a complex interaction between genetics and environment. Many diseases are polygenic, involving more than one gene together with environmental input. Even diseases inherited in an apparently simple Mendelian

Disclosure Statement: Dr P. Watson is employed and paid by the University of Cambridge and Emmanuel College, Cambridge. She has undertaken paid consultancy work for pet food companies (Mars and Eukanuba Europe) and a nutraceutical manufacturer (VetPlus).
Department of Veterinary Medicine, Queen's Veterinary School Hospital, University of Cambridge, Madingley Road, Cambridge CB3 0ES, UK
E-mail address: pjw36@cam.ac.uk

manner involving one gene can be affected by environment and may not be as simple as first thought (see discussion of copper storage disease later).

It is important for clinicians to be aware of breed predispositions for liver disease: this helps with diagnosis because it increases suspicion of disease, although it is also important to remember that not all dogs of that breed with liver disease will necessarily have the breed typical disease. Breed spotting is, therefore, not a substitute for a complete work-up, just an aid. Understanding breed predispositions will also, it is hoped, help us further to elucidate the cause of the diseases through genetic studies and, therefore, help us with more effective treatment as well as informing preventative strategies, now and in the future.

BREED-RELATED CONGENITAL LIVER DISEASES

Congenital portosystemic shunts (CPSS) are one of several congenital liver diseases outlined in **Fig. 1**, which encompass developmental abnormalities in hepatic vascular and ductal plate development of puppies in utero. There is some overlap between the diseases as detailed in **Fig. 2** and even between isolated CPSS and ductal plate abnormalities in the liver as detailed later.

Congenital Portosystemic Shunts

CPSS are relatively common in dogs. A detailed discussion of CPSS is beyond the scope of this article and can be found in other sources, including *Veterinary Clinics of North America*, May 2015. The focus here is to summarize the evidence for inherited CPSS and the relationships between CPSS and other congenital vascular diseases of the liver. Extrahepatic CPSS are most commonly diagnosed in small-breed dogs and intrahepatic CPSS most commonly in large breed dogs. Strong breed associations are reported in the veterinary literature for CPSS, but there is also a geographic variation **(Table 1)**.

Intrahepatic CPSS are common in Irish wolfhounds throughout the world and are most commonly patent ductus venosus, which should be on the left; but not all Irish wolfhounds with CPSS have this form on shunt. Krotscheck and colleagues[1] reported 125 dogs with intrahepatic CPSS from Australia and the United States. Five of these

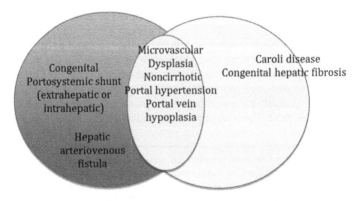

Fig. 1. Congenital liver diseases in dogs. Note that as well as overlapping syndromes, it is possible to have concurrent diseases, for example, congenital portosystemic shunt and microvascular dysplasia (see text for details).

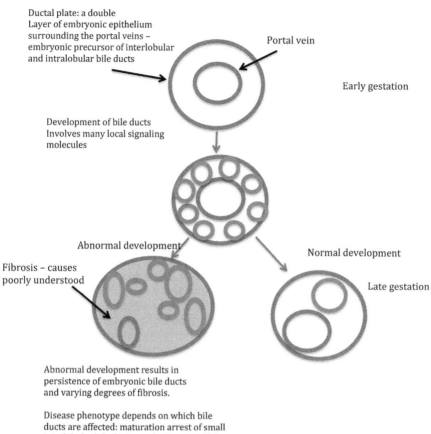

Ductal plate: a double
Layer of embryonic epithelium
surrounding the portal veins –
embryonic precursor of interlobular
and intralobular bile ducts

Portal vein

Early gestation

Development of bile ducts
Involves many local signaling
molecules

Abnormal development

Normal development

Fibrosis – causes
poorly understood

Late gestation

Abnormal development results in
persistence of embryonic bile ducts
and varying degrees of fibrosis.

Disease phenotype depends on which bile
ducts are affected: maturation arrest of small
interlobular bile ducts results in congenital
hepatic fibrosis, whereas maturation arrest of
medium intrahepatic bile ducts results in Caroli
disease

Fig. 2. Development of ductal plate in liver. (*Data from* Shorbagi A. Experience of a single center with congenital hepatic fibrosis: a review of the literature. World J Gastroenterol 2010;16(6):683.)

Table 1
Some published breed relationships for congenital portosystemic shunts in dogs

Intrahepatic Shunt	Extrahepatic Shunt	Microvascular Dysplasia
Irish wolfhounds	Cairn terrier	Cairn terrier
Deerhounds	Yorkshire terrier	Yorkshire terrier
Australian cattle dog	Maltese terrier	Papillon
Golden retriever	Jack Russell terrier	Toy poodle
Labrador retriever	Dachshunds	
Old English sheepdogs	Havanese	
	Dandy dinmont	
	Miniature schnauzer	
	West Highland white terrier	
	Shih tzu	
	Pug	

dogs were Irish wolfhounds of which 4 had the expected left divisional CPSS, but one had an anatomically different right divisional shunt. The same study also showed that the breeds presenting with intrahepatic CPSS varied between countries. For example, Australian cattle dogs are commonly recognized with CPSS in Australia, whereas Labrador retrievers were more commonly diagnosed in the United States. Australian cattle dogs were also more likely to have right divisional shunts than other breeds, as were male dogs. However, the conclusions of this and other studies were that, although it is possible to predict that most large-breed dogs will have intrahepatic as opposed to extrahepatic CPSS, the exact anatomic location of the shunt can vary and imaging is necessary to confirm this. Several studies have investigated the genetics of CPSS in different breeds. In Irish wolfhounds, breeding studies have shown a strong genetic basis but suggested at least 3 or 4 alleles in 2 loci are involved.[2] The occurrence of intrahepatic CPSS was found to be strongly inherited but not the location (right or left divisional).

In small-breeds dogs, studies in Maltese terriers[3] and cairn terriers[4] have demonstrated what seems to be a common, partially penetrant recessive inheritance. There is also an interesting overlap with microvascular dysplasia (MVD) (see next section) with some dogs with MVD producing puppies with CPSS. This evidence and other evidence has led to the suggestion that mutations predisposing to CPSS are in fact mutations that predispose to several abnormalities in development of the liver vasculature and ductal plates and that the exact phenotype inherited depends on other genes and the environment both within and outside the uterus. A compelling theory also suggests poor nutrition and/or placental development of the fetus in utero as a part of this environment, which is supported by documented resorption of puppies in some affected dams.[3]

Microvascular Dysplasia, Portal Vein Hypoplasia, and Noncirrhotic Portal Hypertension

MVD, portal vein hypoplasia, and noncirrhotic portal hypertension are all congenital abnormalities in development of the intrahepatic portal veins. There is likely an overlap between these conditions, and there may or may not be an overlap with other ductal plate abnormalities developmentally (see later discussion). MVD tends to be reported mostly in smaller-breed dogs and is usually not associated with portal hypertension and ascites,[5–7] whereas noncirrhotic portal hypertension is more often reported in large-breed dogs and, as the name suggests, presents with portal hypertension.[8] The histologic appearances of MVD, portal vein hypoplasia, and noncirrhotic portal hypertension are also very similar with a lack of portal vein branches in smaller portal triads being the hallmark. The difference between these diseases (if there is one) is largely related to the response of the liver and the presence or absence of portal hypertension. MVD is in fact physiologically unusual in that there is usually no evidence of portal hypertension and ascites. The portal vasculature is a large parallel, low-resistance circulation (like a tree with multiple branches), so the portal pressure is usually low. A reduction in portal vein branches such as occurs with MVD should result in portal hypertension because of a reduction in the number of parallel vessels and, thus, increase in resistance. The fact that this does not happen argues strongly for a form of intrahepatic shunting that has been demonstrated to occur in other species via vascular shunts from the portal vein to the hepatic vein bypassing the sinusoids. In contrast, in noncirrhotic portal hypertension, it is assumed that these shunts are nonfunctional; therefore, portal hypertension develops.

The liver of a dog with CPSS also has a very similar histologic appearance to these conditions: the presence of a single large shunting vessel diverting blood from the liver results in a reduction in smaller portal vein branches. The only reliable way to differentiate CPSS and MVD is to search for a large shunting vessel. Occasionally, dogs may have concurrent MVD or other microscopic vascular anomalies in addition to a gross shunting vessel; in these dogs, liver function tests fail to normalize after surgical ligation of their CPSS and there may be an increased risk of postoperative portal hypertension.

MVD has been reported as a congenital disorder in several breeds, but particularly cairn terriers and Yorkshire terriers (see **Table 1**). A recent study of histologically confirmed canine liver disease in Japan found MVD was the most common diagnosis, accounting for 29.4% of all diagnoses of liver disease in their population with Yorkshire terriers, papillons, and toy poodles being particularly affected, although the investigators noted that they could not differentiate MVD and portal vein hypoplasia histologically.[5] Studies in cairn terriers have suggested an autosomal recessive inheritance of MVD in the breed.[6] This breed is the only breed whereby genetic studies have been reported. It has been demonstrated that CPSS is inherited in cairn terriers, and there has been speculation that there may be overlap in the genetic factors predisposing to MVD and CPSS, although more work needs to be done to confirm this.[4]

Ductal Plate Abnormalities

Congenital ductal plate abnormalities encompass several developmental abnormalities of the portal triad, including juvenile hepatic fibrosis and Caroli disease. These abnormalities particularly affect the bile ducts. Portal vein hypoplasia and MVD might be separate diseases or might be related to ductal plate abnormalities: in human medicine, incomplete development of the portal vein branches is a recognized consequence of ductal plate abnormalities with an absence of portal vein branches in smaller triads (likened to pollard willows) and embryonic development of bile ducts and portal circulation are known to be linked.[9] **Fig. 2** gives a summary of ductal plate development, demonstrating why abnormalities result in biliary hyperplasia with increased fibrosis. In human medicine, a variety of both recessive and dominant genetic diseases are recognized that predispose to a variety of ductal plate abnormalities, together with a variety of concurrent diseases, such as collagen disorders and polycystic kidneys. In dogs, most of theses diseases appear in the literature as small cases series and very little is understood about the underlying genetics.

Biliary Ductal Plate Malformations (Congenital Hepatic Fibrosis, Caroli Disease)

Brown and others[10] first reported congenital hepatic fibrosis in dogs in 2010 in 5 dogs of a variety of breeds. Reports in the veterinary literature have been sparse since this time, but it is likely that the disease is underrecognized. The experience of this author and also of Pillai and colleagues[11] is that several affected dogs are misdiagnosed on histology as portal fibrosis, cirrhosis, chronic hepatitis, or cholangitis. Increasing reporting of the disease should help improve recognition. This improved recognition is important because affected dogs often do better on long-term management than dogs with cirrhosis or chronic hepatitis. A key histologic finding differentiating the biliary hyperplasia of congenital hepatic fibrosis from the secondary biliary hyperplasia in chronic hepatitis and cirrhosis is the lack of proliferation of the embryonic bile ducts demonstrated by negative staining with immunohistologic stains, such as Ki67.[10,11]

Is congenital hepatic fibrosis a breed-related disease? If it is similar to ductal plate abnormalities in humans, it should be. Pillai and colleagues[11] in 2016 reported 30 boxer dogs from the histology archive at Cornell with ductal plate malformations, suggesting an increased prevalence in this breed, although that has not been confirmed. Interestingly, there was a high prevalence of concurrent congenital hepatic abnormalities, such as atrophy of liver lobes, gallbladder abnormalities, or vascular abnormalities. Two dogs had Caroli disease (see later discussion), but no dog had evidence of cysts in the pancreas or liver. Thirty-five percent of dogs in this study had a significant accumulation of copper in the liver, although the investigators offered no real explanation for this apart from increased dietary copper.

Recent work at the University of Cambridge in the United Kingdom suggests that Skye terrier hepatitis may in fact be a congenital ductal plate abnormality. Skye terrier hepatitis was first reported in 1988 in 9 related dogs from the United Kingdom.[12] It was associated with hepatic copper deposition but did not show features typical of copper storage disease: copper accumulation did not accompany the initial histologic features but seemed rather to be related to the severity of cholestasis suggesting a primary disorder of bile metabolism.

Histologic examination of 3 Skye terriers recently presenting in the United Kingdom with liver disease and repeat examination of a case reported in Glasgow in 2003[13] has demonstrated features suggestive of congenital hepatic fibrosis.[14] Interestingly, there is a suggestion in the breed that some dogs also have renal dysplasia, although this has yet to be confirmed. Work is continuing to further characterize the histology and genetics of the disease in Skye terriers.

Caroli disease describes congenital dilation of the large and segmental bile ducts and seems to occur as a result of maturation arrest of medium intrahepatic bile ducts. Reports in the veterinary literature are sparse. In 2006, 2 golden retriever littermates from South Africa were reported to have this disease and both also had portal fibrosis and renal cysts[15]; 8 affected dogs of a variety of breeds were reported from the Netherlands in 2003[16]; 2 out of 30 boxers with ductal plate abnormalities from Cornell in 2016 were reported to have Caroli disease.[11]

BREED-RELATED ACQUIRED LIVER DISEASES
Breed-Related Idiopathic Chronic Hepatitis

Chronic hepatitis is defined histologically by the World Small Animal Veterinary Association Liver Standardization group as a hepatic mononuclear or mixed inflammatory infiltrate with hepatocyte necrosis and/or apoptosis and varying degrees of fibrosis. It is remarkably common in dogs, with a prevalence of up to 12% at postmortem examination in old dogs. In most cases the cause of chronic hepatitis remains unknown and it remains idiopathic.[17] Increased amounts of copper are found in the liver of some dogs with chronic hepatitis: some have true copper storage disease whereas in others, the copper build up may be secondary to the liver disease. The interpretation of the role of copper in canine chronic hepatitis is complicated and will be discussed separately.

Chronic hepatitis is recognized in a variety of dog breeds and crossbreeds. However, there are strong breed predilections reported in the literature and these seem to have altered with time and geographic location. Breed predilections are summarized in **Table 2**. There are also reported gender and age biases in some breeds in the studies referenced: Andersson and Sevelius noted a male predisposition in American and English cocker spaniels, which were a mean of 5 years old, and a female predisposition in Labradors, which were a mean of 6.9 years old at presentation. Bexfield and colleagues[22] reported a median age for all dogs of 8 years with an overall sex ratio of 1.5 females to 1.0 male. However, Dalmatians, Dobermans, and English springer spaniels (ESS) presented at a significantly younger age than Labrador retrievers, cairn terriers, and English cocker spaniels. There was an overrepresentation of females in the Dalmatians, Dobermans, English cocker spaniels, English springer spaniels, and Labrador retrievers and an overrepresentation of males in the American cocker

Table 2
Reported breed predilections for canine chronic hepatitis

Andersson and Sevelius,[21] 1991[a]	Bexfield et al,[22] 2012[b]	Hirose et al,[5] 2014[c]	Poldervaart et al,[31] 2009[d]	Other Single Breed Reports
Labrador retrievers	Labrador retriever	Labrador retriever	Labrador retriever and golden retriever	—
American cocker spaniel	American cocker spaniel	*American cocker spaniel*	American cocker spaniel	American cocker spaniel[e]
English cocker spaniel	English cocker spaniel	—	English cocker spaniel	—
Doberman pinscher	Doberman pinscher	—	—	—
West Highland white terrier	—	—	West Highland white terrier	West Highland white terrier[f]
Scottish terrier	—	—	—	—
—	Dalmatian	—	—	Dalmatian[g]
—	English springer spaniel	—	—	—
—	—	*Miniature schnauzer*	—	—
—	—	*Pomeranian*	—	—
—	—	*Miniature dachshund*	—	—
—	—	—	—	Skye terrier[h]
—	—	—	German pointer	—

[a] Two-hundred fifty cases of histopathologically confirmed chronic hepatitis in one diagnostic laboratory in Sweden + 49 dogs with histopathologically confirmed chronic hepatitis at the Animal Hospital of Helsingborg 1984 to 1989. Control population: Swedish Kennel Club registrations (representing 60%–70% of all dogs in Sweden).

[b] Five-hundred fifty-one cases histopathologically confirmed chronic hepatitis from 6 histopathology laboratories in the United Kingdom from 2001 to 2008. Control population: microchip data from one company from 2001 and 2008: 175,442 and 311,085 dogs, respectively.

[c] A total of 463 canine liver biopsies at Veterinary Medical Center of University of Tokyo from 2006 to 2012. Odds ratios compared with all cases with chronic hepatitis. A proportion are probably copper storage disease – see text. Dogs with *italics* were classified as cholangiohepatitis.

[d] Retrospective study of histologically confirmed hepatitis at University of Utrecht from 2002 to 2006. Twenty-one acute hepatitis; 67 chronic hepatitis. Control population: total clinic population. Breeds shown had increased risk of chronic hepatitis. Jack Russell terrier also had increased risk of acute hepatitis.

[e] Kanemoto and colleagues[23]; may be some overlap of cases with Hirose and colleagues.[5]

[f] Thornburg and colleagues.[28]

[g] Probably copper storage disease; see relevant section.

[h] Probably ductal plate abnormality; see text.

spaniels. Hirose and colleagues[5] also reported a female predisposition in Labradors and Dobermans with chronic hepatitis in Japan and a strong male predisposition in miniature dachshunds with cholangiohepatitis.

It is very important to realize that several different insults to the liver may produce histologically very similar findings: for example, chronic infectious causes, toxic causes, and autoimmune causes may appear identical on histology. This similarity increases the challenge for clinicians to decide appropriate treatment in affected dogs because, in most cases, the cause is not confirmed. In some cases, breed predilections might help understand the cause; but in many cases it does not because of our currently limited understanding of etiopathogenesis. The hope is that ongoing research in specific dog breeds will help elucidate causes. **Box 1** lists possible reasons for increased prevalence of chronic hepatitis in a particular dog breed. The current state of knowledge of potential causes in individual dog breeds is summarized later. It is clear that there is still much work to be done (**Fig. 3**).

Dobermans

Chronic hepatitis was first reported in Doberman pinschers in the 1980s. Since that time, they have been consistently identified in studies all over the world as having an increased risk of disease, but there has been debate about the cause. Most reports show a strong female predominance, and work from Scandinavia suggests an autoimmune cause with a strong association to dog leukocyte antigen (DLA) class II alleles and haplotypes[18] and increased expression of DLA class II on hepatocytes in affected dogs.[19]

In contrast, studies published from Utrecht have provided strong evidence for a unique form of copper storage disease in Dobermans (see section on copper storage disease). Which is correct? It is very likely that these studies show 2 different subgroups of Doberman pinschers, a proportion of which have autoimmune hepatitis and a proportion of which have copper storage disease. It is known that the Dobermans with copper storage disease respond well to copper chelation, whereas the Dobermans with autoimmune disease do not need this but may respond to immunosuppression: there is no recent direct evidence of a response to steroids in Dobermans with chronic hepatitis, but the original article demonstrating the efficacy of steroids in canine chronic hepatitis included a large number of Dobermans.[20] It is, therefore, very

---

Box 1
Potential reasons for breed-related chronic hepatitis in dogs and comparison with human medicine

Increased susceptibility to infectious causes of chronic hepatitis and/or to chronicity of infection rather than recovery
- No reports for hepatitis in dogs, but known breed predispositions to other diseases (eg, rottweiler and parvovirus)
- In humans, known genetic variations in susceptibility to chronic hepatitis B and other viruses

Susceptibility to autoimmune disease
- Suspected in some Dobermans (see text) and also possibly English springer spaniels and cocker spaniels
- In humans, known genetic variations in susceptibility to autoimmune hepatitis

Mutation of gene coding for protein involved in metal transport/storage/excretion
- Copper storage disease in Bedlington terriers and other breeds (see text)
- In humans, Wilson disease (equivalent to copper storage disease) and also hemochromatosis due to excess iron

Gene mutations resulting in hepatic accumulation of glycoprotein protease inhibitor
- Alpha-1 antitrypsin inhibitor deficiency suspected but never proved in cocker spaniels (see text)
- Alpha-1 antitrypsin inhibitor deficiency well described in humans

Increased susceptibility to chronic hepatic damage with toxic causes
- None described for chronic hepatitis but known susceptibility of Dobermans to acute liver insult from potentiated sulphonamides and suspected susceptibility of Labrador retrievers to carprofen toxicity
- In humans, known genetic predispositions to alcohol-induced chronic hepatitis and cirrhosis

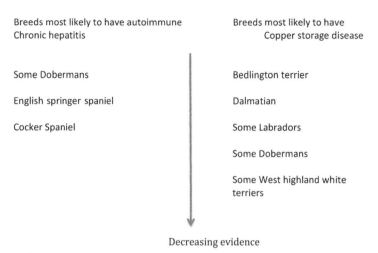

Breeds most likely to have autoimmune Chronic hepatitis	Breeds most likely to have Copper storage disease
Some Dobermans	Bedlington terrier
English springer spaniel	Dalmatian
Cocker Spaniel	Some Labradors
	Some Dobermans
	Some West highland white terriers

Decreasing evidence

Fig. 3. Breed predispositions for copper and autoimmune hepatitis.

important to take a liver biopsy from all affected Dobermans and assess for copper before considering treatment. If copper is not deemed to be the cause, assessing the severity and type of inflammatory cell infiltrate in the liver and checking the dog's DLA class II haplotype may help direct treatment of autoimmune disease.

Cocker spaniels

English and American cocker spaniels have consistently appeared as having increased risk of disease in surveys of dogs with chronic hepatitis (see **Table 2**). One early study showed a strong male predominance in both American and English cockers,[21] whereas a more recent UK study showed a male predominance in American cockers but a female predominance in English cockers[22] and a recent Japanese study of American cocker spaniels showed no sex predisposition.[23] The median age at diagnosis was reported to be 8 years 9 months in English cockers and 5 years 6 months in American cockers in one study[22] and 4 years 6 months in American cockers in another study.[23]

The cause of the disease in cockers remains a matter of debate, and it is unknown whether American and English cocker spaniels have the same or different diseases. Early investigations suggested that some English and American cocker spaniels might suffer from a condition similar to alpha-1 antitrypsin (AAT) deficiency in humans with accumulation of an unusual form of the molecule in hepatocytes. However, this has never been convincingly confirmed. Unlike the very-well-described AAT deficiency in humans, affected dogs did not have deficient circulating AAT and it was unclear if the abnormal form in the hepatocytes was the cause or an effect of the disease.[24] Thirteen American cocker spaniels reported more recently with chronic hepatitis in Japan all had severe fibrosis and cirrhosis with minimal inflammation suggesting that their disease had been subclinical until the end stage. The original cause was unknown, and copper staining ruled out copper storage disease.[23] English cocker spaniels in the United Kingdom have been reported as having a multiorgan duct-centered autoimmune disease similar to a human disease called immunoglobulin G4 (IgG4)-related disease.[25,26] Affected dogs and humans typically have chronic pancreatitis, glomerulonephritis, dry eye and dry mouth. Humans also often have immune attack on the biliary tract.[27] It is plausible this might also occur in a subset of cocker spaniels, although this has not yet been convincingly demonstrated. Interestingly, and unlike many other autoimmune diseases, human IgG4-related disease is more common in older males and is suggested to be a disease predisposed by immune senescence. This finding might explain the male predominance in cockers with chronic hepatitis in some canine studies. It is also interesting to note that Hirose and colleagues reported 5 America cocker spaniels with cholangiohepatitis, stressing involvement of the bile duct.

West Highland white terriers

West Highland white terriers were reported as having an increased risk of chronic hepatitis by Andersson and Sevelius[21] in 1991 and the disease was further investigated by Thornburg and colleagues[28] in 1996 who reported 2 subgroups of affected dogs: one with apparently classic copper storage disease and one with no copper involvement and idiopathic chronic hepatitis. West Highland white terriers were also reported to have an increased risk of hepatitis in a recent retrospective study from Utrecht in which 2 out of 4 dogs with chronic hepatitis had copper-associated disease and 2 out of 4 dogs had idiopathic chronic hepatitis. No further studies have been published on hepatitis in the breed, and a recent epidemiologic study of canine chronic hepatitis in dogs in the United Kingdom did not identify West Highland white terriers as having increased risk of disease.[22]

English springer spaniels

ESS have been identified in the United Kingdom and Norway as having a significantly increased risk of chronic hepatitis, which is more common in dogs from show lines than working lines.[22] A recently published study documents the clinical and histologic signs in 68 affected dogs.[29] There was a marked female predominance, and the median age of affected dogs was younger than most other cases of chronic hepatitis at 3 years 7 months (range 7 months to 8 years 5 months). Clinical signs tend to be severe and the prognosis poor. Half of the dogs were icteric at presentation, and the median survival time was only 189 days, although 12 dogs survived more than a year from diagnosis. None of the dogs had evidence of excessive copper accumulation on histology. The cause remains unclear; but a recent study demonstrated an association with a DLA class II haplotype, suggesting the disease might be infectious or autoimmune.[30] Searches for an infectious cause of disease have so far been fruitless. However, anecdotally, affected ESS respond well to steroid treatment, suggesting the disease may be autoimmune, although more work will be required to confirm this.

To the author's knowledge hepatitis has not yet appeared with increased prevalence in ESS in the United States. However, anecdotally, there is also an increased prevalence of hepatitis in ESS in Norway. Interestingly, Norwegian ESS show dogs are more closely related to UK dogs than North American dogs. There have also been sporadic reports of hepatitis in ESS in Australia, another country that has used largely UK bloodlines. Initial pedigree analysis of affected UK dogs failed to find a common ancestor within 6 generations. All this evidence argues for a disease with some genetic involvement, which emerged relatively recently, probably appearing in UK dogs longer ago than the 6-generation pedigree but after the founder dogs went to North America.

- Dalmatians (see copper section later)
- Labrador retrievers (see copper section later)
- Skye terriers (see ductal plate section earlier)

Breed-Related Copper Storage Disease

Copper storage disease should be considered separately from idiopathic chronic hepatitis, although there is obvious overlap. This disease is another disease whereby there is a clear interaction of genes and environment (**Fig. 4**). Breeds such as the Bedlington terrier with a strong genetic tendency to copper storage disease will develop clinical disease with normal amounts of dietary copper and have to be fed on a low-copper diet lifelong to avoid hepatitis. Other breeds, such as the Labrador retriever, are less susceptible to copper overload but may develop copper storage disease if their diet is high in copper; their genetic susceptibility to this seems to vary between countries and continents. A retrospective study of acute and chronic hepatitis in dogs in Utrecht suggested up to 36% of dogs with chronic hepatitis had copper-associated disease.[31] Any dog of any breed or crossbreed can develop copper-associated hepatitis either with or without dietary copper loading; it is important to rule this out on all liver biopsies specimens, at least semiquantitatively by staining for copper. Clinicians should also remember the potential for ingestion of toxic quantities of copper by any dog, for example, through inadvertent access to high copper calf food or supplements. There is evidence for increased environmental exposure to copper in dogs since the 1980s leading to increased accumulation in the liver, although it is unclear whether this is in the diet itself, dietary supplements used by owners, or both.[32] There is also some evidence that copper in manufactured dog food has become more bioavailable in recent years, potentially increasing the risk of copper storage disease in susceptible dogs.[33]

The traditional definition of copper storage disease relies on several classic histopathologic and clinical findings as detailed in **Table 3**. A more fluid interpretation is presented in **Fig. 4**. In either case, 2 important points are worth noting:

1. Dogs are much more resistant than humans to the buildup of periportal copper secondary to cholestasis. In an experimental study in mixed-breed dogs, the bile ducts were ligated from 21 to 93 days. Liver copper concentrations in the liver only

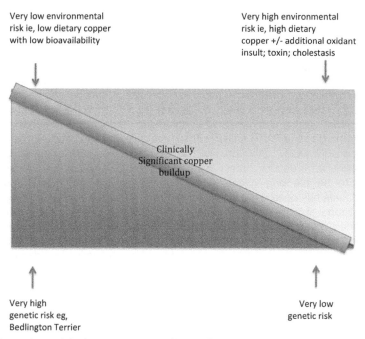

Very low environmental risk ie, low dietary copper with low bioavailability

Very high environmental risk ie, high dietary copper +/- additional oxidant insult; toxin; cholestasis

Clinically Significant copper buildup

Very high genetic risk eg, Bedlington Terrier

Very low genetic risk

Fig. 4. Dynamic model of copper storage disease demonstrating interaction of genes and environment.

Table 3
Traditional criteria for diagnosis of primary copper storage disease

Primary Copper Storage Disease	Copper Deposition Secondary to Cholestasis
Copper accumulates around the central vein (zone 3)	Copper accumulates around the portal triad (zone 1)
Copper accumulation predates inflammation (clear cause and effect)	Copper accumulation comes after inflammation
Copper colocates with inflammation	Copper does not colocate with inflammation
Degree of copper accumulation correlates with degree of liver disease	Copper accumulation is much less than the severity of liver disease
Hepatic copper concentration <400 µg/g dry weight[32]	Hepatic copper concentration >1800 µg/g dry weight[32]

Note comments in text about dogs being relatively resistant to secondary copper accumulation.

increased significantly if the diet was copper loaded, suggesting that dogs are resistant to copper buildup secondary to cholestasis unless they have increased dietary concentrations or a problem with copper excretion. The dogs showed histologic changes typical of chronic cholestasis and early biliary cirrhosis but no significant liver injury in spite of copper concentrations, which were 8 times normal suggesting, that they needed an additional insult, such as oxidant damage, for increased hepatic copper to lead to hepatitis.[34]

2. Serious consideration should be given to copper chelation and a low-copper diet in dogs with more than a small amount of copper identified on histopathology, even if this is thought to be secondary, because of the risk that the copper will result in hepatocyte necrosis in response to an additional insult in the future. Therefore, to an extent it is academic whether the copper deposition is primary or secondary; the most important question is whether it is present in significant amounts.

Bedlington terrier

Bedlington terriers have the most well documented and investigated copper storage disease of any dog breed. Reports demonstrate a clear primary copper storage disease with centrilobular distribution and clear association between the degree of copper buildup and severity of disease. The disease is confined to the liver, but dogs with marked copper buildup can have acute hepatocyte damage and hemolysis. The disease seems to be inherited as an autosomal recessive trait and had a high prevalence in the breed previously, although this has been reducing with selective breeding. Studies identified a genetic defect associated with the disease, which was initially assumed to be the only cause, a deletion in the COMMD1 gene (previously MURR1)[35]; this has been used for screening for breeding. However, Bedlington terriers with copper storage disease but without a COMMD1 deletion have been reported in the United States, United Kingdom, and Australia (Coronado and colleagues,[36] 2003; Haywood,[37] 2006; Hyun and Filippich,[38] 2004), suggesting that there are additional mutations involved in the breed. One of these has recently been identified in homozygous COMMD1 negative Bedlington terriers with copper storage disease in the United Kingdom where a mutation has been found in the ABCA12 gene, which encodes for an ATP-binding cassette, a divalent metal transporter protein.[39] Hepatic copper excretion is a complex process; it seems likely that multiple genes are involved such that, as Bedlingtons with COMMD1 deletions have been selectively removed from the population, other genetic defects contributing to copper storage disease have become more prevalent.

Dalmatians

Copper-associated hepatitis has been reported in several young Dalmatian dogs in the United States and Canada.[40,41] Dogs usually presented as young adults (mean 6 years in one study) with acute onset gastrointestinal signs and marked elevation in liver enzymes. Hepatic histology was very supportive of primary copper storage disease with centrilobular distribution of copper and very high concentrations. Prognosis was poor with a mean time from diagnosis to death of 80 days suggesting dogs present in end-stage disease. There have been no published reports of copper storage disease in Dalmatians in the United Kingdom, but the breed was reported as having an increased prevalence of chronic hepatitis in one UK study[22]; the author has anecdotally heard reports of cases in the United Kingdom.

Doberman pinschers

Several Dutch studies have demonstrated without doubt that a proportion of Doberman pinschers have a form of copper storage disease. The copper seems to buildup in zone 3 in most cases, and there is clinical response to copper chelators.[42,43] A recent study in Dutch Dobermans showed reduced expression of genes associated with copper efflux and reduce glutathione in affected dogs.[44] However, as discussed in the previous section, not all Doberman pinschers with chronic hepatitis have copper storage disease, so it is very important to take a liver biopsy from affected dogs before initiating treatment.

Labrador retrievers

Published reports from Utrecht and the United States suggested that copper storage disease was the predominant cause of chronic hepatitis in this breed.[45–48] However, until recently, copper storage disease was not recognized in Labradors with chronic hepatitis in the United Kingdom, even though Labradors are predisposed to disease in this country.[22] More recently, the author has identified individual Labradors with high concentrations of hepatic copper, but this remains uncommon. This finding is interesting because it does suggest a difference in genetics between UK Labradors and those in the United States or the Netherlands and underlines the fact that chronic hepatitis is a diverse disease with several potential causes and potential reasons for increased breed susceptibilities. There may be a change in prevalence with time: more recently, Poldervaart and colleagues[31] reported 16 Labradors in their study of hepatitis in dogs in the Netherlands, of which 11 were idiopathic and only 5 associated with copper.

Affected dogs tend to be middle aged at presentation; histologic findings are supportive of primary copper storage disease with a centrilobular pattern and colocalization with inflammatory cells, together with high concentrations of copper (see **Table 3**).[45,46] A genetic predisposition is further supported by finding evidence of increased copper in the livers of clinically normal relatives.[48] Affected dogs respond to treatment with copper chelators and low-copper diet, although the long-term response to diet seems to vary depending on the severity of the phenotype.[48,49]

Breed-Related Vacuolar Hepatopathies

The term *vacuolar hepatopathy* is used to describe a variety of causes of vacuolated hepatocytes, which are generally considered to be secondary to other diseases, particularly endocrine disease. Vacuoles may result from hepatocytes being full of fat (steatosis) or glycogen or water (hepatocellular swelling or cloudy swelling). Hyperadrenocorticism typically results in glycogen vacuolation, and diabetes mellitus and hypothyroidism typically result in fat deposition. However, there are many other causes of vacuolation, including hepatocyte injury with toxins, which may be primary rather than secondary hepatopathies. The different types of vacuolation can to some extent be distinguished by their patterns on light microscopy; but this can be challenging in some cases, and special stains may be necessary.

Vacuolar hepatopathies are very common and generally are not considered to be breed related but with 2 notable exceptions, which are discussed here.

Vacuolar hepatopathy in Scottish terriers

An apparently breed-related glycogen vacuolar hepatopathy has been reported in Scottish terriers in the United States and France.[50–52] Affected dogs present with a marked increase in serum alkaline phosphatase and an apparently increased risk of developing hepatocellular carcinoma. The median age at presentation was 8 years for hepatopathy and older for carcinoma. The pathogenesis remains poorly understood. Some affected dogs show clinical features suggestive of hyperadrenocorticism, but results of adrenal function testing are inconsistent; in one study, 5 out of 7 dogs tested had normal urine cortisol/creatinine ratios.[50] Gallbladder mucocele has been reported in 16% of cases. Dogs show a poor response to treatments for hyperadrenocorticism, and management is currently supportive.

Familial hypertriglyceridemia in miniature schnauzers

Familial hypertriglyceridemia (FHTG) is very common in miniature schnauzers, and the prevalence increases with age. In a recent study of 192 miniature schnauzers in the United States, 32.8% showed increased serum triglycerides and more than 75% of dogs were more than 9 years of age.[53] Pancreatitis is the most clinically significant clinical consequence of FHTG; but liver disease is also very common in affected dogs, with vacuolar hepatopathy and gallbladder mucocele being the commonest pathologies.

In human medicine, FHTG is known to be a polygenic disease, involving the interaction of genes with environmental factors, such as fat concentration of the diet, concurrent endocrine disease, and liver disease.[54] Individuals with FHTG have delayed clearance of dietary fats by the liver, which becomes more clinically significant with age because of hepatocyte aging. A recent study in dogs demonstrated reduction in expression of genes involved in hepatic cholesterol trafficking with age in dogs, supporting this theory in dogs as well as humans.[55]

Candidate gene studies in miniature schnauzers for mutations in single genes involved in fat metabolism (lipoprotein lipase and apolipoprotein C-II) have failed to find a difference between affected and unaffected dogs.[56]

Gallbladder Mucocele

A gallbladder mucocele is cystic mucinous hyperplasia of the gallbladder wall with accumulation of thick mucus. A mucocele can be an incidental finding on diagnostic imaging or postmortem examination but can cause secondary obstruction of the biliary tract or even gallbladder wall pressure necrosis and rupture. The cause is poorly understood, but there does seem to be a relationship with hyperlipidemia. There is a suggestion in the literature of breed relationships, with an increased incidence in small-breed dogs. Aguirre and colleagues[57] (2007) reported gallbladder mucocele in 38 Shetland sheepdogs; Malek and colleagues[58] (2013) reported gallbladder mucocele in 43 dogs, including 10 cocker spaniels, 5 Shetland sheepdogs, and 4 miniature schnauzers. A Japanese case-control study of gallbladder mucocele showed a significant association with increased cholesterol or triglycerides, and miniature schnauzers were one of the breeds predisposed to mucocele.[59] There is conflicting evidence that mutation of the gene ABCB4, which encodes a membrane transporter protein, is associated with gallbladder mucoceles in Shetland sheep dogs. An initial study found such an association,[60] but in a subsequent study this result was not reproduced in this or other breeds of dog.[61] The investigators of the latter study concluded their findings do not rule out the possibility that *ABCB4* dysfunction may be one of many contributors in a multifactorial cause.[61]

REFERENCES

1. Krotscheck U, Adin CA, Hunt GB, et al. Epidemiologic factors associated with the anatomic location of intrahepatic portosystemic shunts in dogs. Vet Surg 2007; 36(1):31–6.
2. Van Steenbeek FG, Leegwater PAJ, van Sluijs FJ, et al. Evidence of inheritance of intrahepatic portosystemic shunts in Irish wolfhounds. J Vet Intern Med 2009; 23(4):950–2.
3. O'Leary CA, Parslow A, Malik R, et al. The inheritance of extra-hepatic portosystemic shunts and elevated bile acid concentrations in Maltese dogs. J Small Anim Pract 2013;55(1):14–21.
4. Van Straten G, Leegwater PAJ, De Vries M, et al. Inherited congenital extrahepatic portosystemic shunts in cairn terriers. J Vet Intern Med 2005;19(3):321–4.
5. Hirose N, Uchida K, Kanemoto H, et al. A retrospective histopathological survey on canine and feline liver diseases at the University of Tokyo between 2006 and 2012. J Vet Med Sci 2014;76(7):1015–20.
6. Schermerhorn T, Center SA, Dykes NL, et al. Characterization of hepatoportal microvascular dysplasia in a kindred of cairn terriers. J Vet Intern Med 1996; 10(4):219–30.
7. Christiansen JS, Hottinger HA, Allen L, et al. Hepatic microvascular dysplasia in dogs: a retrospective study of 24 cases (1987-1995). J Am Anim Hosp Assoc 2000;36(5):385–9.
8. Bunch SE, Johnson SE, Cullen JM. Idiopathic noncirrhotic portal hypertension in dogs: 33 cases (1982-1998). J Am Vet Med Assoc 2001;218(3):392–9.
9. Shorbagi A. Experience of a single center with congenital hepatic fibrosis: a review of the literature. World J Gastroenterol 2010;16(6):683.
10. Brown DL, Van Winkle T, Cecere T, et al. Congenital hepatic fibrosis in 5 dogs. Vet Pathol 2010;47(1):102–7.
11. Pillai S, Center SA, McDonough SP, et al. Ductal plate malformation in the liver of boxer dogs: clinical and histological features. Vet Pathol 2016;53(3):602–13.
12. Haywood S, Rutgers HC, Christian MK. Hepatitis and copper accumulation in Skye terriers. Vet Pathol 1988;25(6):408–14.
13. McGrotty YL, Ramsey IK, Knottenbelt CM. Diagnosis and management of hepatic copper accumulation in a Skye terrier. J Small Anim Pract 2003;44(2):85–9.
14. Watson PJ, Reading MR, Constantino-Casas F. Skye terrier hepatitis re-appraised: is this a congenital ductal plate abnormality? Proceedings of the ECVIM Congress. Liverpool, United Kingdom, September 2013.
15. Last RD, Hill JM, Roach M, et al. Congenital dilatation of the large and segmental intrahepatic bile ducts (Caroli's disease) in two golden retriever littermates. J S Afr Vet Assoc 2006;77(4):210–4.
16. Görlinger S, Rothuizen J, Bunch S, et al. Congenital dilatation of the bile ducts (Caroli's disease) in young dogs. J Vet Intern Med 2003;17(1):28–32.
17. Watson PJ, Roulois AJA, Scase TJ, et al. Prevalence of hepatic lesions at post-mortem examination in dogs and association with pancreatitis. J Small Anim Pract 2010;51(11):566–72.

18. Dyggve H, Kennedy LJ, Meri S, et al. Association of Doberman hepatitis to canine major histocompatibility complex II. Tissue Antigens 2010;77(1):30–5.
19. Speeti M, Ståhls A, Meri S, et al. Upregulation of major histocompatibility complex class II antigens in hepatocytes in Doberman hepatitis. Vet Immunol Immunopathol 2003;96(1–2):1–12.
20. Strombeck DR, Miller LM, Harrold D. Effects of corticosteroid treatment on survival time in dogs with chronic hepatitis: 151 cases (1977-1985). J Am Vet Med Assoc 1988;193(9):1109–13.
21. Andersson M, Sevelius E. Breed, sex and age distribution in dogs with chronic liver disease: a demographic study. J Small Anim Pract 1991;32(1):1–5.
22. Bexfield NH, Buxton RJ, Vicek TJ, et al. Breed, age and gender distribution of dogs with chronic hepatitis in the United Kingdom. Vet J 2012;193(1):124–8.
23. Kanemoto H, Sakai M, Sakamoto Y, et al. American cocker spaniel chronic hepatitis in Japan. J Vet Intern Med 2013;7(5):1041–8.
24. Sevelius E, Andersson M, Jönsson L. Hepatic accumulation of alpha-1-antitrypsin in chronic liver disease in the dog. J Comp Pathol 1994;111(4):401–12.
25. Watson PJ, Roulois A, Scase T, et al. Characterization of chronic pancreatitis in English cocker spaniels. J Vet Intern Med 2011;25(4):797–804.
26. Coddou MF. An investigation of polysystemic immune-mediated disease in the English cocker spaniel. [MPhil Thesis]. University of Cambridge; 2015.
27. Bateman AC, Deheragoda MG. IgG4-related systemic sclerosing disease - an emerging and under-diagnosed condition. Histopathology 2009;55(4):373–83.
28. Thornburg LP, Rottinghaus G, Dennis G, et al. The relationship between hepatic copper content and morphologic changes in the liver of West Highland white terriers. Vet Pathol 1996;33(6):656–61.
29. Bexfield NH, Andres-Abdo C, Scase TJ, et al. Chronic hepatitis in the English springer spaniel: clinical presentation, histological description and outcome. Vet Rec 2011;169(16):415.
30. Bexfield NH, Watson PJ, Aguirre-Hernandez J, et al. DLA class II alleles and haplotypes are associated with risk for and protection from chronic hepatitis in the English springer spaniel. PLoS One 2012;7(8):e42584. Shoukry NH, ed.
31. Poldervaart JH, Favier RP, Penning LC, et al. Primary hepatitis in dogs: a retrospective review (2002-2006). J Vet Intern Med 2009;23(1):72–80.
32. Johnston AN, Center SA, McDonough SP, et al. Hepatic copper concentrations in Labrador retrievers with and without chronic hepatitis: 72 cases (1980–2010). J Am Vet Med Assoc 2013;242(3):372–80.
33. Gagné JW, Wakshlag JJ, Center SA, et al. Evaluation of calcium, phosphorus, and selected trace mineral status in commercially available dry foods formulated for dogs. J Am Vet Med Assoc 2013;243(5):658–66.
34. Azumi N. Copper and liver injury–experimental studies on the dogs with biliary obstruction and copper loading. Hokkaido Igaku Zasshi 1982;57(3):331–49.
35. Forman OP, Boursnell MEG, Dunmore BJ, et al. Characterization of the COMMD1 (MURR1) mutation causing copper toxicosis in Bedlington terriers. Anim Genet 2005;36(6):497–501.
36. Coronado VA, Damaraju D, Kohijoki R, et al. New haplotypes in the Bedlington terrier indicate complexity in copper toxicosis. Mamm Genome 2003;14(7):483–91.
37. Haywood S. Copper toxicosis in Bedlington terriers. Vet Rec 2006;159(20):687.
38. Hyun C, Filippich LJ. Inherited canine copper toxicosis in Australian Bedlington terriers. J Vet Sci 2004;5(1):19–28.

39. Haywood S, Boursnell M, Loughran MJ, et al. Copper toxicosis in non-COMMD1 Bedlington terriers is associated with metal transport gene ABCA12. J Trace Elem Med Biol 2016;35:83–9.
40. Webb CB, Twedt DC, Meyer DJ. Copper-associated liver disease in Dalmatians: a review of 10 dogs (1998-2001). J Vet Intern Med 2002;16(6):665–8.
41. Cooper VL, Carlson MP, Jacobson J, et al. Hepatitis and increased copper levels in a Dalmatian. J Vet Diagn Invest 1997;9(2):201–3.
42. Mandigers PJJ, van den Ingh TSGAM, Bode P, et al. Association between liver copper concentration and subclinical hepatitis in Doberman pinschers. J Vet Intern Med 2004;18(5):647–50.
43. Mandigers PJJ, van den Ingh TSGAM, Bode P, et al. Improvement in liver pathology after 4 months of D-penicillamine in 5 Doberman pinschers with subclinical hepatitis. J Vet Intern Med 2005;19(1):40–3.
44. Spee B, Mandigers PJ, Arends B, et al. Differential expression of copper-associated and oxidative stress related proteins in a new variant of copper toxicosis in Doberman pinschers. Comp Hepatol 2005;4(1):3.
45. Hoffmann G, Ingh TSGAM, Bode P, et al. Copper-associated chronic hepatitis in Labrador retrievers. J Vet Intern Med 2006;20(4):856–61.
46. Smedley R, Mullaney T, Rumbeiha W. Copper-associated hepatitis in Labrador retrievers. Vet Pathol 2009;46(3):484–90.
47. Shih JL, Keating JH, Freeman LM, et al. Chronic hepatitis in Labrador retrievers: clinical presentation and prognostic factors. J Vet Intern Med 2007;21(1):33–9.
48. Fieten H, Biourge VC, Watson AL, et al. Dietary management of Labrador retrievers with subclinical hepatic copper accumulation. J Vet Intern Med 2015;29(3):822–7.
49. Fieten H, Biourge VC, Watson AL, et al. Nutritional management of inherited copper-associated hepatitis in the Labrador retriever. Vet J 2014;199(3):429–33.
50. Cortright CC, Center SA, Randolph JF. Clinical features of progressive vacuolar hepatopathy in Scottish terriers with and without hepatocellular carcinoma: 114 cases (1980–2013). J Am Vet Med Assoc 2014;245(7):797–808.
51. Peyron C, Lecoindre P, Chevallier M, et al. Vacuolar hepatopathy in 43 French Scottish terriers: a morphological study. Revue Méd. Vét 2015;166:7–8, 176-84.
52. Zimmerman KL, Panciera DL, Panciera RJ, et al. Hyperphosphatasemia and concurrent adrenal gland dysfunction in apparently healthy Scottish terriers. J Am Vet Med Assoc 2010;237(2):178–86.
53. Xenoulis PG, Suchodolski JS, Levinski MD, et al. Investigation of hypertriglyceridemia in healthy miniature schnauzers. J Vet Intern Med 2007;21(6):1224–30.
54. Brahm A, Hegele R. Hypertriglyceridemia. Nutrients 2013;5(3):981–1001.
55. Kil DY, Vester Boler BM, Apanavicius CJ, et al. Age and diet affect gene expression profiles in canine liver tissue. PLoS One 2010;5(10):e13319. Kowaltowski AJ, ed.
56. Xenoulis PG, Suchodolski JS, Ruaux CG, et al. Association between serum triglyceride and canine pancreatic lipase immunoreactivity concentrations in miniature schnauzers. J Am Anim Hosp Assoc 2010;46(4):229–34.
57. Aguirre AL, Center SA, Randolph JF, et al. Gallbladder disease in Shetland sheepdogs: 38 cases (1995–2005). J Am Vet Med Assoc 2007;231(1):79–88.
58. Malek S, Sinclair E, Hosgood G, et al. Clinical findings and prognostic factors for dogs undergoing cholecystectomy for gallbladder mucocele. Vet Surg 2013;42(4):418–26.

59. Kutsunai M, Kanemoto H, Fukushima K, et al. The association between gall-bladder mucoceles and hyperlipidaemia in dogs: a retrospective case control study. Vet J 2013;199:76–9.
60. Mealey KL, Minch JD, White SN, et al. An insertion mutation in ABCB4 is associated with gallbladder mucocele formation in dogs. Comp Hepatol 2010;9:6.
61. Cullen JM, Willson CJ, Minch JD, et al. Lack of association of ABCB4 insertion mutation with gallbladder mucoceles in dogs. J Vet Diagn Invest 2014;26(3): 434–6.

Feline Hepatic Lipidosis

Chiara Valtolina, DVM*, Robert P. Favier, DVM, PhD

KEYWORDS

- Feline • Hepatic lipidosis • Cats • Liver • Triglyceride • Obesity • VLDL • TG

KEY POINTS

- The primary metabolic abnormalities leading to triglyceride (TG) accumulation in the hepatocytes are not yet completely understood.
- The presumptive diagnosis of feline hepatic lipidosis (FHL) is based on patient history, clinical presentation, clinicopathologic findings, and ultrasonographic appearance of the liver; however, history and clinical and clinicopathologic presentation are not specific for lipidosis and any underlying disease process can confound them.
- Nutrition should be initiated on the day of admission to reverse the negative energy balance and catabolic state typical of FHL; early nutrition is the cornerstone of treatment in FHL.

INTRODUCTION

Feline hepatic lipidosis (FHL), the most common hepatobiliary disease in cats,[1–5] is characterized by the accumulation of excessive triglycerides (TGs) in more than 80% of the hepatocytes, resulting in a greater than 50% increase in liver weight,[2,6,7] secondary impairment of liver function, and intrahepatic cholestasis.[2,6,8,9] A specific geographic distribution of the disease has been suggested based on the available reports of FHL from different areas, including North America, Great Britain, Japan, and Western Europe. The higher prevalence of FHL in these areas might be secondary to feeding habits of cat owners and a high incidence of obesity in the feline population.[1]

The pathophysiology of FHL is complex. The primary metabolic abnormalities leading to TG accumulation in the hepatocytes are not yet completely understood, but they could consist of alterations of the pathways of uptake, synthesis, degradation, and secretion of fatty acids (FAs). Nonetheless, the variability in reported historical, physical, and clinicopathologic findings in cats with naturally occurring hepatic lipidosis (HL) suggests that this is a syndrome with many causative factors.

A negative energy balance, usually caused by anorexia, is considered the primary cause for initiating FHL. In an experimental model of FHL, lipidosis occurs within

The authors have nothing to disclose.
Department of Clinical Sciences of Companion Animals, Faculty of Veterinary Medicine, Utrecht University, Yalelaan 108, 3584 CM, Utrecht, The Netherlands
* Corresponding author.
E-mail address: c.valtolina@uu.nl

2 weeks of the development of anorexia.[8,10] In a clinical setting, FHL has been seen to develop after a period of anorexia that ranges from 2 to 14 days.[1,6] FHL is classified as primary or secondary. In primary FHL, anorexia occurs in a healthy animal secondary to decreased food availability, administration of nonpalatable food,[7,8] or decreased food intake secondary to a stressful event. Secondary lipidosis occurs in animals that develop anorexia as a consequence of underlying disease. Secondary lipidosis is the most common form of lipidosis described, occurring in approximately 95% of cases. The diseases associated with the development of lipidosis are numerous and include diabetes mellitus, pancreatitis, inflammatory hepatobiliary disease, gastrointestinal disease, renal failure, and neoplasia.[1,2]

Because the cat is a pure a carnivore, its lipid and protein metabolism[11–14] make it dependent on obligatory essential FAs (EFAs), amino acids, and vitamins, which become deficient after a period of prolonged anorexia. These deficiencies are considered important cofounding factors for the development of FHL.[2,12]

The development of HL after a period of anorexia has also been described in other strict carnivores, such as the European polecat (*Mustela putorius*) and the American mink (*Neovison vison*).[15,16] The in-depth study of the pathophysiologic mechanisms behind the development of HL in these other obligated carnivores could help better understand the pathophysiology of FHL in cats.

PATHOPHYSIOLOGY

Due to evolutionary pressure, cats have developed unique adaptations of lipid and protein metabolism reflecting a strict carnivorous state,[12–14,17–19] which has an impact on cats' requirements for EFA and essential amino acids.[2,13,20] Like other mammals, cats are unable to synthesize EFAs, like linoleic acid (18:2n-6) and α-linoleic acid (18:3n-3). In addition, unlike other mammals, cats have a limited capacity to synthesize the long-chain polyunsaturated FA (LCPUFA), arachidonic acid (AA) (20:4n-6) from linoleic acid, and eicosapentaenoic acid (20:3n-3) and docosahexaenoic acid (22:6n-3) from α-linoleic acid (18:3n-3). The explanation for this peculiarity is that cats have a severely decreased activity of the enzymes Δ5-desaturase and Δ6-desaturase, enzymes involved in the formation of LCPUFA from EFA.[21–24] Recently, Trevizan and colleagues[11] revealed that cats have an active Δ5-desaturase and that they are able to synthetize AA from γ-linolenic acid via bypassing the Δ6-desaturase step but not in an amount allows them to store this LCPUFA in condition of anorexia.

LCPUFAs are involved in numerous processes. Increased levels of LCPUFAs are well known to protect against the development of HL via the so-called fuel partitioning action of LCPUFA.[25,26] LCPUFAs, n-3 LCPUFA species (ie, docosahexaenoic acid) rather than the n-6 LCPUFA (ie, AA), favor FA oxidation over TG storage and they direct glucose away from FA synthesis by facilitating glycogen synthesis.[27,28] LCPUFAs down-regulate sterol regulatory element binding protein-1 expression and impair its processing, resulting in an inhibition of the transcription of lipogenic and glycolytic genes.[28–30] Furthermore, n-3 LCPUFA species act as ligand activators of the peroxisome proliferator-activated receptor-α (PPAR-α) present in liver and adipose tissue, up-regulating the expression of genes encoding enzymes involved in FA oxidation.[28,31]

Cats possess limited ability to adapt their protein metabolic pathways for conserving nitrogen and they rapidly develop essential amino acid deficiency and protein malnutrition after a period of prolonged anorexia. In both experimentally induced and spontaneous FHL, plasma concentrations of alanine, arginine, citrulline, taurine, and methionine become markedly reduced (>50% reduction from baseline).[2,12,32]

Cats with FHL show changes in carbohydrate metabolism that resemble those seen in critically ill cats. Cats with HL, compared with healthy subjects, have higher circulating concentrations of glucose, lactate, glucagon, and nonesterified FAs (NEFAs) and have lower circulating concentrations of insulin.[33,34]

Although the exact pathophysiologic mechanism of FHL remains elusive, there is an imbalance between the influx of NEFAs derived from peripheral fat stores, de novo synthesis of FAs, the rate of hepatic FA oxidation for energy, and the dispersal of hepatic TGs via excretion of very low-density lipoproteins (VLDLs).

Influx of Free Fatty Acid from Peripheral Fat Stores

FHL is considered a negative energy balance state and it is characterized by increased circulating concentrations of the counter-regulatory hormones (glucagon, growth hormone, cortisol, and catecholamines) that lead to an increased activity of hormone-sensitive lipase, promoting lipolysis and mobilization of NEFAs from the visceral adipose tissue (VAT). Increased levels of counter-regulatory hormones and decreased circulating concentrations of insulin lead to increased hormone-sensitive lipase activity, resulting in decreased lipogenesis, increased peripheral insulin resistance by decreased activity of the glucose transport protein-4, and impaired glucose tolerance.[35] High concentrations of circulating free FAs (FFAs) also contribute to peripheral insulin resistance.[1,2,36,37]

NEFAs are released from the adipose tissue and transported to the liver via the portal circulation. The predominant lipid that accumulates within the hepatocyte is TG.[4] A higher concentration of palmitate (16:0) was found in liver tissue from cats with FHL compared with control subjects that mirrored the increased concentrations of palmitate in the adipose tissue of the same animals.[4] This finding confirmed the hypothesis that FFAs in livers of cats with FHL are derived from VAT.[2,4,12,33] Besides adipose tissue being the major site for storage of excess energy as TGs during a positive energy balance state, it has also an important endocrine function by secreting multiple adipokines, including adiponectin, leptin, chemokines, and cytokines.[38,39] These adipokines are involved in energy homeostasis and inflammation and might be responsible for the development of peripheral insulin resistance.[38–40] Common inflammatory cytokines reported to be elevated in obese cats compared with lean individuals are tumor necrosis factor α and interleukin.[41,42] Adiponectin exerts a profound insulin-sensitizing effect as well as anti-inflammatory and antiatherosclerotic effects. Leptin is a regulator of adipose tissue mass and regulates insulin sensitivity.[39] The adipose tissue of FHL cats had markedly increased tumor necrosis factor α concentrations compared with that of healthy subjects.[43] In cats with FHL, both the serum concentrations of adiponectin and leptin were found increased compared with healthy subjects, but only leptin was significantly increased in cats with FHL compared with cats with other liver diseases.[39] Obesity predisposes cats to FHL during a period of anorexia, because of the quantity of FAs that can be rapidly released from peripheral fat stores and VAT, release of inflammatory adipokines from the adipose tissue, and the insulin resistance associated with obesity.[1,2,37,42,44]

De Novo Lipogenesis

De novo lipid (DNL) synthesis in cats occurs mainly in the adipose tissue, followed by the liver, mammary glands, and muscle. This differs from human and rodents where the liver is the primary site for DNL synthesis.[45–47] Although glucose is the precursor for DNL in humans, in cats acetate resulting from incomplete FA oxidation (ie, ketogenesis), typically increased in FHL, is the substrate for the formation of the FFA palmitate (16:0).[2,36,46,48] Palmitate is found both in the adipose tissue and liver of cats with FHL, whereas it is not in healthy cats.[4] It cannot be ruled out that palmitate accumulation is the result of the de novo lipogenesis contributing to HL. Similarly in the mink, an animal that has metabolic similarities with the domestic cat,[19,46] DNL from acetate in HL may be accompanied by the adipogenic transformation of hepatocytes, as is seen in human nonalcoholic fatty liver disease (NAFLD), where the liver begins to express gene profiles characteristic of healthy adipose tissue.[46,49,50] To date, the concept of adipogenic transformation of hepatocytes has not been evaluated in cats.

Once having reached the liver, FFAs can enter 2 pathways: either they undergo β-oxidation in the mitochondria or they can be esterified to TG and secreted via the VLDL pathway.

Hepatic β-Oxidation

Mitochondrial β-oxidation is the main oxidative pathway for the disposal of FA under normal physiologic conditions.[51] Short-chain NEFAs and medium-chain NEFAs freely enter the mitochondria, whereas the activity of the enzyme carnitine palmitoyl transferase-1 regulates the entry of the long-chain FAs. Oxidation of FA produces acetyl coenzyme A, which can be used to provide energy via the tricarboxylic acid (Krebs) cycle to provide energy and/or to form ketone bodies. L-Carnitine is part of the 2 enzymes that regulate transport of FA from the circulation into the mitochondria and from the hepatic cytosol back into plasma.

Ketone body formation is increased in cats with FHL, suggesting an enhanced rate of β-oxidation of FA.[1,2,32,36,37] It is unknown, however, if the rate of β-oxidation is adapted to compensate for the greatly increased FA accumulation in the hepatocytes. The increase of ketone bodies in cases of lipidosis is most likely the result of the more complex catabolic state, increased insulin resistance, and decreased tolerance to glucose that develops in these patients than being the result of an increased rate of β-oxidation.[12,34,36]

In human medicine, abnormal β-oxidation from mitochondrial dysfunction has been suggested and reported as a potential cause for lipid accumulation in hepatocytes during NAFLD.[51] Center and colleagues[52] reported that in FHL hepatocyte mitochondria were reduced in number and markedly abnormal, suggesting that mitochondrial dysfunction could also occur in FHL.

There is a lot of discussion about the role of carnitine in FHL. Because L-carnitine is essential for the transportation of FA into the mitochondria, L-carnitine deficiency has been proposed as one of the main pathophysiologic mechanisms for the accumulation of FAs in the liver.[2,32,53,54] Measurement of L-carnitine concentrations in different tissues (liver, kidney, and blood) from cats affected with FHL, however, failed to support this hypothesis.[53,55,56] On the other hand, there is also evidence that supplementation of L-carnitine in experimental lipidosis dramatically reduces hepatic lipid accumulation[57] and increases the rate of β-oxidation in obese cats.[53,54,58] Furthermore, a protective effect of L-carnitine was demonstrated in fasting cats and in cats with HL where supplementation of L-carnitine reduced the increase of plasma FA concentrations compared with control cats.[53] Therefore, it is possible that in a situation of anorexia and an increased catabolic state tissue concentrations of L-carnitine are insufficient to meet demand and supplementation might be beneficial.

Methionine is an essential amino acid fundamental for numerous methylation reactions and an important thiol donor involved in the synthesis of glutathione. Glutathione is an important oxygen free radical scavenger and is involved in the hepatocellular protection against oxidative injury and its hepatic concentrations are reduced in cats with liver disease.[59] Because methionine and its coenzyme S-adenosylmethionine together are precursors of carnitine, methionine deficiency might contribute to inefficient levels of L-carnitine.[2,12,32,55]

Dispersal of Hepatic Triglycerides via Very Low-Density Lipoprotein Excretion

Once in the hepatocyte, NEFAs can be esterified to TG. TGs usually accumulate in vacuoles within hepatocytes or can be incorporated into VLDLs to be excreted into the peripheral circulation.

Rapid onset of protein malnutrition and deficiency of essential amino acids are thought to be important pathophysiologic mechanisms for the development of FHL. A lack of apolipoprotein B100, a major component of the VLDL, was proposed as a reason for the diminished ability to excrete TGs from the liver.[3,6] Cats with HL, however, are known to have increased levels of TG in plasma, with greatest distribution in the VLDL fraction (approximately 62% vs 25% in healthy, lean cats),[60] and increased serum concentrations of VLDL, with the VLDL fraction representing approximately 19% of the total lipoprotein mass compared with 2% in healthy lean cats. This suggests that VLDL secretion seems enhanced and not deficient in FHL.[20,60–62] Despite hepatic VLDL secretion increased in cats with FHL, this increase might not be sufficient to prevent the lipid overload of hepatocytes, in face of a dramatic increase of NEFA transport to the liver.

Arginine and taurine deficiency in cats with FHL could also compromise lipid metabolism and excretion of TG via the VLDL excretion pathway. Arginine is an important urea cycle substrate, and arginine deficiency has been associated with the development of hyperammonemia and hepatic encephalopathy (HE) in cats with FHL.[63,64] Taurine deficiency has been shown to increase lipolysis in peripheral tissues and has been linked to secondary accumulation of NEFAs in the liver.[12,65] Supplementation of taurine in experimental cats during initial weight gain followed by weight loss was associated with decreased hepatic lipid accumulation.[12,62]

As discussed previously, HL in the American mink and the European polecat, other obligatory carnivores, shares numerous clinical, clinicopathologic, and pathophysiologic characteristics with FHL in domestic cats.[16,46,48,66,67] Both the American mink and the European polecat have been used as animal models to investigate the pathophysiology of NAFLD in people.[16] In the American mink and European polecat, FA data of various adipose tissue depots and liver tissue showed a decrease in the n-3 LCPUFAs.[16,48,67–69] The depletion of n-3 PUFAs during food deprivation could be partly due to the mechanisms of selective FA mobilization: the location of the first double bond from the methyl end affects the fractional mobilization of LCPUFAs and n-3 substrates are often preferred over n-6 ones in FA desaturation reactions and β-oxidation.[70] The decrease in n-3 LCPUFAs causes an increase in the n-6/n-3 PUFA ratio. NAFLD in human seems to be the result of an unfavorable n-6/n-3 PUFA ratio, with an increase in the n-6 LCPUFAs.[26,27] n-3 LCPUFAs are more potent activators of the PPAR-α receptors than n-6 LCPUFAs, and a depletion of n-3 PUFA has been proposed to favor FA and TG synthesis over hydrolysis and FA oxidation and may impair lipid export from the liver by suppressing VLDL secretion.[28,48] An increase in the n-6 LCPUFA concentration in response to food deprivation has been associated with increased inflammation and oxygen free radical formation and n-6 LCPUFAs are considered a key contributor to the pathophysiology and progression of liver steatosis in NAFLD, in the American mink and in the European polecat.[16,27,28,48] A lower concentration of both total n-6 and total n-3 PUFAs was noted in adipose tissue of cats with FHL compared with controls. The n-6/n-3 PUFA ratio was not statistically assessed, but a study from Hall and colleagues[4] suggest that a derangement in the n-6/n-3 PUFA ratio might occur in FHL compared with healthy control cats. Due to the limiting nature of the Δ5-desaturase and especially Δ6-desaturase activities, the LCPUFA status, especially the n-3 LCPUFA status, of domestic cats may be severely compromised during food deprivation and/or rapid weight loss contributing to the pathogenesis of FHL.

Recently, research has been performed in experimental animals and in humans on the immunomodulatory role of circulating bile acids and on their role in suppressing the hypothalamic-pituitary-adrenal (HPA) axis. In humans, the link between critical illness–related corticosteroid insufficiency (CIRCI) and high circulating bile acid concentrations has been established.[71,72] High levels of circulating conjugated or unconjugated bile acids in critical illness has been shown to inhibit glucocorticoids metabolizing enzyme and to inhibit the release of corticotropin-releasing hormone and corticotropin from the HPA axis.[71–73] The hallmark of CIRCI is hemodynamic instability that manifests itself as refractory hypotension despite fluid resuscitation and levels of corticosteroids that are insufficient for the severity of the underlying illness.[74,75] To evaluate if CIRCI also is present in cats with cholestasis, a pilot study was performed.[76] Basal serum cortisol and delta cortisol (the difference between basal and postcorticotropin cortisol) concentrations were evaluated in 20 cats with cholestasis. Cats with refractory hypotension had a lower mean delta cortisol than cats with normal blood pressure, but this was not statistically significant.[76] From human medicine, however, it is known that delta cortisol is not a specific indicator of the HPA axis and adrenal function because it does not take into consideration cortisol breakdown and its availability at the cellular level.[72] Therefore, CIRCI should be suspected in a subpopulation of cats with FHL and refractory hypotension.

HISTORICAL AND CLINICAL FINDINGS

Although FHL is mainly reported in middle-aged cats (median age 7 years), cats of any age can be affected.[1,2,6] There seems to be no clear breed or gender predilection, although in some studies female cats seem to be overrepresented.[6,33] Actual (body condition 4/5) or historical obesity has been mentioned by several investigators as a predisposing factor for the development of FHL.[1,2,4,6,12] Cats affected with HL present with a history of anorexia and weight loss. Other reported clinical signs include icterus, dehydration, vomiting, nausea and ptyalism, constipation or diarrhea, and a poor hair coat (**Figs. 1** and **2**).[2,6] The mentation of cats with FHL can be severely altered if hypokalemia HE are present. In cats with FHL, HE is associated with arginine deficiency and can be worsened by hypokalemia and decreased liver function, which further impairs the urea cycle.[63,64,77] Cats with HE can present with severe mental depression, ptyalism, and severe nausea.[2,6,78] The plasma ammonia concentration should be measured in patients with severely altered mental states. Ammonia tolerance testing is not recommended in cats with FHL.[2] Ventroflexion of the neck, often seen in cats

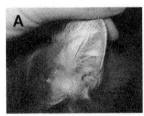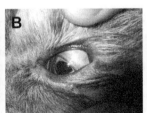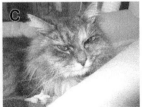

Fig. 1. Cat with FHL. Note the visible icterus of (*A*) skin and (*B*) sclera and (*C*) poor kept hair coat.

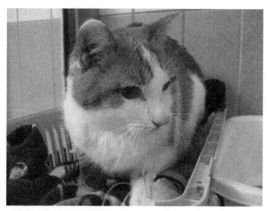

Fig. 2. Ptyalism secondary to nausea in a cat with FHL.

with FHL, and severe muscle weakness can be secondary to the concurrent presence of severe hypokalemia.

SERUM BIOCHEMISTRY

FHL is characterized by an increased bilirubin concentration and increased serum activities of alkaline phosphatase and alanine aminotransferase compared with healthy cats and cats with other liver disease (ie, cholangitis).[2,6,79] Hyperglycemia is often present and is due to insulin resistance and an increase in the counter-regulatory hormones.[2,34,37] Hypoglycemia, when present, indicates severely decreased or even end-stage liver function.

Mild hypoalbuminemia is often reported in FHL secondary to anorexia and decreased hepatic function. Blood urea nitrogen was found decreased in 51% of cats as consequence of chronic anorexia and/or insufficient urea-cycle function.[1,2,6] Commonly reported electrolyte alterations include hypokalemia (30% of cats with FHL), hypomagnesemia (28%), and hypophosphatemia (17%) that can be present at admission or can develop after administration of fluid therapy to correct dehydration.[6] Hypokalemia and hypophosphemia have been associated with an increased morbidity and mortality in FHL.[6] Hypokalemia can increase the encephalopathic effects of ammonia and cause muscle weakness, paralytic ileus, and anorexia; hypophosphatemia can cause severe hemolysis resulting in the need for a blood transfusion.[1,2,6] Cats with HL often have higher serum concentrations of β-hydroxybutyric acid (BHBA) compared with normal cats as reflection of their negative energy balance.[10,36,60] High serum BHBA concentrations are the result of stimulation of the increased lipolysis with mobilization of NEFA, leading to increased hepatic β-oxidation and production of ketone bodies. Clinical signs associated with increased serum BHBA concentrations are usually vague and include anorexia, lethargy, cachexia, and weight loss. Serum BHBA has been suggested as a marker for FHL.[36]

HEMATOLOGY

The complete blood cell count (CBC) is often normal in cats with FHL, but, in some cases, a mild nonregenerative anemia and mild leukocytosis might be present. Underlying inflammatory, infectious, or neoplastic disease could result in an inflammatory leukogram. Heinz bodies can be detected on blood smear evaluation both on admission and during recovery.[1,2,6] Thrombocytopenia does not occur frequently in cats with HL, unless they are suffering from disseminated intravascular coagulation.[6,33,80-84]

TESTS OF COAGULATION

Coagulation abnormalities and clinical bleeding tendencies are reported to be common (45%–73%) in cats with FHL, especially during venipuncture or catheter placement or if invasive procedures, such as esophageal feeding tube placement or liver biopsy, are performed.[2,81-83] Lisciandro and colleagues[83] reported that prolongation of prothrombin time was the most common abnormality (found in 77% of cats with FHL), whereas factor VII activity was reduced in 68% and activated partial thromboplastin time was prolonged in 55% in a population of cats affected with liver disease. In a study by Center and colleagues[82] in cats with HL, 75% had increased proteins invoked by vitamin K absence clotting times, whereas only a minimal percentage had prolonged prothrombin time or activated partial thromboplastin time (4% and 25%, respectively). More recently, Dircks and colleagues[81] found that 40% of cats affected with liver disease had a significant prolongation of the activated partial thromboplastin time compared with healthy cats. Protein C was also decreased in 44% of cats with liver disease, whereas fibrinogen was increased compared with health controls. No significant difference was found for vitamin K–dependent clotting factors (II, VII, IX, and X) between healthy controls and cats with liver disease. The most consistent abnormalities in cats with FHL were an increased factor V activity and D-dimer concentrations, with 54% of cats having values above the reference range for both parameters. Furthermore, 31% of cats with FHL had a severely decreased factor XIII (fibrin stabilizing factor) activity.[81] Not only decreased production but also activation of hemostasis with secondary increased consumption of coagulation factors could be responsible for the bleeding tendencies of patients with FHL.

DIAGNOSIS OF FELINE HEPATIC LIPIDOSIS

The presumptive diagnosis of FHL is based on patient history, clinical presentation, clinicopathologic findings, and ultrasonographic appearance of the liver. History and clinical and clinicopathologic presentation, however, are not specific for lipidosis and any underlying disease process can confound them.

On ultrasound examination, the liver in cats with FHL appears enlarged and diffusely hyperechoic liver compared with the falciform fat.[78] Using these criteria, abdominal ultrasound performed by 3 board-certified radiologists had an accuracy of 70% for diagnosing lipidosis in cats.[85] Comparable ultrasonographic findings of a diffusely hyperechoic liver can be found in healthy obese cats.[86]

The definitive diagnosis is usually made by cytologic evaluation of a fine-needle aspirate and in some cases by histologic evaluation of a liver biopsy.[1,2,87-89] Cytology of the liver has been advocated because it is considered a safer procedure. It often does not require general anesthesia and it is associated with few minor complications compared with liver biopsy.[1,2,88,90] The hallmark of lipidosis on cytology is the presence of steatosis, which can be macrovesicular or microvesicular.[1,2,52] Although vacuolar hepatopathy was the category with the highest percentage of agreement between liver cytology and liver histology, only 51% of feline cases had overall agreement between cytologic and histologic diagnosis of FHL.[87] Furthermore, Willard and colleagues[89] reported 4 cases of cats diagnosed with FHL based on cytology where the underlying liver disease (cholangitis or lymphoma) was missed. Cats that are sick tend to accumulate lipid in their liver, often mimicking FHL, and for this reason a definitive diagnosis of FHL can only be made when greater than 80% of the hepatocytes are affected.[2,6]

Liver biopsy requires general anesthesia and assessment of a patient's hemostatic system (see Jonathan A. Lidbury's article, "Getting the Most Out of Liver Biopsy," in this issue). Thrombocytopenia (<80,000 platelets/μL) and elevated activated partial thromboplastin time (>1.5 times the upper limit of the reference range) were the 2 reported abnormalities that had the strongest association with severe bleeding.[91] Furthermore, liver biopsy collection using Tru-Cut rapid-firing automatic biopsy needles has been associated with the development of vagotonic shock in cats, characterized by bradycardia and cardiovascular collapse up to 30 minutes after the biopsy was performed.[90] These are the reasons why a majority of investigators do not recommend liver biopsies as the initial tool to diagnose FHL. Cats with FHL present a series of cardiovascular, metabolic, and coagulation derangements that make them unsuitable for undergoing general anesthesia and liver biopsy. Liver biopsy should be considered in subjects that despite appropriate treatment fail to improve or if they have a history, clinical finding, or clinicopathologic findings suggestive of a possible underlying hepatic disease other than HL.[1,2]

The use of non–contrast-enhanced CT has been advocated in human medicine as a more reliable and repeatable method for the detection fatty hepatic infiltration in patients with NAFLD compared with cytologic and histologic assessment of the liver.[92,93] Fatty infiltration of organs is associated with x-ray attenuation on CT[94] and level of attenuation of adipose tissue in human medicine is inversely correlated with hepatic fat content.[92,95,96] CT has been used to detect VAT deposition in cats and CT evaluation of total body fat seems to correlate well with the body condition score.[97] Two recent studies evaluated the use of CT to detect liver fatty deposition in FHL but yielded contrasting results. The first experimental study by Nakamura and colleagues[98] evaluated a colony of adult healthy cats where the mean hepatic fat attenuation was 54 Hounsfield units (HU) (range: 43.5–65.9 HU). HL was then experimentally induced and, when CT images of the liver were evaluated, decreased hepatic x-ray attenuation was observed (<35 HU). In a more recent study, Lamb and colleagues[99] evaluated x-ray attenuation in the liver and kidneys of a population of client-owned cats with suspected FHL. Cats were divided into 3 different groups based on the risk of suffering from mild lipidosis, moderate lipidosis, or severe lipidosis. The study however, failed to highlight any differences between groups and the values obtained for x-ray attenuation of the liver were different from the previously published ones. The conclusion of Lam and colleagues[99] was that hepatic CT attenuation of the liver might be of limited value in detecting FHL in patients at risk for lipidosis and that values obtained for hepatic x-ray attenuation could vary between CT scanners. Based on the results of these 2 studies and the need for sedation or anesthesia in a clinically compromised patient, the routine use of CT to diagnose lipidosis cannot yet be recommended and further studies are necessary.

TREATMENT
Fluid and Electrolyte Therapy

Cats presented with FHL can suffer from differing degrees of hypoperfusion secondary to vomiting, anorexia, and adipsia. Hypoperfusion in cats is characterized by tachycardia (heart rate >220 bpm) or inappropriate bradycardia (heart rate <140 bpm), pale mucous membranes, prolonged capillary refill time, often hypothermia, and mild hypotension. Dehydration is a common abnormality seen in cats with FHL. Initial fluid therapy should be directed to correct hypoperfusion if it is present.

A balanced isotonic crystalloid infusion (0.9% NaCl, lactated Ringer solution, or Ringer acetate solution) is the fluid type of choice. Small volume resuscitation, with a 5 mL/kg to 10 mL/kg intravenous (IV) bolus given over 30 minutes should be instituted in hypovolemic cats while slow rewarming is implemented. Repeated examination of the cardiovascular system helps decide if further fluid administration is necessary to achieve euvolemia. Fluid therapy to provide for maintenance requirements and correct deficits according to the estimated percentage of dehydration should then be started (**Tables 1** and **2**) and the total volume is usually administered over 24 hours. There is a lot of debate on what is the best fluid to administer in patients with FHL. Due to poor hepatic function, lactate clearance might not be appropriate in cats with FHL. Therefore, the administration of lactate-based solutions might worsen hyperlactatemia in these patients.[1,2] This seems to only be a theoretic concern, however, because lactated Ringer solution has been used without major complication in cats with FHL.[1] Fluids containing glucose should be avoided in cats with FHL to avoid worsening glucose intolerance and concurrent hyperglycemia.[37] The fluid therapy plan should be re-evaluated and adjusted at least once a day based on the cat's new requirements and clinical condition. The newly formulated plan should take into consideration the fluid balance and the body weight of the patient, percentage of dehydration, and if ongoing losses (vomiting and diarrhea) are still occurring. If enteral or parenteral feeding is implemented, the amount of fluid administered with the nutritional plan should be deducted from the calculated rate of fluid infusion to avoid fluid overload.

Correction of electrolytes abnormalities should take place in the initial phase of hospitalization and before nutrition is started, because insulin release can cause a further decrease in serum/plasma potassium and phosphate concentrations. Abnormalities of potassium and phosphate should be adequately corrected (**Tables 3** and **4**) and these electrolytes should be checked at least twice daily in the beginning of hospitalization. The rate of potassium administration must not exceed 0.5 mEq/kg/h. If hypokalemia is difficult to correct, the serum/plasma magnesium concentration should be

Table 1 Clinical estimation of dehydration	
Estimated Dehydration (% of Body Weight)	**Physical Examination Findings**
<5	Normal (history consistent with excessive fluid loss compared with intake)
5–6	Skin turgor is mildly reduced; mucous membranes are dry.
7–8	Skin turgor is moderately reduced; mucous membranes are dry.
8–10	Skin turgor is severely reduced; mucous membranes are dry; eyes sunken in the orbit.
10–12	Skin turgor is severely reduced; mucous membranes are dry; eyes sunken in the orbit; initial signs of shock (mild tachycardia, pale/pink mucous membranes, slightly prolonged CRT, weak peripheral pulse)
12–15	Clinical signs consistent with shock (tachycardia, pale mucous membranes, weak peripheral pulse, prolonged capillary refill time)

Percentage of dehydration is evaluated based on physical evaluation of the turgor, mucous membranes, and position of the eyes in the orbit. The estimated percentage is used to calculate the amount of fluid necessary for the correction of dehydration in the fluid therapy plan (**Table 2**).

Table 2	
Fluid requirements for a hospitalized cat	
Maintenance fluid therapy	40–60 mL/kg/d
Correction of dehydration	Deficit in mL (to be administered in 12–24 h) = % dehydration $\times$ 10 $\times$ body weight (kg)
Ongoing fluid losses	Based observed fluid loss • Minimal fluid loss: 2 mL/kg/h • Moderate fluid loss: 4 mL/kg/h • Severe fluid loss: 6 mL/kg/h

Based on the cat fluid balance, the fluid therapy plan takes into consideration maintenance fluid therapy plus the correction of dehydration (based on the estimated percentage of dehydration) and the ongoing fluid losses (via vomiting, diarrhea, or polyuria).

also measured and if needed this electrolyte should be supplemented (**Table 5**), as hypomagnesemia can worsen renal wasting of potassium.

Nutritional Management of Feline Hepatic Lipidosis

The cornerstone of treatment in FHL is early nutrition. Nutrition should be initiated on the day of admission to reverse the negative energy balance and catabolic state typical of FHL. The only reason to delay nutrition is the presence of cardiovascular instability (hypoperfusion or hypotension) and severe electrolyte abnormalities. Nutrition can be provided via the enteral or parenteral routes. Wherever possible, enteral feeding is preferred over parenteral nutrition because it helps maintaining intestinal structure and function.[100] In cases of intractable vomiting or because of minimal tolerance to enteral feeding, however, the parenteral route should be taken into consideration.[100] Partial parenteral nutrition could be easily administered via a peripheral catheter and does not require a central venous access, which might initially not be advisable due to coagulation abnormalities.

The ideal diet for FHL should be high in protein (30%–40% of the metabolizable energy), moderate in lipids (approximately 50% of the metabolizable energy), and poor in carbohydrate (approximately 20% of the metabolizable energy).[1,2] Glucose should be used as carbohydrate source because it does not require digestion and can be used by enterocytes as an energy source.[1] In critically ill cats, 6 g of protein/100 kcal (or 25%–35% of their total energy requirements) is considered enough to support their unique metabolism.[100] In FHL, a diet with a protein content of 25% of the metabolizable energy was shown to attenuate but not to ameliorate HL, whereas a diet with a

Table 3		
Guide to potassium supplementation		
Serum Potassium Concentration (mEq/L)	**Milliequivalent of Potassium Added to 1 Liter of Fluid**	**Maximum Fluid Infusion Rate (mL/kg/h)[a]**
<2.0	80	6
2.1–2.5	60	8
2.6–3.0	40	12
3.1–3.5	28	18
3.6–5.0	20	25

[a] So as not exceed a potassium supplementation of 0.5 mEq/kg/h.

Adapted from Greene RW, Scott RC. Lower urinary tract disease. In: Ettinger SJ, editor. Textbook of veterinary internal medicine. Philadelphia: WB Saunders; 1975.

Table 4
Guide to phosphate supplementation

Supplement	Dose/Route	Comments
Potassium phosphate	0.01–0.03 mEq/kg/h IV as a CRI for 6 h or 0.12 mEq/kg/h for severe deficits IV as a CRI	Use a dedicated line and syringe pump. Ensure that this line is not flushed. It is important to consider the amount of potassium administered via phosphate correction and subtract it from the potassium correction.
Potassium phosphate (alternative method)	Calculate the amount of potassium (in milliequivalents) that should be added to 1 L of fluid using **Table 3**; provide half this as potassium chloride and half with potassium phosphate.	This method is simple but it does not allow phosphate supplementation to be adjusted independently of total potassium supplementation. Do not administer potassium phosphate with calcium-containing fluids, for example, lactated Ringer solution.

higher protein content (35%–45% of the metabolizable energy) was shown to reverse the catabolic state and improve clinical signs associated with FHL.[7,32] A majority of the veterinary commercial diets formulated for recovery in cats meet these requirements.

The calorie requirements of these patients can be estimated using the formula:

$$RER = 70 \times (body\ weight\ in\ kg)^{0.75}$$

The use of an illness factor, typically ranging from 1.0 to 2.0, by which the resting energy requirement (RER) is multiplied to meet the increased caloric needs of critically ill patients is no longer recommended.[101] The use of illness factor leads to overfeeding and has been associated with hyperglycemia and gastrointestinal dysfunction as well as hepatic dysfunction. The development of hyperglycemia is especially concerning (particularly during parenteral nutrition) because it is associated with an increased rate of complications and a worse outcome.[102]

Forced enteral feeding should never be considered in a sick cat with FHL because of the risk of the development of food aversion[2] and because it is usually difficult to administer cats enough food to meet their energy requirements. Feeding tubes (nasoesophageal, esophageal, and gastric) allow clinicians to provide enteral nutrition without excessive stress to the patient (**Table 6**). The preferred initial feeding tube

Table 5
Guide to magnesium supplementation

Supplement	Dose/Route	Comments
Magnesium sulfate or Magnesium chloride	Rapid replacement: 0.75–1 mEq/kg/d IV as a CRI for first 24 h Slow replacement: 0.3–0.5 mEq/kg/d IV as a CRI for 2–3 d	Administered as 20% solution diluted in 5% dextrose

Table 6			
Type and characteristics of available feeding tubes for enteral nutrition in cats			
Feeding Tube for Enteral Nutrition	**Size**	**Advantages**	**Disadvantages**
Nasoesophageal	7–8 French	No anesthesia required; easy to place; inexpensive	Short-term solution; only allows administration of a liquid diet
Esophageal	14 French	Easy to place, inexpensive; most diets can be administered; suitable for longer duration feeding	Anesthesia is required; hemorrhage is a potential risk; cellulitis is a potential complication.
Gastric	14–18 French	Suitable for longer duration feeding; most diets can be administered.	Anesthesia is required; tube displacement can result in peritonitis.

choice of the authors and others[1,2] for cats with FHL is the nasoesophageal feeding tube. The introduction of a nasoesophageal feeding tube does not require general anesthesia or heavy sedation and is noninvasive (**Fig. 3**). Cats with FHL are often unstable on admission to undergo general anesthesia and are often coagulopathic. For these reasons, the insertion of esophagostomy and gastrostomy tubes should be considered potentially unsafe in these patients and should be delayed until fluid and coagulation abnormalities have been addressed and the cat is considered stable enough to undergo anesthesia (**Fig. 3**).

Typically, sufficient amounts of a commercial high protein recovery food to provide one-third of the calculated RER is fed on the first day followed by a slow incremental increase in the amount over the next 2 to 3 days until the total RER is provided. The slow increase of the caloric load should decrease the risk of refeeding syndrome. Refeeding syndrome is characterized by severe hypophosphatemia, hypokalemia, and hyperglycemia, with clinical signs of vomiting, diarrhea, and/or shock.[103,104] It is the consequence of a rapid caloric administration to a starved patient in a chronic negative catabolic state, causing rapid insulin release.[103–105]

Cats with FHL are considered feeding volume sensitive and the amount of food they can tolerate per meal might be drastically reduced.[1] The total volume of food required each day should be initially divided into 6 to 8 portions, or administered as a constant rate infusion (CRI). The authors prefer to administer food as a CRI because it seems to reduce nausea, gastric discomfort, and vomiting associated with gastric distension after intermittent food administration. The food should always be administered

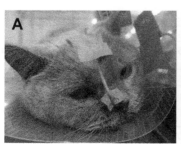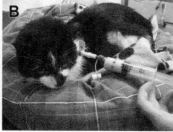

Fig. 3. Cats with (*A*) nasoesophageal and (*B*) esophageal feeding tubes.

lukewarm and, if the intermittent administration is chosen, it should be administered over 10 to 15 minutes. If any signs of discomfort, retching, or vomiting is present, the administration of food should be interrupted.

Antiemetics and gastroprotectants should be considered in cats that are nauseated and/or vomit. Metoclopramide (0.2 mg/kg IV 4 times a day or 1 mg/kg/d IV as a CRI), ondansetron (0.1–0.5 mg/kg IV 2–3 times per day), and maropitant[106] (1 mg/kg subcutaneously [SQ] once a day) can be used alone or in combination to decrease vomiting and nausea. Metoclopramide is not a potent antiemetic in cats but has some prokinetic effect and can facilitate gastric emptying.[107] Omeprazole (1 mg/kg orally twice a day) or ranitidine (2.5 mg/kg IV twice a day) can be used to prevent reflux esophagitis in animals with frequent emesis.[107] The use of appetite stimulants has been discouraged in cats with FHL.[1,2,100,108]

Vitamin K_1 should be administered in cats with impaired coagulation and some clinicians routinely administer it to all cats with FHL. Because the absorption of vitamin K_1 from the gastrointestinal tract might be compromised by cholestasis, 0.5 mg/kg to 1.5 mg/kg SQ at 12-hour intervals for 3 to 4 doses has been recommended.[2]

Other medications and supplements are often suggested for the treatment of FHL (**Table 7**) but their efficacy has not been adequately demonstrated to make definitive recommendations regarding their use.[54,58,59,109,110] L-carnitine supplementation has received more interest than any other food supplements and there are experimental and clinical studies that highlight its benefits. In an experimental study in overweight cats undergoing rapid weight loss, dietary L-carnitine supplementation increased the rate of FFA β-oxidation and decreased TG accumulation in the liver.[53,54,58,62] Furthermore, clinical observation of improvement of the clinical signs and probability of survival in cats with FHL when supplemented with L-carnitine suggests that carnitine should be considered an important addition to nutrition support.[2] A dose of 250 mg/cat/d to 500 mg/cat/d orally has been suggested.[1,2]

PROGNOSIS

If appropriately and rapidly treated with nutritional support and in the absence of a serious underlying disease, cats with FHL have a reported recovery rate of 80% to 85%.[2,10] Reported positive prognostic factors were a younger age and a higher median serum potassium concentration and hematocrit.[2,6] A low albumin concentration on admission was associated with a worse prognosis in a population of cats affected with FHL (C. Valtolina and R.P. Favier, unpublished data, 2016).

Table 7		
Medications and nutraceuticals suggested by the treatment of feline hepatic lipidosis		
Medications or Nutraceuticals	**Route of Administration**	**Dosage**
L-carnitine	PO	250–500 mg total daily dose
Vitamin B_{12}	SQ	250 μg/injection once weekly for 6 wk, once every 2 wk for 6 wk, and then monthly
Taurine	PO	250 mg total daily dose during the first 7–10 d
N-acetylcysteine	IV, PO	Initial first dose 140 mg/kg (20% solution diluted 1:4 or greater with saline) over 30 min, followed by 70 mg/kg every 8–12 h
S-adenosylmethionine	PO	20 mg/kg/d Give at least 1 h before meals

REFERENCES

1. Armstrong PJ, Blanchard G. Hepatic lipidosis in cats. Vet Clin North Am Small Anim Pract 2009;39(3):599–616.
2. Center SA. Feline hepatic lipidosis. Vet Clin North Am Small Anim Pract 2005; 35(1):225–69.
3. Dimski DS. Feline hepatic lipidosis. Semin Vet Med Surg (Small Anim) 1997; 12(1):28–33.
4. Hall JA, Barstad LA, Connor WE. Lipid composition of hepatic and adipose tissues from normal cats and from cats with idiopathic hepatic lipidosis. J Vet Intern Med 1997;11(4):238–42.
5. Lund EM, Armstrong PJ, Kirk CA, et al. Health status and population characteristics of dogs and cats examined at private veterinary practices in the united states. J Am Vet Med Assoc 1999;214(9):1336–41.
6. Center SA, Crawford MA, Guida L, et al. A retrospective study of 77 cats with severe hepatic lipidosis: 1975-1990. J Vet Intern Med 1993;7(6):349–59.
7. Biourge VC, Massat B, Groff JM, et al. Effects of protein, lipid, or carbohydrate supplementation on hepatic lipid accumulation during rapid weight loss in obese cats. Am J Vet Res 1994;55(10):1406–15.
8. Biourge VC, Groff JM, Munn RJ, et al. Experimental induction of hepatic lipidosis in cats. Am J Vet Res 1994;55(9):1291–302.
9. Postic C, Girard J. The role of the lipogenic pathway in the development of hepatic steatosis. Diabetes Metab 2008;34(6 Pt 2):643–8.
10. Blanchard G, Paragon BM, Serougne C, et al. Plasma lipids, lipoprotein composition and profile during induction and treatment of hepatic lipidosis in cats and the metabolic effect of one daily meal in healthy cats. J Anim Physiol Anim Nutr (Berl) 2004;88(3–4):73–87.
11. Trevizan L, de Mello Kessler A, Brenna JT, et al. Maintenance of arachidonic acid and evidence of Delta5 desaturation in cats fed gamma-linolenic and linoleic acid enriched diets. Lipids 2012;47(4):413–23.
12. Verbrugghe A, Bakovic M. Peculiarities of one-carbon metabolism in the strict carnivorous cat and the role in feline hepatic lipidosis. Nutrients 2013;5(7): 2811–35.
13. Zoran DL. The carnivore connection to nutrition in cats. J Am Vet Med Assoc 2002;221(11):1559–67.
14. MacDonald ML, Rogers QR, Morris JG. Nutrition of the domestic cat, a mammalian carnivore. Annu Rev Nutr 1984;4:521–62.
15. Mustonen AM, Pyykonen T, Paakkonen T, et al. Adaptations to fasting in the American mink (mustela vison): carbohydrate and lipid metabolism. Comp Biochem Physiol A Mol Integr Physiol 2005;140(2):195–202.
16. Nieminen P, Mustonen AM, Karja V, et al. Fatty acid composition and development of hepatic lipidosis during food deprivation–mustelids as a potential animal model for liver steatosis. Exp Biol Med (Maywood) 2009;234(3):278–86.
17. Morris JG. Idiosyncratic nutrient requirements of cats appear to be diet-induced evolutionary adaptations. Nutr Res Rev 2002;15(1):153–68.
18. Verbrugghe A, Hesta M, Daminet S, et al. Nutritional modulation of insulin resistance in the true carnivorous cat: a review. Crit Rev Food Sci Nutr 2012;52(2): 172–82.
19. Eisert R. Hypercarnivory and the brain: protein requirements of cats reconsidered. J Comp Physiol B 2011;181(1):1–17.

20. Szabo J, Ibrahim WH, Sunvold GD, et al. Effect of dietary protein quality and essential fatty acids on fatty acid composition in the liver and adipose tissue after rapid weight loss in overweight cats. Am J Vet Res 2003;64(3):310–5.

21. Hassam AG, Rivers JP, Crawford MA. The failure of the cat to desaturate linoleic acid; its nutritional implications. Nutr Metab 1977;21(5):321–8.

22. Rivers JP, Sinclair AJ, Craqford MA. Inability of the cat to desaturate essential fatty acids. Nature 1975;258(5531):171–3.

23. Rivers JP, Sinclair AJ, Moore DP, et al. The abnormal metabolism of essential fatty acids in the cat [proceedings]. Proc Nutr Soc 1976;35(2):66A–7A.

24. Pawlosky R, Barnes A, Salem N Jr. Essential fatty acid metabolism in the feline: Relationship between liver and brain production of long-chain polyunsaturated fatty acids. J Lipid Res 1994;35(11):2032–40.

25. Mahfouz MM, Smith TL, Kummerow FA. Effect of dietary fats on desaturase activities and the biosynthesis of fatty acids in rat-liver microsomes. Lipids 1984; 19(3):214–22.

26. Clarke SD. Nonalcoholic steatosis and steatohepatitis. I. molecular mechanism for polyunsaturated fatty acid regulation of gene transcription. Am J Physiol Gastrointest Liver Physiol 2001;281(4):G865–9.

27. Araya J, Rodrigo R, Videla LA, et al. Increase in long-chain polyunsaturated fatty acid n - 6/n - 3 ratio in relation to hepatic steatosis in patients with non-alcoholic fatty liver disease. Clin Sci (Lond) 2004;106(6):635–43.

28. Videla LA, Rodrigo R, Araya J, et al. Oxidative stress and depletion of hepatic long-chain polyunsaturated fatty acids may contribute to nonalcoholic fatty liver disease. Free Radic Biol Med 2004;37(9):1499–507.

29. Matsuzaka T, Shimano H, Yahagi N, et al. Dual regulation of mouse delta(5)- and delta(6)-desaturase gene expression by SREBP-1 and PPARalpha. J Lipid Res 2002;43(1):107–14.

30. Yoshikawa T, Shimano H, Yahagi N, et al. Polyunsaturated fatty acids suppress sterol regulatory element-binding protein 1c promoter activity by inhibition of liver X receptor (LXR) binding to LXR response elements. J Biol Chem 2002; 277(3):1705–11.

31. Osborne TF. Sterol regulatory element-binding proteins (SREBPs): Key regulators of nutritional homeostasis and insulin action. J Biol Chem 2000;275(42): 32379–82.

32. Biourge V, Groff JM, Fisher C, et al. Nitrogen balance, plasma free amino acid concentrations and urinary orotic acid excretion during long-term fasting in cats. J Nutr 1994;124(7):1094–103.

33. Brown B, Mauldin GE, Armstrong J, et al. Metabolic and hormonal alterations in cats with hepatic lipidosis. J Vet Intern Med 2000;14(1):20–6.

34. Chan DL, Freeman LM, Rozanski EA, et al. Alteration in carbohydrate metabolism in critically ill cats. J Vet Emerg Crit Care 2006;16(Suppl 2):S7–13.

35. Knieriem M, Otto CM, Macintire D. Hyperglycemia in critically ill patients. Compend Contin Educ Vet 2007;29(6):360–2, 364–72; [quiz: 372].

36. Aroch I, Shechter-Polak M, Segev G. A retrospective study of serum beta-hydroxybutyric acid in 215 ill cats: clinical signs, laboratory findings and diagnoses. Vet J 2012;191(2):240–5.

37. Biourge V, Nelson RW, Feldman EC, et al. Effect of weight gain and subsequent weight loss on glucose tolerance and insulin response in healthy cats. J Vet Intern Med 1997;11(2):86–91.

38. Hoenig M, Thomaseth K, Waldron M, et al. Insulin sensitivity, fat distribution, and adipocytokine response to different diets in lean and obese cats before and after weight loss. Am J Physiol Regul Integr Comp Physiol 2007;292(1):R227–34.

39. Mazaki-Tovi M, Abood SK, Segev G, et al. Alterations in adipokines in feline hepatic lipidosis. J Vet Intern Med 2013;27(2):242–9.

40. Jung UJ, Choi MS. Obesity and its metabolic complications: the role of adipokines and the relationship between obesity, inflammation, insulin resistance, dyslipidemia and nonalcoholic fatty liver disease. Int J Mol Sci 2014;15(4): 6184–223.

41. Hoenig M, McGoldrick JB, deBeer M, et al. Activity and tissue-specific expression of lipases and tumor-necrosis factor alpha in lean and obese cats. Domest Anim Endocrinol 2006;30(4):333–44.

42. Hoenig M, Wilkins C, Holson JC, et al. Effects of obesity on lipid profiles in neutered male and female cats. Am J Vet Res 2003;64(3):299–303.

43. Miller C, Bartges J, Cornelius L, et al. Tumor necrosis factor-alpha levels in adipose tissue of lean and obese cats. J Nutr 1998;128(Suppl 12):2751S–2S.

44. Hoenig M. The cat as a model for human nutrition and disease. Curr Opin Clin Nutr Metab Care 2006;9(5):584–8.

45. Richard MJ, Holck JT, Beitz DC. Lipogenesis in liver and adipose tissue of the domestic cat (felis domestica). Comp Biochem Physiol B 1989;93(3):561–4.

46. Rouvinen-Watt K, Harris L, Dick M, et al. Role of hepatic de novo lipogenesis in the development of fasting-induced fatty liver in the American mink (neovison vison). Br J Nutr 2012;108(8):1360–70.

47. Bergen WG, Mersmann HJ. Comparative aspects of lipid metabolism: Impact on contemporary research and use of animal models. J Nutr 2005;135(11): 2499–502.

48. Rouvinen-Watt K, Mustonen AM, Conway R, et al. Rapid development of fasting-induced hepatic lipidosis in the American mink (neovison vison): effects of food deprivation and re-alimentation on body fat depots, tissue fatty acid profiles, hematology and endocrinology. Lipids 2010;45(2):111–28.

49. Pardina E, Baena-Fustegueras JA, Llamas R, et al. Lipoprotein lipase expression in livers of morbidly obese patients could be responsible for liver steatosis. Obes Surg 2009;19(5):608–16.

50. Westerbacka J, Kolak M, Kiviluoto T, et al. Genes involved in fatty acid partitioning and binding, lipolysis, monocyte/macrophage recruitment, and inflammation are overexpressed in the human fatty liver of insulin-resistant subjects. Diabetes 2007;56(11):2759–65.

51. Wei Y, Rector RS, Thyfault JP, et al. Nonalcoholic fatty liver disease and mitochondrial dysfunction. World J Gastroenterol 2008;14(2):193–9.

52. Center SA, Guida L, Zanelli MJ, et al. Ultrastructural hepatocellular features associated with severe hepatic lipidosis in cats. Am J Vet Res 1993;54(5): 724–31.

53. Blanchard G, Paragon BM, Milliat F, et al. Dietary L-carnitine supplementation in obese cats alters carnitine metabolism and decreases ketosis during fasting and induced hepatic lipidosis. J Nutr 2002;132(2):204–10.

54. Center SA, Harte J, Watrous D, et al. The clinical and metabolic effects of rapid weight loss in obese pet cats and the influence of supplemental oral L-carnitine. J Vet Intern Med 2000;14(6):598–608.

55. Biourge V, Groff JM, Morris JG, et al. Long-term voluntary fasting in adult obese cats: Nitrogen balance, plasma amino acid concentrations and urinary orotic acid excretion. J Nutr 1994;124(Suppl 12):2680S–2S.

56. Jacobs G, Cornelius L, Keene B, et al. Comparison of plasma, liver, and skeletal muscle carnitine concentrations in cats with idiopathic hepatic lipidosis and in healthy cats. Am J Vet Res 1990;51(9):1349–51.

57. Armstrong PJ. Feline hepatic lipidosis. In proceeding of the 7th annual ACVIM forum. San Diego (CA), May 1989. p. 335–7.

58. Center SA, Warner KL, Randolph JF, et al. Influence of dietary supplementation with (L)-carnitine on metabolic rate, fatty acid oxidation, body condition, and weight loss in overweight cats. Am J Vet Res 2012;73(7):1002–15.

59. Center SA, Warner KL, Erb HN. Liver glutathione concentrations in dogs and cats with naturally occurring liver disease. Am J Vet Res 2002;63(8):1187–97.

60. Pazak HE, Bartges JW, Cornelius LC, et al. Characterization of serum lipoprotein profiles of healthy, adult cats and idiopathic feline hepatic lipidosis patients. J Nutr 1998;128(Suppl 12):2747S–50S.

61. Ibrahim WH, Szabo J, Sunvold GD, et al. Effect of dietary protein quality and fatty acid composition on plasma lipoprotein concentrations and hepatic triglyceride fatty acid synthesis in obese cats undergoing rapid weight loss. Am J Vet Res 2000;61(5):566–72.

62. Ibrahim WH, Bailey N, Sunvold GD, et al. Effects of carnitine and taurine on fatty acid metabolism and lipid accumulation in the liver of cats during weight gain and weight loss. Am J Vet Res 2003;64(10):1265–77.

63. Lidbury JA, Cook AK, Steiner JM. Hepatic encephalopathy in dogs and cats. J Vet Emerg Crit Care (San Antonio) 2016;26(4):471–87.

64. Morris JG, Rogers QR. Ammonia intoxication in the near-adult cat as a result of a dietary deficiency of arginine. Science 1978;199(4327):431–2.

65. Cantafora A, Blotta I, Rossi SS, et al. Dietary taurine content changes liver lipids in cats. J Nutr 1991;121(10):1522–8.

66. Dick MF, Hurford J, Lei S, et al. High feeding intensity increases the severity of fatty liver in the American mink (neovison vison) with potential ameliorating role for long-chain n-3 polyunsaturated fatty acids. Acta Vet Scand 2014;56:5.

67. Mustonen AM, Puukka M, Rouvinen-Watt K, et al. Response to fasting in an unnaturally obese carnivore, the captive european polecat mustela putorius. Exp Biol Med (Maywood) 2009;234(11):1287–95.

68. Nieminen P, Kakela R, Pyykonen T, et al. Selective fatty acid mobilization in the American mink (mustela vison) during food deprivation. Comp Biochem Physiol B Biochem Mol Biol 2006;145(1):81–93.

69. Mustonen AM, Kakela R, Nieminen P. Different fatty acid composition in central and peripheral adipose tissues of the American mink (mustela vison). Comp Biochem Physiol A Mol Integr Physiol 2007;147(4):903–10.

70. Nieminen P, Rouvinen-Watt K, Collinsb D, et al. Fatty acid profiles and relative mobilization during fasting in adipose tissue depots of the American marten (martes Americana). Lipids 2006;41(3):231–40.

71. McNeilly AD, Macfarlane DP, O'Flaherty E, et al. Bile acids modulate glucocorticoid metabolism and the hypothalamic-pituitary-adrenal axis in obstructive jaundice. J Hepatol 2010;52(5):705–11.

72. Boonen E, Van den Berghe G. Understanding the HPA response to critical illness: novel insights with clinical implications. Intensive Care Med 2015;41(1):131–3.

73. Quinn M, Ueno Y, Pae HY, et al. Suppression of the HPA axis during extrahepatic biliary obstruction induces cholangiocyte proliferation in the rat. Am J Physiol Gastrointest Liver Physiol 2012;302(1):G182–93.

74. Fede G, Spadaro L, Tomaselli T, et al. Adrenocortical dysfunction in liver disease: a systematic review. Hepatology 2012;55(4):1282–91.

75. Marik PE, Pastores SM, Annane D, et al. Recommendations for the diagnosis and management of corticosteroid insufficiency in critically ill adult patients: consensus statements from an international task force by the American college of critical care medicine. Crit Care Med 2008;36(6):1937–49.

76. Webster CRL. Metabolic consequences of cholestasis in cats. Society of Comparative Hepatology 25th Ecvim-Ca Congress. Lisbon, Portugal, September 10–12, 2015.

77. Rothuizen J. Important clinical syndromes associated with liver disease. Vet Clin North Am Small Anim Pract 2009;39(3):419–37.

78. Larson MM. Ultrasound imaging of the hepatobiliary system and pancreas. Vet Clin North Am Small Anim Pract 2016;46(3):453–80.

79. Center SA, Baldwin BH, Dillingham S, et al. Diagnostic value of serum gamma-glutamyl transferase and alkaline phosphatase activities in hepatobiliary disease in the cat. J Am Vet Med Assoc 1986;188(5):507–10.

80. Gagne JM, Armstrong PJ, Weiss DJ, et al. Clinical features of inflammatory liver disease in cats: 41 cases (1983-1993). J Am Vet Med Assoc 1999;214(4):513–6.

81. Dircks B, Nolte I, Mischke R. Haemostatic abnormalities in cats with naturally occurring liver diseases. Vet J 2012;193(1):103–8.

82. Center SA, Warner K, Corbett J, et al. Proteins invoked by vitamin K absence and clotting times in clinically ill cats. J Vet Intern Med 2000;14(3):292–7.

83. Lisciandro SC, Hohenhaus A, Brooks M. Coagulation abnormalities in 22 cats with naturally occurring liver disease. J Vet Intern Med 1998;12(2):71–5.

84. Kavanagh C, Shaw S, Webster CR. Coagulation in hepatobiliary disease. J Vet Emerg Crit Care (San Antonio) 2011;21(6):589–604.

85. Feeney DA, Anderson KL, Ziegler LE, et al. Statistical relevance of ultrasonographic criteria in the assessment of diffuse liver disease in dogs and cats. Am J Vet Res 2008;69(2):212–21.

86. Nicoll RG, O'Brien RT, Jackson MW. Qualitative ultrasonography of the liver in obese cats. Vet Radiol Ultrasound 1998;39(1):47–50.

87. Wang KY, Panciera DL, Al-Rukibat RK, et al. Accuracy of ultrasound-guided fine-needle aspiration of the liver and cytologic findings in dogs and cats: 97 cases (1990-2000). J Am Vet Med Assoc 2004;224(1):75–8.

88. Weiss DJ, Moritz A. Liver cytology. Vet Clin North Am Small Anim Pract 2002; 32(6):1267–91, vi.

89. Willard MD, Weeks BR, Johnson M. Fine-needle aspirate cytology suggesting hepatic lipidosis in four cats with infiltrative hepatic disease. J Feline Med Surg 1999;1(4):215–20.

90. Rothuizen J, Twedt DC. Liver biopsy techniques. Vet Clin North Am Small Anim Pract 2009;39(3):469–80.

91. Bigge LA, Brown DJ, Penninck DG. Correlation between coagulation profile findings and bleeding complications after ultrasound-guided biopsies: 434 cases (1993-1996). J Am Anim Hosp Assoc 2001;37(3):228–33.

92. Oliva MR, Mortele KJ, Segatto E, et al. Computed tomography features of nonalcoholic steatohepatitis with histopathologic correlation. J Comput Assist Tomogr 2006;30(1):37–43.

93. Pickhardt PJ, Park SH, Hahn L, et al. Specificity of unenhanced CT for non-invasive diagnosis of hepatic steatosis: implications for the investigation of the natural history of incidental steatosis. Eur Radiol 2012;22(5):1075–82.

94. Roldan-Valadez E, Favila R, Martinez-Lopez M, et al. Imaging techniques for assessing hepatic fat content in nonalcoholic fatty liver disease. Ann Hepatol 2008;7(3):212–20.

95. Kodama Y, Ng CS, Wu TT, et al. Comparison of CT methods for determining the fat content of the liver. AJR Am J Roentgenol 2007;188(5):1307–12.

96. Ma X, Holalkere NS, Kambadakone RA, et al. Imaging-based quantification of hepatic fat: methods and clinical applications. Radiographics 2009;29(5): 1253–77.

97. Lee P, Mori A, Takemitsu H, et al. Lipogenic gene expression in abdominal adipose and liver tissues of diet-induced overweight cats. Vet J 2011;190(2): e150–3.

98. Nakamura M, Chen HM, Momoi Y, et al. Clinical application of computed tomography for the diagnosis of feline hepatic lipidosis. J Vet Med Sci 2005;67(11): 1163–5.

99. Lam R, Niessen SJ, Lamb CR. X-ray attenuation of the liver and kidney in cats considered at varying risk of hepatic lipidosis. Vet Radiol Ultrasound 2014;55(2): 141–6.

100. Chan DL. The inappetent hospitalised cat: Clinical approach to maximising nutritional support. J Feline Med Surg 2009;11(11):925–33.

101. Freeman LM, Chan DL. Total parenteral nutrition. In: DiBartola SP, editor. Fluid, electrolyte, and acid-base disorders in small animal practice. 3rd edition. St Louis (MO): Elsevier; 2006. p. 584–601.

102. Pyle SC, Marks SL, Kass PH. Evaluation of complications and prognostic factors associated with administration of total parenteral nutrition in cats: 75 cases (1994-2001). J Am Vet Med Assoc 2004;225(2):242–50.

103. Brenner EA, Salazar AM, Zabotina OA, et al. Characterization of european forage maize lines for stover composition and associations with polymorphisms within O-methyltransferase genes. Plant Sci 2012;185–186:281–7.

104. Justin RB, Hohenhaus AE. Hypophosphatemia associated with enteral alimentation in cats. J Vet Intern Med 1995;9(4):228–33.

105. Adams LG, Hardy RM, Weiss DJ, et al. Hypophosphatemia and hemolytic anemia associated with diabetes mellitus and hepatic lipidosis in cats. J Vet Intern Med 1993;7(5):266–71.

106. Hickman MA, Cox SR, Mahabir S, et al. Safety, pharmacokinetics and use of the novel NK-1 receptor antagonist maropitant (cerenia) for the prevention of emesis and motion sickness in cats. J Vet Pharmacol Ther 2008;31(3):220–9.

107. Trepanier L. Acute vomiting in cats: rational treatment selection. J Feline Med Surg 2010;12(3):225–30.

108. Delaney SJ. Management of anorexia in dogs and cats. Vet Clin North Am Small Anim Pract 2006;36(6):1243–9, vi.

109. Center SA. Metabolic, antioxidant, nutraceutical, probiotic, and herbal therapies relating to the management of hepatobiliary disorders. Vet Clin North Am Small Anim Pract 2004;34(1):67–172, vi.

110. Webster CR, Cooper J. Therapeutic use of cytoprotective agents in canine and feline hepatobiliary disease. Vet Clin North Am Small Anim Pract 2009;39(3): 631–52.

Feline Cholangitis

Lara Boland, MANZCVS (Feline Medicine)*,
Julia Beatty, BVetMed, PhD, FANZCVS (Feline Medicine)

KEYWORDS

- Feline • Cat • Cholangitis • Liver • Lymphocytic • Neutrophilic • Inflammation
- Fluke

KEY POINTS

- Inflammatory liver disease (cholangitis) is common in cats.
- Three major forms are recognized: neutrophilic, lymphocytic, and chronic cholangitis. Results of diagnostic modalities, including hematology, biochemistry, abdominal ultrasound, and fecal analysis, can assist in ranking differentials.
- Liver biopsy and/or bile analysis (cytology and bacterial culture) are necessary for definitive diagnosis.
- Empiric antibiotic and other supportive treatments are indicated in clinically unstable cases of suspected neutrophilic cholangitis in which invasive diagnostics carry an unacceptable risk.
- Neutrophilic cholangitis and chronic cholangitis can usually be cured with appropriate treatment. Lymphocytic cholangitis can be managed and some cats have long survival times.

INTRODUCTION

Inflammatory liver disease is reported to be the most common, or second most common, abnormality detected in feline liver biopsies.[1,2] Hirose and colleagues[2] (2014) diagnosed inflammatory liver disease in 50% of abnormal biopsies submitted to a teaching hospital in Japan. In the United States, 25.7% of cases had inflammatory disease, whereas 49.7% had hepatic lipidosis.[1]

The term cholangitis to describe inflammatory liver disease is favored over cholangiohepatitis. Cholangitis most accurately reflects the histopathological abnormalities that are centered on the biliary tract with secondary, if any, involvement of the hepatic parenchyma. The World Small Animal Veterinary Association standardization committee recognizes 3 forms of feline cholangitis: neutrophilic, lymphocytic, and chronic, the latter associated with liver fluke.[3]

Disclosure Statement: The authors have nothing to disclose.
Faculty of Veterinary Science, Valentine Charlton Cat Centre, School of Life and Environmental Sciences, The University of Sydney, 65 Parramatta Road, Sydney, New South Wales 2006, Australia
* Corresponding author.
E-mail address: lara.boland@sydney.edu.au

vetsmall.theclinics.com

This article reviews the etiopathogenesis, clinical findings, risks, and benefits of diagnostic investigations, comorbidities, treatment, and outcomes of feline cholangitis.

NEUTROPHILIC CHOLANGITIS

Except in liver fluke endemic regions, neutrophilic cholangitis is the most commonly reported form in most studies, making up 56.3% to 90% of cases of inflammatory liver disease.[2,4,5]

CAUSES

Most cases of neutrophilic cholangitis result from bacterial infection.[6,7] Comorbid disease is common, in particular pancreatitis, either alone or with inflammatory bowel disease (IBD) in a syndrome known as triaditis, and may increase the risk of ascending bacterial infection.[5,6,8,9] In the cat, the common bile duct and pancreatic duct usually enter the duodenum together at the major duodenal papilla. Conversely, pancreatitis and IBD may be a consequence of neutrophilic cholangitis.[2]

The role of *Helicobacter* spp in feline neutrophilic cholangitis and/or triaditis is unclear. Although *Helicobacter* spp are detected by polymerase chain reaction (PCR) in the liver and bile of cats with neutrophilic and lymphocytic cholangitis, they are also detected in cats with noninflammatory liver disease and clinically healthy cats.[4,6,10]

SIGNALMENT

No consistent age, breed, or sex predispositions for neutrophilic cholangitis in cats have been identified.[5,11,12]

HISTORY

A short history of illness, usually less than 2 weeks, is typical.[7,12] Common historical findings include:[5,11,12]

- Lethargy
- Inappetence
- Anorexia
- Vomiting
- Diarrhea
- Recent weight loss

PHYSICAL EXAMINATION

Physical examination findings include lethargy, dehydration, jaundice, pyrexia, cranial abdominal pain, ptyalism, and hepatomegaly (**Fig. 1**).[5,7,11,12] Ptyalism can occur secondary to nausea or hepatic encephalopathy (see Adam G. Gow's article "Hepatic Encephalopathy," in this issue). Jaundice can be intrahepatic or posthepatic secondary to partial or complete common bile duct obstruction from biliary tract inflammation or inflammatory debris, concurrent cholelithiasis, or pancreatitis.[7]

LABORATORY FINDINGS

Laboratory changes can support a diagnosis of neutrophilic cholangitis. Hematological and biochemical abnormalities in cats with neutrophilic cholangitis are summarized in **Table 1**.

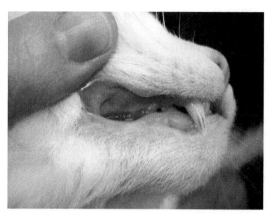

Fig. 1. Marked jaundice of the mucous membranes and skin of a cat.

Neutrophilia ranges from severe with a left shift and toxic changes to absent. Of note, neutrophilic cholangitis is not always accompanied by liver enzyme elevations.[5] Compared with lymphocytic cholangitis, cases of neutrophilic cholangitis have higher segmental and band neutrophil counts, as well as increases in alanine aminotransferase (ALT) activity and total bilirubin.[11] Inappetence, dehydration, vomiting, and diarrhea can precipitate prerenal azotemia, hypokalemia, hyponatremia, and hypochloremia.

Coagulation times (prothrombin time, activated partial thromboplastin time, activated clotting time) can be prolonged and must be evaluated before invasive

Table 1
Abnormalities reported in hematology and biochemical analysis in cats with neutrophilic cholangitis

Hematology	Prevalence (%)	Biochemistry	Prevalence (%)
Lymphopenia	66.6	Hyperbilirubinemia	68.8–83.3
Leukocytosis	33.3	Increased ALT activity	56.7–100
Neutrophilia ± left shift	25.0–33.3	Increased ALP activity	33.3–48.3
Mild nonregenerative or poorly regenerative anemia	32.3	Increased AST activity	95.5–100
Leukopenia	16.6	Hyperglobulinemia	56.3
Neutropenia	16.6	Prerenal azotemia	33.3
		Hyperglycemia	33.3
		Increased GGT activity	22.2
		Hyponatremia	33.3
		Hypochloremia	33.3
		Hypokalemia	Not reported
		Hypoglycemia	Not reported
		Hypoalbuminemia	Not reported
		Hypercholesterolemia or hypocholesterolemia	Not reported

Abbreviations: ALP, alkaline phosphatase; ALT, alanine aminotransferase; AST, aspartate aminotransferase; GGT, gamma-glutamyltransferase.
    Data from Refs.[5,7,11–13]

diagnostics such as liver biopsy[11,13] (see also Cynthia R.L. Webster's article "Hemostatic Disorders Associated with Hepatobiliary Disease," in this issue). Hepatic dysfunction may result in hyperammonemia and liver function should be evaluated before anesthesia. Preprandial and postprandial serum bile acid concentrations may be abnormal or may not be interpretable due to the presence of hyperbilirubinemia[11] (see also Yuri A. Lawrence and Jörg M. Steiner's article "Laboratory Evaluation of the Liver," in this issue).

Hypocobalaminemia or hypercobalaminemia can be present in cats with neutrophilic cholangitis and/or in cats with concurrent pancreatitis or IBD.[14,15] Elevated feline pancreas-specific lipase immunoreactivity concentrations raise suspicion for concurrent pancreatitis. One study showed that biochemical and hematological parameters did not assist in identifying concurrent pancreatitis.[5]

DIAGNOSTIC IMAGING

Imaging findings can support a diagnosis of neutrophilic cholangitis but normal findings do not exclude the diagnosis. Abdominal radiographs may reveal mild hepatomegaly or cholecystoliths.[11] Abdominal ultrasound may reveal increased thickness and irregularity of the gall bladder wall, dilation and tortuosity of the cystic and common bile ducts, diffuse hyperechogenicity of the liver parenchyma, hepatomegaly, hyperechoic gall bladder contents, gall bladder distention, and choleliths if present (**Figs. 2** and **3**).[5,11,16] Marolf and colleagues[16] (2012) found no significant differences in ultrasonographic changes between cats with neutrophilic versus lymphocytic cholangitis.

Ultrasonographic changes associated with concurrent pancreatitis, including hypoechogenicity of the pancreas, peripancreatic fluid accumulation, irregular pancreatic margins, and hyperechoic peripancreatic fat, may be present.[5,17] Concurrent IBD may manifest as intestinal wall thickening with preserved layering.[5,18]

BACTERIAL CULTURE

Ascending infection via the biliary tree is thought to be the most common route. Ascending bacterial infection is supported by frequent culture of enteric bacteria

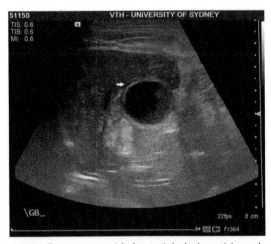

Fig. 2. Ultrasound image from a cat with bacterial cholecystitis and common bile duct obstruction. The gall bladder is distended with a thickened wall (*white arrow*) and echogenic content. (*Courtesy of* Dr Joanna Pilton, The University of Sydney, Sydney, Australia.)

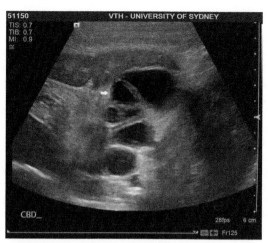

Fig. 3. Ultrasound image from a cat with bacterial cholecystitis and common bile duct obstruction. The common bile duct (CBD) (*white arrow*) is markedly distended and tortuous, and has a thickened wall and echogenic intraluminal material. (*Courtesy of* Dr Joanna Pilton, The University of Sydney, Sydney, Australia.)

from bile or liver biopsies from affected cats (**Box 1**).[5,8,19–21] A single bacterial species is cultured from more than 80% of cases, with *Escherichia coli* being the most common isolate.[5,6,8,12,19,20] Other possible routes of infection include hematogenous seeding, enteric mucosal translocation, or entry via the portal system.[6,8,12,19]

Normally, bile in cats is sterile although transient bactibilia with enteric bacteria has been reported.[20,21] Risk factors for the development of persistent biliary infection include cholelithiasis, biliary tract obstruction, hepatic neoplasia, congenital abnormalities, extrahepatic disease (eg, pancreatitis, IBD, triaditis), or pre-existing inflammatory liver disease.[6,8,20,22]

Box 1
Bacteria cultured from bile, liver, and choleliths in cats

Bacteria

- *Escherichia coli*

- *Enterococcus* spp
  - *Enterococcus faecalis*

- *Streptococcus* spp
  - *Streptococcus viridans*

- *Clostridium* spp
  - *Clostridium perfringens*

- *Bacterioides* spp

- *Salmonella enterica* serovar Typhimurium

- *Pseudomonas* spp
  - *Pseudomonas fluorescens*

- *Staphylococcus* spp

- *Acinetobacter* spp

Data from Refs.[5–8,19,20,23,24]

DIAGNOSTIC SAMPLE COLLECTION

If neutrophilic cholangitis is suspected, samples for bacterial culture obtained by minimally invasive percutaneous ultrasound-guided cholecystocentesis are recommended. Obtaining bile rather than liver tissue for culture is more likely to return a positive culture result (36% vs 14%).[19] Other methods for obtaining samples for culture are described in **Table 2**.

Bile collected from cats with neutrophilic cholangitis can be grossly purulent and malodourous (**Fig. 4**). Abnormal bile (ie, affected by inflammation and/or bacterial infection) is more likely when white blood cell counts and gamma-glutamyltransferase activity are increased.[8]

Cytology should be routinely performed alongside bile culture to guide first-line therapy and to support culture results (**Fig. 5**). Some bacteria are difficult to culture or may be overgrown by *Escherichia coli*.[8] Negative cultures can also result from previous antibiotic administration or a bacteriostatic effect of bile.[8] Failure to culture some bacterial species present in cats with neutrophilic cholangitis can have treatment

Table 2
Diagnostic sample collection for cytology, bacterial culture, and histopathology

Method	Benefits	Risks	Tests	Comments
Percutaneous ultrasound-guided cholecystocentesis	Minimally invasive Optimal sample for culture	Gall bladder rupture Septic peritonitis Hemorrhage	Cytology Bacterial culture	Ultrasound equipment and experience required
Cholecystocentesis at exploratory laparotomy	Good visualization	Invasive Gall bladder rupture Septic peritonitis Hemorrhage	Cytology Bacterial culture	—
Ultrasound-guided hepatic biopsy	Minimally invasive	Hemorrhage	Cytology Bacterial culture Histopathology	Coagulation testing essential Ultrasound equipment and experience required
Hepatic wedge biopsy at exploratory laparotomy or laparoscopy	Good visualization and hemostasis Larger biopsy (more representative)	Invasive Hemorrhage	Cytology Bacterial culture Histopathology	Coagulation testing essential Shorter recovery following laparoscopy
Hepatic fine-needle aspirate	Minimally invasive	Hemorrhage (unlikely)	Cytology Bacterial culture	Ultrasound equipment required Cytology may not be representative of the disease process Bacterial culture less likely to be positive than bile culture

Data from Refs.[5,6,8,19,25]

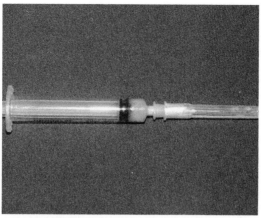

Fig. 4. Grossly purulent bile aspirated from the gall bladder of a cat with bacterial cholecystitis. (*From* Brain PH, Barrs VR, Martin P, et al. Feline cholecystitis and acute neutrophilic cholangitis: clinical findings, bacterial isolates, and response to treatment in six cases. J Feline Med Surg 2006;8:95; with permission.)

implications. Nonbacterial pathogens are rare in feline cholangitis and bile cytology can assist in identifying these.[8]

HEPATIC FINE-NEEDLE ASPIRATE CYTOLOGY

Fine-needle aspirate cytology may reveal neutrophilic inflammation but this is a nonspecific finding and bacteria are rarely seen. Cytology can, however, support a diagnosis of concurrent hepatic lipidosis or lymphoma.

LIVER BIOPSY

Histopathology of liver biopsy samples is required for definitive diagnosis. Biopsy may not be possible, for example, in unstable or deteriorating patients or if financial

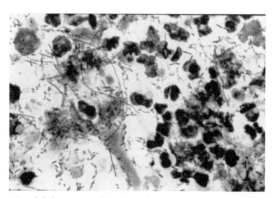

Fig. 5. Diff-Quik stained bile smear showing degenerate neutrophilic inflammation and pleomorphic bacterial rods and cocci from a cat with bacterial cholecystitis. (*From* Brain PH, Barrs VR, Martin P, et al. Feline cholecystitis and acute neutrophilic cholangitis: clinical findings, bacterial isolates, and response to treatment in six cases. J Feline Med Surg 2006;8:96; with permission.)

restrictions exist. In these cases, treatment is based on a presumptive diagnosis of neutrophilic cholangitis, ideally supported by bile cytology and culture results. Inflammatory diseases are distributed unevenly throughout the hepatic parenchyma so the collection of multiple biopsies is preferred (see **Table 2**).[5]

Histopathological features of neutrophilic cholangitis (**Fig. 6**) are summarized in **Table 3**. Neutrophilic cholangitis may be subclassified as acute or chronic based on the inflammatory infiltrate and clinical presentation, although treatment recommendations are unaffected.

COMORBIDITIES

Pancreatitis and IBD are commonly recognized comorbidities. Other comorbidities, including hepatic lipidosis, cholelithiasis, gall bladder congenital abnormalities, hepatic or intestinal neoplasia, extrahepatic biliary obstruction, and exocrine pancreatic insufficiency, have been reported in cats with neutrophilic cholangitis.[5,12,23,31,32] Neutrophilic cholangitis can also develop as a complication of cholecystoduodenostomy or choledochal stenting.[32] No association with feline immunodeficiency virus (FIV) or feline leukemia virus (FeLV) infection is recognized.[7]

TREATMENT

Antibiotics and supportive care are the mainstays of treatment of neutrophilic cholangitis (**Table 4**).[7,11,12]

Antibiotic Selection

Antibiotic selection is ideally based on the results of bacterial culture and sensitivity testing. Empiric antibiotic therapy is required, at least until culture results are received. Unless cytologic findings support alternate choices, empiric therapy should provide

Table 3
Summary of liver histologic features of neutrophilic, lymphocytic, and chronic cholangitis in cats

Neutrophilic Cholangitis	Lymphocytic Cholangitis	Chronic Cholangitis Associated with Liver Fluke
• Portal neutrophilic infiltrates • Lower numbers of lymphocytes and plasma cells in portal areas • Neutrophilic infiltrates can extend into the hepatic parenchyma • Dilated intrahepatic biliary ducts • Neutrophils within biliary duct lumens and infiltrating duct walls • Bile duct proliferation, hyperplasia and epithelial degeneration • Variable degrees of fibrosis • Periportal necrosis	• Moderate to marked aggregates of small lymphocytes infiltrating portal areas and around bile ducts • Biliary hyperplasia • Biliary ductular proliferation • Variable degrees of portal fibrosis • Lymphocytes can penetrate the lumen of biliary ducts and infiltrate biliary epithelium leading to ductopenia • Lymphocytic infiltrates can extend into the hepatic parenchyma	• Periductal and portal inflammatory infiltrates, which can extend into the hepatic parenchyma (lymphocytes, macrophages, plasma cells, eosinophils, and neutrophils) • Dilation and adenomatous hyperplasia of biliary ducts • Periportal and periductal fibrosis • Hyperplastic adenomatous or ulcerative cholecystitis can be present • Adult liver flukes or eggs are often not identified

Data from Refs.[1,5,11,22,26–30]

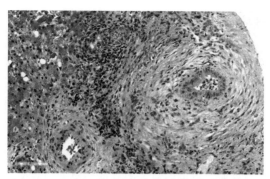

Fig. 6. Liver biopsy from a cat with chronic neutrophilic cholangitis. There is pronounced periductal concentric fibrosis with mild edema and biliary hyperplasia. A mixed periportal inflammatory infiltrate and intraductal neutrophils are present (3'3-diaminobenzidine and hematoxylin). (*Courtesy of* Dr Mark Krockenberger, The University of Sydney, Sydney, Australia.)

coverage for gram-positive and negative aerobes and anaerobes.[7,11,12] Bactericidal antibiotics that achieve therapeutic levels in bile and do not require hepatic activation or excretion are ideal. Appropriate choices include a fluoroquinolone, penicillin and metronidazole, or a fluoroquinolone together with a potentiated penicillin/ clindamycin.[5,7]

Intravenous (IV) antibiotic therapy is indicated initially. The duration of antibiotic treatment should ideally be based on follow-up culture results but this is often not practical or affordable. Empiric antibiotic therapy for 4 to 6 weeks duration is suggested.[7]

Supportive Care

Hospitalization periods range from a few days to a week or more.[7] IV fluid therapy is used for rehydration and correction of electrolyte abnormalities (see **Table 4**). Hypo-kalemia should be identified and treated. Analgesia can be safely provided by the use of opioids. Nonsteroidal anti-inflammatory drugs are contraindicated in cats with dehydration, inappetence, vomiting, and diarrhea because of the risk of severe adverse effects such as nephrotoxicity and gastrointestinal ulceration. Antiemetics and appetite stimulants may be required.[33,34] Other medications that may benefit cats with neutrophilic cholangitis include S-adenosylmethionine, silybin, and urso-deoxycholic acid (UDCA).[35–37]

Vitamin K_1 deficiency can occur in conditions causing biliary obstruction and can contribute to coagulation abnormalities in cats with liver disease (see Cynthia R.L. Webster's article, "Hemostatic Disorders Associated with Hepatobiliary Disease," in this issue). Laboratory assessment of coagulation and/or supplementation of vitamin K_1 should be completed before hepatic sampling. Cats with hypocobalaminemia should be supplemented. Nutrition may be provided for anorexic cats by the use of nasoesophageal, esophageal, or gastric feeding tubes.[11]

Treatment of Concurrent Disease

Pancreatitis is treated with the supportive care recommendations previously discussed (see **Table 4**). Following resolution of bacterial infection and inappetence, treatment of IBD with hydrolyzed protein diet trials and/or immunosuppressive medications such as prednisolone, may be indicated in individual cases.[11]

Table 4
Drugs used for the treatment of neutrophilic cholangitis, lymphocytic cholangitis, and liver fluke infections in cats

Drug	Drug Group and Proposed Action	Indication	Dose and Route	Side Effects
Amoxicillin-clavulanate	Antibiotic Potentiated aminopenicillin	Neutrophilic cholangitis Anaerobes Gram-positive aerobes	8.75 mg/kg (combined constituents) SC SID 12.5–25 mg/kg PO BID–TID	Gastrointestinal side effects Hypersensitivity reactions
Ticarcillin-clavulanate	Antibiotic Potentiated penicillin	Neutrophilic cholangitis Anaerobes Gram-positive aerobes	50 mg/kg IV TID	Gastrointestinal side effects Hypersensitivity reactions
Amoxicillin	Antibiotic Aminopenicillin	Neutrophilic cholangitis Anaerobes Gram-positive aerobes	10–20 mg/kg IV TID or PO BID–TID	Gastrointestinal side effects Hypersensitivity reactions
Metronidazole	Antibiotic Synthetic nitroimidazole	Neutrophilic cholangitis Anaerobes	10 mg/kg IV or PO BID	Gastrointestinal side effects Hepatotoxicity Neurotoxicity
Chloramphenicol	Antibiotic	Neutrophilic cholangitis Gram-positive aerobes Anaerobes	10–20 mg/kg IV, SC, or PO BID	Gastrointestinal side effects Bone marrow suppression
Clindamycin	Antibiotic Lincosamide	Neutrophilic cholangitis Gram-positive aerobes Anaerobes	10–12.5 mg/kg IV or PO BID Follow PO dosing with food or water	Gastrointestinal side effects Esophagitis, esophageal stricture
Marbofloxacin	Antibiotic Fluoroquinolone	Neutrophilic cholangitis Gram-negative aerobes	2 mg/kg IV, SC, or PO SID	Gastrointestinal side effects Potential for cartilage abnormalities in young animals
Enrofloxacin	Antibiotic Fluoroquinolone	Neutrophilic cholangitis Gram-negative aerobes	2.5 mg/kg SC or PO BID	Gastrointestinal side effects Retinal blindness Potential for cartilage abnormalities in young animals
Gentamicin	Antibiotic Aminoglycoside	Neutrophilic cholangitis Gram-negative aerobes	5–8 mg/kg IV or SC SID Administer with IV fluid therapy	Nephrotoxicity Ototoxicity

Drug	Category/Mechanism	Disease	Dose	Side effects
Buprenorphine	Analgesia; Opiate partial agonist	Neutrophilic cholangitis	0.01–0.03 mg/kg IV, IM, or sublingually QID–TID	Sedation; Dose-dependent cardiorespiratory depression
Methadone	Analgesia; Opiate agonist	Neutrophilic cholangitis	0.1–0.2 mg/kg IV or IM q4-6 h; IV CRI: 0.1 mg/kg/h	Sedation; Dose-dependent cardiorespiratory depression
Fentanyl	Analgesia; Opiate agonist	Neutrophilic cholangitis	IV CRI: 1–6 μg/kg/h	Sedation; Dose-dependent cardiorespiratory depression
Potassium chloride or gluconate	Electrolyte	Neutrophilic cholangitis	Chloride: IV CRI do not exceed 0.5 mmol/kg/h; Gluconate: 2–6 mEq/d PO	Hyperkalemia; Phlebitis
Phytomenadione (K_1)	Vitamin	Neutrophilic cholangitis; Lymphocytic cholangitis	0.5–1 mg/kg SC BID–TID	—
Cyanocobalamin (B_{12})	Vitamin	Neutrophilic cholangitis	250 μg SC q 7 d for 4–6 wk then monthly	—
Maropitant	Antiemetic; Neurokinin receptor antagonist	Neutrophilic cholangitis	1 mg/kg SC or PO SID	Injection site pain
Metoclopramide	Antiemetic	Neutrophilic cholangitis	0.2–0.5 mg/kg IM, SC, or PO TID; IV CRI: 1–2 mg/kg/d	Sedation; Disorientation
Ondansetron	Antiemetic; 5-HT3 receptor antagonist	Neutrophilic cholangitis	0.5 mg/kg IV or PO SID–BID; IV CRI: 0.5 mg/kg/h for 6 h	Constipation; Sedation
Mirtazapine	Appetite stimulant; Tetracyclic antidepressant; 5-HT3 receptor antagonist	Neutrophilic cholangitis; Lymphocytic cholangitis	1.875–3.75 mg/cat PO q2-3 d	Sedation; Vocalization; Disorientation; Ptyalism
S-adenosylmethionine	Hepatoprotectant; Reduce inflammation; Reduce apoptosis; Promote cell regeneration	Neutrophilic cholangitis	90 mg PO SID	—

(continued on next page)

Table 4
(continued)

Drug	Drug Group and Proposed Action	Indication	Dose and Route	Side Effects
Silybin	Hepatoprotectant Antioxidant Free radical scavenger Anti-inflammatory Stimulates bile flow and production of hepatoprotective bile acids	Neutrophilic cholangitis	9 mg PO SID	—
Ursodeoxycholic acid	Bile acid Increased bile flow Possible cytoprotective properties	Neutrophilic cholangitis Lymphocytic cholangitis	10–15 mg/kg PO SID	—
Prednisolone	Glucocorticoid Anti-inflammatory Immunosuppressant	Lymphocytic cholangitis	1 mg/kg SID IV, PO	Polyphagia Polydipsia Polyuria Skin fragility Poor fur regrowth Weight gain Gastrointestinal ulceration Diabetes mellitus
Praziquantel	Anticestodal antiparasitic	Liver fluke	10–25 mg/kg SC or PO SID for 3–5 d	Injection site reaction Gastrointestinal side effects

Abbreviations: CRI, continuous rate infusion; IM, intramuscular; IV, intravenous; SC, subcutaneous.
Data from Refs.[7,11,12,30,33–38]

COMPLICATIONS

Complications are uncommon. Those reported include partial or complete common bile duct obstruction secondary to inflammation or cholelithiasis, gall bladder necrosis, and hepatic abscess formation.[5,7,8,39] Gall bladder resection, choledochal stenting, or cholecystoduodenostomy may be indicated (**Fig. 7**).[7,13,24,32]

PROGNOSIS

Most cats recover with appropriate treatment and recurrence is rare with reported survival times of several years.[7,11] Concurrent disease may affect long-term outcome in some cats.[11]

LYMPHOCYTIC CHOLANGITIS

There are conflicting data regarding the prevalence of lymphocytic cholangitis in cats. This disease accounted for only 0.17% of cats presenting to a university referral hospital and 6.8% of all cats with inflammatory liver disease in a necropsy study.[1,40] However, a recent study of cats in Greece reported a higher prevalence with 18 per 27 symptomatic and 14 per 20 asymptomatic cats having histopathological evidence of cholangitis. Of these, 25 had lymphocytic and 5 had chronic neutrophilic cholangitis.[41] Histologic severity scores were not significantly different between symptomatic and asymptomatic cats. Possible explanations for this higher prevalence may include regional differences, sample size, differences in study design, and histopathology classification or interpretation. The significance of histopathologically identified cholangitis in asymptomatic cats is unclear and requires further investigation.

CAUSES

Lymphocytic hepatic infiltrates on histopathology, often marked, are most consistent with an immune-mediated cause.[22,27] Some investigators suggest transient bacterial

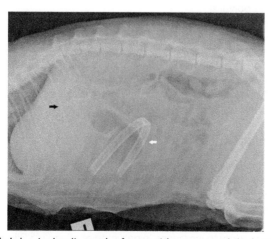

Fig. 7. Left lateral abdominal radiograph of a cat with a common bile duct (CBD) obstruction postoperatively. A radiopaque stent (*black arrow*) is located within the CBD and duodenum. A Jackson-Pratt abdominal drain (Mila International, Inc, Kentucky) is also present (*white arrow*). (*Courtesy of* Dr Joanna Pilton, The University of Sydney, Sydney, Australia.)

infection as a trigger for progressive immune-mediated hepatic inflammation, although clinically significant or persistent bacterial infection has not been clearly associated with lymphocytic cholangitis.[22,42] Culture of bile or liver, fluorescence in situ hybridization, and PCR demonstrated enteric bacterial species in some cases.[5,22,42] Their significance is unclear, especially because bacteria were also identified in control cats. Reported bacterial species include: *Escherichia coli*, *Enterococcus* spp, *Helicobacter* spp, *Micrococcus* spp, *Streptococcus* spp, *Jeotgallicoccus pinnipedialis*, *Citrococcus* spp, and *Brevibacterium casei*.[5,22,42] The role, if any, of *Helicobacter* spp infections in cats with lymphocytic cholangitis is also controversial.[22,42,43] Antibiotic treatment of cats with lymphocytic cholangitis is, therefore, not recommended unless indicated by bacterial culture and sensitivity testing in individual cases.

SIGNALMENT

Cats of any age, breed, or sex can be affected. Some studies report an increased risk in young cats and others in older cats.[26,40,44] A male predisposition is inconsistently reported.[26,27,40] Persian or Norwegian Forest cats are overrepresented in studies from the United Kingdom and the Netherlands, respectively.[26,40]

HISTORY

A protracted history of slowly progressive illness over weeks to months is typical for lymphocytic cholangitis.[26,27,45] In contrast to cats with neutrophilic cholangitis, they may be bright, alert, and responsive at presentation. Commonly reported historical findings include:[11,26,27,40]

- Weight loss
- Polyphagia
- Anorexia
- Vomiting
- Lethargy
- Polydipsia and polyuria

PHYSICAL EXAMINATION

Physical examination findings include poor body condition, jaundice, hepatomegaly, ascites, and lethargy.[11,26,27,40] Less commonly reported are generalized lymphadenomegaly and hepatic encephalopathy.[26,27] In contrast to neutrophilic cholangitis, pyrexia is rarely reported.

LABORATORY FINDINGS

Abnormalities on hematology and biochemistry in cats with lymphocytic cholangitis are summarized in **Table 5**. Laboratory changes can support a diagnosis of lymphocytic cholangitis. In comparison with cats with neutrophilic cholangitis, hematology is usually within reference range and ALT activity and total bilirubin increases tend to be of a lower magnitude.[11,26,45] Hypoalbuminemia is usually mild and hyperglobulinemia may be marked secondary to increases in gammaglobulins.[26,40] Bile acids and resting ammonia levels may be increased.[26,40] Coagulation times (prothrombin time, activated partial thromboplastin time, activated clotting time) are prolonged in some cats.[11] No retroviral association is identified.[26,40]

Table 5
Abnormalities in hematology and biochemical analysis in cats with lymphocytic cholangitis

Hematology	Prevalence (%)	Biochemistry	Prevalence (%)
Mild nonregenerative or poorly regenerative anemia	0–66.6	Increased ALT activity	52–57.1
		Increased ALP activity	32–57.1
		Hyperglobulinemia	42.9–48
		Hypoalbuminemia	0–33.3
		Hyperbilirubinemia	28–28.6

Abbreviation: ALP, alkaline phosphatase; ALT, alanine aminotransferase.
Data from Refs.[11,26,40,44–46]

ABDOMINAL FLUID ANALYSIS

Affected cats can develop moderate to marked ascites. Abdominal fluid analysis typically reveals a high protein content with increased globulin levels, small lymphocytes, nondegenerate neutrophils, and other inflammatory cell types.[26,45]

DIAGNOSTIC IMAGING

Hepatomegaly and/or ascites may be detected radiographically. Findings on abdominal ultrasound and/or exploratory laparotomy include normal hepatic parenchyma or coarse to nodular echotexture, hepatomegaly, ascites, and abdominal lymphadenomegaly, which can be marked.[11,26,45] Abnormalities involving the gall bladder or extrahepatic biliary tree are uncommon, in contrast to neutrophilic cholangitis.[26]

LIVER BIOPSY

Histopathological features of lymphocytic cholangitis (**Fig. 8**) are summarized in **Table 3**. Portal lymphocytes are reported to be predominantly CD3+ T cells.[27]

History, physical examination, biochemistry, fluid analysis, and abdominal ultrasound findings in cats with lymphocytic cholangitis can mimic those of lymphoma or feline infectious peritonitis.[22,26] Liver histopathology is required for definitive

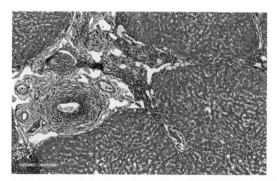

Fig. 8. Liver biopsy from a cat with marked chronic lymphocytic cholangitis. There is moderate periductal fibrosis with a variably intense portal lymphocytic infiltrate with widespread moderate hepatocellular nodular hyperplasia (3′3-diaminobenzidine and hematoxylin). (*Courtesy of* Dr Mark Krockenberger, The University of Sydney, Sydney, Australia.)

diagnosis. The histologic findings of bile duct targeting, ductopenia, peribiliary fibrosis, portal B-cell aggregates, portal lipogranulomas, and in some cases the results of polyclonal PCR for T-cell receptor gene rearrangement can assist in differentiating lymphocytic cholangitis from lymphoma.[22]

Distinct from lymphocytic cholangitis, lymphocytic portal hepatitis is a common, progressive, age-related change in healthy cats characterized by low-level portal lymphocyte and plasma cell infiltration, bile duct proliferations, and fibrosis.[1,47] Lymphocytic portal hepatitis is not associated with pancreatitis or IBD.

COMORBIDITIES

The potential role of comorbid diseases in the etiopathogenesis of lymphocytic cholangitis is less well elucidated than for neutrophilic cholangitis.[22,40,41,45] Weiss and colleagues[9] (1996) found no significant difference in the prevalence of pancreatitis or IBD in 36 cats that they classified as having lymphocytic portal hepatitis compared with 24 cats without inflammatory hepatic disease. Fragkou and colleagues[41] (2016) reported that 16 per 18 symptomatic cats with cholangitis had comorbid disease (triaditis, 8; IBD, 6; pancreatitis, 2) and 10 per 14 asymptomatic cats with cholangitis had comorbid enteritis on histopathology. This study also found that the IBD histopathology severity score had a positive correlation with the number of comorbidities. Warren and colleagues[22] (2011) found that 5 per 10 cats with lymphocytic cholangitis had comorbid IBD and 3 per 17 had comorbid nonhepatic lymphoma. Direct comparison of these studies is difficult due to factors such as sample size, differences in study design, and histopathology classifications or interpretation.

TREATMENT

Treatments for lymphocytic cholangitis include immunosuppressive doses of prednisolone and/or UDCA (see **Table 4**).[11,26,40,45] Supportive care such as feeding tubes and therapeutic abdominocentesis may be indicated.[11,26] Further investigation is required to determine optimal treatment, drug dosages, and treatment length required for cats with lymphocytic cholangitis. One retrospective study found that prednisolone treatment was significantly associated with longer survival times compared with UDCA treatment alone.[40] There was no difference in survival times between cats treated with 1 or 2 mg/kg/d of prednisolone. In another study, the same investigators found a greater improvement in histologic evidence of hepatic inflammation in cats treated with prednisolone compared with UDCA.[44] However, the UDCA-treated group had less severe initial histopathological changes and only 9 cats were studied.

PROGNOSIS

Resolution of ascites and median and mean survival times of 26 to 36 months with treatment are reported in studies with small numbers of cats.[11,26,40,45]

CHRONIC CHOLANGITIS ASSOCIATED WITH LIVER FLUKE INFESTATION

Liver flukes reported to infect cats are trematodes belonging to the families Dicrocoeliidae (*Platynosomum* spp) and Opisthorchiidae (*Opisthorchis* spp, *Clonorchis* spp, *Metorchis* spp, and *Amphimerus* spp). There is lack of consensus on the classification of individual species, some of which may be synonymous.[48,49]

DISTRIBUTION

Feline liver fluke infestation has been reported throughout the world with different regional prevalences.[48,49] The Opisthorchiidae family also infect humans who acquire infection from eating undercooked fish. Cats, as well as many other mammals, including dogs, may act as reservoir hosts in endemic regions.[50,51] Most reports in the English language of clinical disease in cats describe *Platynosomum* spp infections.

LIFECYCLE

Trematodes have complex life cycles involving 2 to 4 hosts and many larval stages.

Platynosomum spp fluke lifecycles are incompletely understood but are thought to involve:[48,52]

- First intermediate host: land snail species ingest eggs and shed sporocysts into the environment
- Second intermediate host: terrestrial isopods (crustaceans) ingest sporocysts
- Paratenic host: lizard and amphibian species are infected by eating isopods
- Definitive host: cats are infected by eating lizards. The flukes migrate to the liver and eggs are shed in feces

The Opisthorchiidae fluke life cycles involve:[49]

- First intermediate host: aquatic snail species ingest eggs and shed redia into the environment
- Second intermediate host: fish of the family Cyprinidae are infected when cercaria penetrate their epithelium
- Definitive host: cats are infected by eating raw fish. The flukes migrate to the liver and eggs are shed in feces

Platynosomum fastosum

Platynosomum spp are found in tropical and subtropical regions where they can cause lizard poisoning in cats. In endemic regions, the prevalence of *P fastosum* infestation can exceed 80% among free roaming cats.[48,53–55] The flukes reside in the gall bladder and biliary ducts causing inflammation and obstruction.

SIGNALMENT

An inconsistent female predisposition has been reported. Free roaming cats more than 2 years of age are overrepresented.[54,56]

HISTORY

Most liver fluke infections in cats are asymptomatic.[57] If clinical signs occur, historical findings include chronic or acute[28,57–60]

- Inappetence
- Lethargy
- Weight loss
- Vomiting
- Diarrhea

Acute presentations may be associated with extrahepatic biliary obstruction. Disease severity may be affected by parasite burden, repeated infection, and/or chronicity.[30]

PHYSICAL EXAMINATION

Physical examination findings include poor body condition, dehydration, jaundice, hepatomegaly, abdominal pain, and ascites.[28,30,57,58,60]

LABORATORY FINDINGS

Laboratory findings reported in cats with liver fluke infections are summarized in **Table 6**. Most cases for which FIV and FeLV status has been reported are negative.[30,59]

Fecal analysis to identify fluke eggs can assist in diagnosis.[29,55,61] Negative fecal analysis does not rule out infection. The accuracy of fecal analysis is influenced by intermittent shedding of eggs, low parasite burdens, low numbers of eggs per gram of feces, and the fecal analysis method.[29,55,61] Formalin-ether sedimentation is a sensitive technique. Repeated fecal analysis combined with other laboratory and imaging findings may be required for diagnosis. Fecal PCR tests have been developed for some liver fluke species.

Köster and colleagues[29] (2016) reported that analysis of bile obtained by percutaneous ultrasound-guided cholecystocentesis contained a significantly higher fluke egg count than fecal analysis. This technique may assist in cases if liver fluke infestation is suspected but not confirmed by fecal analysis.

DIAGNOSTIC IMAGING

Abdominal radiographs and ultrasound examination are often unremarkable in cats infected with liver fluke. Nonspecific abnormalities, which may be precipitated by chronic infections or high parasite burden, include distended and tortuous common bile ducts, periductal hyperechogenicity, intrahepatic biliary dilation, hyperechoic and thickened gall bladder walls, gall bladder sludge, gall bladder distention, hepatomegaly, irregular liver margins, hyperechoic and heterogeneous hepatic parenchyma, and diffuse cystic hepatic changes.[28–30,56,59]

COMORBIDITIES

Bacterial cholangitis (*Escherichia coli*) associated with liver fluke infestation was reported in 6 per 13 cats.[29] However, all cats in this study were FIV positive. The incidence of clinically significant bacterial cholecystitis in liver fluke infested cats requires further investigation. Liver fluke infections have rarely been associated with cholangiocarcinoma in cats.[62]

Table 6 Abnormalities in hematology and biochemical analysis reported in liver fluke infections (*Platynosomum* spp) in cats	
Hematology	Biochemistry
Mild nonregenerative anemia	Hyperbilirubinemia
Eosinophilia	Increased ALT activity
Lymphocytosis	Increased ALP activity
	Increased AST activity

Abbreviations: ALP, alkaline phosphatase; ALT, alanine aminotransferase; AST, aspartate aminotransferase.
   Data from Refs.[28,30,57,59,61]

LIVER BIOPSY

Gross postmortem and exploratory laparotomy findings in cats infected with liver fluke may include gallbladder distension; wall thickening and necrosis; enlarged bile ducts; thickened, dilated, and tortuous common bile and cystic ducts; obstruction of the cystic or common bile duct; presence of liver flukes within the gall bladder and biliary tree; and mild to moderate hepatomegaly.[30,57,58,62]

Histopathological features of chronic cholangitis associated with liver fluke infections are summarized in **Table 3**.

TREATMENT

Praziquantel is effective against liver flukes.[30,48] Treatment of concurrent neutrophilic cholangitis may be indicated in individual cases (see **Table 4**).

PROGNOSIS

Although most cats remain asymptomatic, liver fluke infestation can be fatal.

Opisthorchiidae

Opisthorchiidae (*Opisthorchis* spp, *Clonorchis* spp, *Metorchis* spp, and *Amphimerus* spp) occur worldwide and prevalences of 30% to 50% in free roaming cats are common.[50,51] Reports of clinical disease in cats are rare but this may be underreported.

Clinical, laboratory and histopathology findings in cats infected with *Opisthorchis* spp, *Metorchis* spp, *Clonorchis* spp, and *Amphimerus* spp mirror those of *P fastosum* infections.[50,63–65] Treatment with praziquantel is effective.

SUMMARY AND DISCUSSION

Feline cholangitis includes diverse inflammatory liver diseases. Diagnosis of cholangitis, which underpins appropriate treatment, can be achieved by a logical step-wise approach to the patient. Prognosis depends on the disease process and individual patient factors but many cases can be rewarding to treat.

REFERENCES

1. Gagne JM, Weiss DJ, Armstrong PJ. Histopathologic evaluation of feline inflammatory liver disease. Vet Pathol 1996;33(5):521–6.
2. Hirose N, Uchida K, Kanemoto H, et al. A retrospective histopathological survey on canine and feline liver diseases at the University of Tokyo between 2006 and 2012. J Vet Med Sci 2014;76(7):1015–20.
3. Van den Ingh TSGAM, Cullen JM, Twedt DC, et al. Morphological classification of biliary disorders of the canine and feline liver. In: Rothuizen J, Bunch SE, Charles JA, et al, editors. WSAVA standards for clinical and histological diagnosis of canine and feline liver disease. World Small Animal Veterinary Association standardization group. Edinburgh (Scotland): Saunders Elsevier; 2006. p. 61–76.
4. Greiter-Wilke A, Scanziani E, Soldati S, et al. Association of *Helicobacter* with cholangiohepatitis in cats. J Vet Intern Med 2006;20:822–7.
5. Callahan Clark JE, Haddad JL, Brown DC, et al. Feline cholangitis: a necropsy study of 44 cats (1986-2008). J Feline Med Surg 2011;13(8):570–6.
6. Twedt DC, Cullen J, McCord K, et al. Evaluation of fluorescence in situ hybridization for the detection of bacteria in feline inflammatory liver disease. J Feline Med Surg 2014;16(2):109–17.

7. Brain PH, Barrs VR, Martin P, et al. Feline cholecystitis and acute neutrophilic cholangitis: clinical findings, bacterial isolates and response to treatment in six cases. J Feline Med Surg 2006;8:91–103.

8. Peters LM, Glanemann B, Garden OA, et al. Cytological findings of 140 bile samples from dogs and cats and associated clinical pathological data. J Vet Intern Med 2016;30:123–31.

9. Weiss DJ, Gagne JM, Armstrong PJ. Relationship between inflammatory hepatic disease and inflammatory bowel disease, pancreatitis and nephritis in cats. J Am Vet Med Assoc 1996;209(6):1114–6.

10. Sjödin S, Trowald-Wigh G, Fredriksson M. Identification of Helicobacter DNA in feline pancreas, liver, stomach, and duodenum: Comparison between findings in fresh and formalin-fixed paraffin-embedded tissue samples. Res Vet Sci 2011;91:e28–30.

11. Gagne JM, Armstrong PJ, Weiss DJ, et al. Clinical features of inflammatory liver disease in cats: 41 cases (1983-1993). J Am Vet Med Assoc 1999;214(4):513–6.

12. Hirsch VM, Doige CE. Suppurative cholangitis in cats. J Am Vet Med Assoc 1983; 182(11):1223–6.

13. Shaker EH, Zawie DA, Garvey MS, et al. Suppurative cholangiohepatitis in a cat. J Am Anim Hosp Assoc 1991;27:148–50.

14. Trehy MR, German AJ, Silvestrini P, et al. Hypercobalaminaemia is associated with hepatic and neoplastic disease in cats: a cross sectional study. BMC Vet Res 2014;10(1):1–16.

15. Simpson KW, Fyfe J, Cornetta A, et al. Subnormal concentrations of serum cobalamin (vitamin B12) in cats with gastrointestinal disease. J Vet Intern Med 2001; 15(1):26–32.

16. Marolf AJ, Leach L, Gibbons DS, et al. Ultrasonographic findings of feline cholangitis. J Am Anim Hosp Assoc 2012;48(1):36–42.

17. Oppliger S, Hartnack S, Reusch CE, et al. Agreement of serum feline pancreas-specific lipase and colorimetric lipase assays with pancreatic ultrasonographic findings in cats with suspicion of pancreatitis: 161 cases (2008-2012). J Am Vet Med Assoc 2014;244(9):1060–5.

18. Daniaux LA, Laurenson MP, Marks SL, et al. Ultrasonographic thickening of the muscularis propria in feline small intestinal small cell T-cell lymphoma and inflammatory bowel disease. J Feline Med Surg 2014;16(2):89–98.

19. Wagner KA, Hartmann FA, Trepanier LA. Bacterial culture results from liver, gallbladder, or bile in 248 dogs and cats evaluated for hepatobiliary disease: 1998–2003. J Vet Intern Med 2007;21:417–24.

20. Sung JY, Leung JWC, Olson ME, et al. Demonstration of transient bacterobilia by foreign body implantation in feline biliary tract. Dig Dis Sci 1991;36(7):943–8.

21. Sung JY, Olson ME, Leung JWC, et al. The sphincter of Oddi is the boundary of bacterial colonization of the feline biliary and the gastrointestinal tract. Microb Ecol Health Dis 1990;3:199–207.

22. Warren A, Center S, McDonough S, et al. Histopathologic features, immunophenotyping, clonality, and eubacterial fluorescence in situ hybridization in cats with lymphocytic cholangitis/cholangiohepatitis. Vet Pathol 2011;48(3):627–41.

23. Eich CS, Ludwig LL. The surgical treatment of cholelithiasis in cats: a study of nine cases. J Am Anim Hosp Assoc 2002;38:290–6.

24. Mayhew PD, Holt DE, McLear RC, et al. Pathogenesis and outcome of extrahepatic biliary obstruction in cats. J Small Anim Pract 2002;43(6):247–53.

25. Savary-Bataille KCM, Bunch SE, Spaulding KA, et al. Percutaneous ultrasound-guided cholecystocentesis in healthy cats. J Vet Intern Med 2003;17:298–303.

26. Lucke VM, Davies JD. Progressive lymphocytic cholangitis in the cat. J Small Anim Pract 1984;25:249–60.
27. Day MJ. Immunohistochemical characterization of the lesions of feline progressive lymphocytic cholangitis/cholangiohepatitis. J Comp Pathol 1998;119(2): 135–47.
28. Xavier FG, Morato GS, Righi DA, et al. Cystic liver disease related to high *Platynosomum fastosum* infection in a domestic cat. J Feline Med Surg 2007;9(1): 51–5.
29. Köster L, Shell L, Illanes O, et al. Percutaneous ultrasound-guided cholecystocentesis and bile analysis for the detection of *Platynosomum* spp.-induced cholangitis in cats. J Vet Intern Med 2016;30:787–93.
30. Haney DR, Christiansen JS, Toll J. Severe cholestatic liver disease secondary to liver fluke (*Platynosomum concinnum*) infection in three cats. J Am Anim Hosp Assoc 2006;42(3):234–7.
31. Costa Devoti C, Murtagh K, Batchelor D, et al. Exocrine pancreatic insufficiency with concurrent pancreatitis, inflammatory bowel disease and cholangiohepatitis in a cat. Vet Rec Case Rep 2015;3:e000237.
32. Mayhew PD, Weisse CW. Treatment of pancreatitis-associated extrahepatic biliary tract obstruction by choledochal stenting in seven cats. J Small Anim Pract 2008;49(3):133–8.
33. Batchelor DJ, Devauchelle P, Elliott J, et al. Mechanisms, causes, investigation and management of vomiting disorders in cats: a literature review. J Feline Med Surg 2013;15(4):237–65.
34. Quimby JM, Lunn KF. Mirtazapine as an appetite stimulant and anti-emetic in cats with chronic kidney disease: a masked placebo-controlled crossover clinical trial. Vet J 2013;197(3):651–5.
35. Center SA, Randolph JF, Warner KL, et al. The effects of S-adenosylmethionine on clinical pathology and redox potential in the red blood cell, liver, and bile of clinically normal cats. J Vet Intern Med 2005;19(3):303–14.
36. Avizeh R, Najafzadeh H, Razijalali M, et al. Evaluation of prophylactic and therapeutic effects of silymarin and N-acetylcysteine in acetaminophen-induced hepatotoxicity in cats. J Vet Pharmacol Ther 2010;33(1):95–9.
37. Nicholson BT, Center SA, Randolph JF, et al. Effects of oral ursodeoxycholic acid in healthy cats on clinicopathological parameters, serum bile acids and light microscopic and ultrastructural features of the liver. Res Vet Sci 1996;61(3):258–62.
38. Plumb DC. Plumb's veterinary drug handbook. 8th edition. New York: John Wiley & Sons Inc; 2015.
39. Sergeeff JS, Armstrong PJ, Bunch SE. Hepatic abscesses in cats: 14 cases (1985–2002). J Vet Intern Med 2004;18:295–300.
40. Otte CMA, Penning LC, Rothuizen J, et al. Retrospective comparison of prednisolone and ursodeoxycholic acid for the treatment of feline lymphocytic cholangitis. Vet J 2013;195(2):205–9.
41. Fragkou FC, Adamama-Moraitou KK, Poutahidis T, et al. Prevalence and clinicopathological features of triaditis in a prospective case series of symptomatic and asymptomatic cats. J Vet Intern Med 2016;30(4):1031–45.
42. Otte CMA, Pérez Gutiérrez O, Favier RP, et al. Detection of bacterial DNA in bile of cats with lymphocytic cholangitis. Vet Microbiol 2012;156(1–2):217–21.
43. Boomkens SY, Kusters JG, Hoffmann G, et al. Detection of *Helicobacter pylori* in bile of cats. FEMS Immunol Med Microbiol 2004;42:307–11.

44. Otte CMA, Rothuizen J, Favier RP, et al. A morphological and immunohistochemical study of the effects of prednisolone or ursodeoxycholic acid on liver histology in feline lymphocytic cholangitis. J Feline Med Surg 2014;16(10):796–804.

45. Prasse KW, Mahaffey EA, DeNovo R, et al. Chronic lymphocytic cholangitis in three cats. Vet Pathol 1982;19(2):99–108.

46. Nakayama H, Uchida K, Lee S, et al. Three cases of feline sclerosing lymphocytic cholangitis. J Vet Med Sci 1992;54(4):769–71.

47. Weiss DJ, Gagne JM, Armstrong PJ. Characterization of portal lymphocytic infiltrates in feline liver. Vet Clin Pathol 1995;24(3):91–5.

48. Basu AK, Charles RA. A review of the cat liver fluke *Platynosomum fastosum* Kossack, 1910 (Trematoda: Dicrocoeliidae). Vet Parasitol 2014;200(1–2):1–7.

49. King S, Scholz T. Trematodes of the family Opisthorchiidae: a minireview. Korean J Parasitol 2001;39(3):209–21.

50. Aunpromma S, Tangkawattana P, Papirom P, et al. High prevalence of *Opisthorchis viverrini* infection in reservoir hosts in four districts of Khon Kaen Province, an opisthorchiasis endemic area of Thailand. Parasitol Int 2012;37(1):60–4.

51. Lin R, Tang J, Zhou D, et al. Prevalence of *Clonorchis sinensis* infection in dogs and cats in subtropical southern China. Parasit Vectors 2011;4(0):180.

52. Pinto HA, Mati VLT, de Melo AL. New insights into the life cycle of *Platynosomum* (Trematoda: Dicrocoeliidae). Parasitol Res 2014;113:2701–7.

53. Krecek RC, Moura L, Lucas H, et al. Parasites of stray cats (*Felis domesticus* L., 1758) on St. Kitts, West Indies. Vet Parasitol 2010;172:147–9.

54. Rodríguez-Vivas RI, Williams JJ, Quijao-Novelo AG, et al. Prevalence, abundance and risk factors of liver fluke (*Platynosomum concinnum*) infection in cats in Mexico. Vet Rec 2004;154(22):693–4.

55. Rocha NO, Portela RW, Camargo SS, et al. Comparison of two coproparasitological techniques for the detection of *Platynosomum* spp. infection in cats. Vet Parasitol 2014;204(3–4):392–5.

56. Salomão M, Souza-Dantas LM, Mendes-de-Almeida F, et al. Ultrasonography in hepatobiliary evaluation of domestic cats (*Felis catus*, L., 1758) infected by *Platynosomum looss*, 1907. Int J Appl Res Vet Med 2005;3(3):271–9.

57. Taylor D, Perri SF. Experimental infection of cats with the liver fluke *Platynosomum concinnum*. Am J Vet Res 1977;38(1):51–4.

58. Powell KW. Liver fluke infection in a cat. J Am Vet Med Assoc 1970;156(2):218.

59. Barriga OO, Caputo CA, Weisbrode SE. Liver flukes (*Platynosomum concinnum*) in an Ohio cat. J Am Vet Med Assoc 1981;179(9):901–3.

60. Soto JA, Villalobos A, Arraga de Alvarado CM, et al. Obstructive biliary cirrhosis in a cat due to *Platynosomum fastosum* infection. Revista Cientifica 1991;1(2): 16–9.

61. Ramos RAN, Lima VFS, Monteiro MFM, et al. New insights into diagnosis of *Platynosomum fastosum* (Trematoda: Dicrocoeliidae) in cats. Parasitol Res 2016; 115:479–82.

62. Andrade RLFS, Dantas AFM, Pimentel LA, et al. *Platynosomum fastosum*-induced cholangiocarcinomas in cats. Vet Parasitol 2012;190:277–80.

63. Watson TG, Croll NA. Clinical changes caused by the liver fluke *Metorchis conjunctus* in cats. Vet Pathol 1981;18(6):778–85.

64. Lewis DT, Malone JB, Taboada J, et al. Cholangiohepatitis and choledochectasia associated with *Amphimerus pseudofelineus* in a cat. J Am Anim Hosp Assoc 1991;27(2):156–62.

65. Chang HP. Pathological changes in the intrahepatic bile ducts of cats (*Felis catus*) infested with *Clonorchis sinensis*. J Pathol Bacteriol 1965;89(0):357–64.

Hepatobiliary Neoplasia

Laura E. Selmic, MPH

KEYWORDS

- Biliary • Dog • Cat • Hepatic • Hepatobiliary • Liver • Neoplasia

KEY POINTS

- Hepatobiliary neoplasia is uncommon in dogs and cats.
- Metastatic neoplasia arises more commonly than primary hepatobiliary neoplasia.
- Older animals are generally affected and may show nonspecific clinical signs.
- Ultrasound imaging can help to characterize liver lesions and guide sampling with fine needle aspiration. Treatment for massive liver tumor morphology involves liver lobectomy.
- Prognosis depends on the tumor morphology, type, and stage, but can be good for cats and dogs with massive hepatocellular tumors; animals experience prolonged survival and low recurrence rates.

INTRODUCTION

Based on necropsy studies hepatobiliary neoplasia is uncommon in dogs and cats, representing only 0.6% to 1.3% and 1.5% to 2.3% of all cancer in dogs and cats, respectively.[1,2] Tumors found in the hepatobiliary system may be primary (arising in the liver, gallbladder, or bile ducts) or secondary (arising in other organs and metastasizing to the liver). In dogs and cats, metastatic liver tumors are diagnosed more commonly than primary tumors.[3,4] In dogs, malignant tumors of the gastrointestinal tract, spleen and pancreas can commonly spread to the liver owing to its blood supply from the portal venous system draining these organs. Primary tumors can arise from different cell types present in the hepatobiliary system and the resultant tumors be classified as being hepatocellular, bile duct, neuroendocrine (or carcinoid), or mesenchymal (**Box 1**). These primary tumors can be malignant or benign. Other processes can affect the liver including lymphoma, disseminated systemic histiocytosis, mastocytosis and myelolipomas.

Primary liver tumors can be classified morphologically, as being

1. Massive: a single large tumor involving only one liver lobe;
2. Nodular: multiple tumors located in different liver lobes; or
3. Diffuse: either multifocal nodular changes in different liver lobes or diffuse changes throughout the liver.

The author has nothing to disclose.
Department of Veterinary Clinical Medicine, College of Veterinary Medicine, University of Illinois Urbana-Champaign, 1008 West Hazelwood Drive, Urbana, IL 61802, USA
E-mail address: lselmic@illinois.edu

Vet Clin Small Anim 47 (2017) 725–735
http://dx.doi.org/10.1016/j.cvsm.2016.11.016
0195-5616/17/© 2016 Elsevier Inc. All rights reserved.

Box 1
Primary hepatobiliary tumor types and examples

1. Hepatocellular
   a. Hepatic adenoma
   b. Hepatocellular carcinoma
   c. Hepatoblastoma

2. Biliary
   a. Biliary adenoma (or cystadenoma)
   b. Biliary carcinoma

3. Neuroendocrine
   a. Neuroendocrine carcinoma or carcinoid

4. Mesenchymal
   a. Hemangiosarcoma
   b. Leiomyosarcoma
   c. Fibrosarcoma
   d. Osteosarcoma
   e. Malignant mesenchymoma
   f. Chondrosarcoma

The tumor type, morphologic classification, and disease staging results help to determine treatment options and prognosis.

HISTORY AND PHYSICAL EXAMINATION

The majority of dogs and cats diagnosed with malignant hepatobiliary tumors are greater than 10 years old.[1,5] This is in contrast with the findings of 1 study, where dogs with liver carcinoids are more frequently diagnosed when younger than 10 years.[1] There have been no sex or breed predispositions identified for hepatocellular carcinoma (HCC) in dogs, but some studies have indicated overrepresentation of male dogs.[1,6,7] A recent case-control study has suggested vacuolar hepatopathy in Scottish Terriers could be linked to adrenal steroidogenesis and predispose dogs to HCC.[8]

Many dogs and cats with hepatobiliary neoplasia have clinical signs at diagnosis; clinical signs are more likely to be present if there is malignant disease. Clinical signs of hepatobiliary tumors may be vague and nonspecific and include anorexia, weight loss, lethargy, polydipsia, polyuria, ascites, vomiting, and diarrhea.[1–7,9–12] In cats, alopecia has been reported to be associated with hepatocellular and bile duct carcinomas.[13,14] Other, more specific clinical signs can be present including hepatomegaly and icterus.[1–4,6,7,9–12] Icterus can be seen more commonly in dogs with extrahepatic biliary carcinomas and diffuse neuroendocrine carcinomas.[1,11] Seizures, weakness, and ataxia uncommonly arise and might be owing to hepatic encephalopathy, a paraneoplastic syndrome causing hypoglycemia, or metastases to the central nervous system.[1,6,15] Additionally, lethargy, weakness, and ataxia could result from hemoperitoneum owing to rupture of the liver mass.[16,17] Although the physical examination may be unremarkable in some cases, a cranial abdominal mass may be palpable in up to 75% of dogs and cats if a massive primary liver tumor is present.[1–4,6,7,9–12] However, the absence of a cranial abdominal mass cannot be used to rule out hepatobiliary neoplasia because liver masses can be contained within the costal arch in deep-chested breeds and not be palpable, or alternatively nodular or diffuse disease could be present without palpable abnormality.[1–4,6,7,9–12]

DIAGNOSTIC EVALUATION
Laboratory Test Findings

It is common for dogs and cats with hepatobiliary neoplasia to have hematologic and biochemical abnormalities; however, often the changes are nonspecific. Anemia may be present in up to 57% of dogs and leukocytosis with neutrophilia in up to 90% of dogs and 28% of cats with hepatic neoplasia.[1,7,9] Leukocytosis may result from inflammation and necrosis that can occur with massive liver tumors. Most often, the anemia is mild and nonregenerative.[1,7] Possible causes could include cancer-associated anemia or anemia of chronic disease, sequestration, microangiopathic destruction, or iron deficiency.[18] Anemia can commonly occur in combination with thrombocytopenia in dogs and cats with hemangiosarcoma,[19] whereas thrombocytosis (>500 × 10^3/µL) has been reported in 46% of dogs with HCC.[7]

Coagulation profile abnormalities have been reported in dogs; it follows that it is advisable to evaluate this laboratory parameter before invasive diagnostic or therapeutic procedures.[7,20] Liver enzymes are increased frequently at presentation, but are not specific for hepatobiliary neoplasia.[1,3,7,21–23] In cats, 1 study found higher serum alanine aminotransferase activities, aspartate aminotransferase activities, and total bilirubin concentrations in cats with malignant compared with benign tumors, although this finding has not been evaluated further or replicated and thus cannot be used to differentiate benign and malignant disease.[10] Other biochemical abnormalities can be present, including hypoalbuminemia, hyperglobulinemia, and increased serum bile acid cocontrations.[1,3,7,22,24,25] In addition, increased total serum bilirubin is present in up to 20% of dogs with hepatic neoplasia.[1] Hypoglycemia has been documented rarely in association with HCC, hepatic leiomyosarcoma, or hemangiosarcoma in dogs.[1,6,15] Azotemia was a common biochemical abnormality in cats with hepatic neoplasia in 1 report and may be a reflection of the age of the cats at diagnosis.[9] In addition, other concurrent disorders have been reported to confound the clinicopathologic findings in cats with HCC.[5]

IMAGING FINDINGS

Abdominal radiography may indicate the presence of a cranial abdominal mass in dogs or cats with massive liver tumor morphology or other cranial abdominal organ masses.[26] Abdominal ultrasound imaging is more useful than abdominal radiography for identification and characterization of hepatobiliary neoplasia. Ultrasound examination can determine the morphology (massive, nodular, or diffuse) and size of tumors, the affected side of the liver, and the proximity of lesions to the gallbladder and vena cava in cats and dogs.[7,27] The ability of ultrasound imaging distinguish between benign liver disease and tumors has been evaluated, and many studies have shown marked variability in the ultrasonographic appearance of all diagnoses (malignant and benign), with no specific features that were consistent across all studies.[28–32] Enhanced ultrasound techniques such as harmonic ultrasound examination have been evaluated to see if they can help to differentiate between malignant and benign neoplasia.[33–36] Histopathologic assessment remains the gold standard for the diagnosis of hepatobiliary malignancy.

Ultrasound imaging can be used for abdominal staging to evaluate for metastases. The likelihood of metastases to local lymph nodes, peritoneum, and lungs depends on the tumor type. For all malignant epithelial tumors, local lymph node spread can occur. Spread to other organs in the abdomen is possible and splenic metastases are seen most often from sarcomas.[1] Peritoneal carcinomatosis occurs most commonly with biliary carcinoma and carcinoids.[1] Thoracic radiography (3-view) or computed tomography scanning is indicated after the detection of a liver mass to rule out pulmonary metastases. Central nervous system metastases have also been reported in dogs.[1]

Ultrasound imaging can also be used to guide fine needle aspiration or needle core biopsy of a liver mass to obtain cells or tissue for diagnosis of hepatobiliary neoplasia.[32,37,38] This should only be performed after the evaluation of platelets and coagulation profile given mild to moderate bleeding is a complication that can occur in 5% of cases.[37] Fine needle aspiration can help to differentiate between benign and malignant liver processes. It has been reported to provide an accurate diagnosis in up to 60% of cases; this may be owing in part to the fact that malignant neoplasms differ in their exfoliative nature (round cell tumors and epithelial tumors being more exfoliative than mesenchymal tumors).[39] If the cytologic result indicates neoplasia, clinicians can have a high confidence in the diagnosis, but in the absence of this result neoplasia cannot be ruled out.[38] Percutaneous needle core biopsies are more invasive, but are associated with a greater likelihood of correct diagnosis (up to 90%).[37] Other, more invasive biopsy techniques such as laparoscopic or keyhole laparotomy can be performed to obtain larger liver biopsy specimens (see Jonathan A. Lidbury's article, "Getting the Most Out of Liver Biopsy," in this issue). Liver biopsy is not always indicated before surgery for treatment of a massive hepatic tumors given excisional biopsy can be performed for diagnosis and treatment.

Advanced imaging techniques, such as computed tomography and MRI, can be used to characterize the liver lesion(s). These imaging techniques have the benefit of being able to establish position of liver lesions in relation to important anatomic features, which is beneficial for surgical planning for the resection of massive hepatocellular tumors (**Fig. 1**). It is possible that additional lesions could be detected. It is important that patients are not deemed to be unsuitable candidates for surgery based

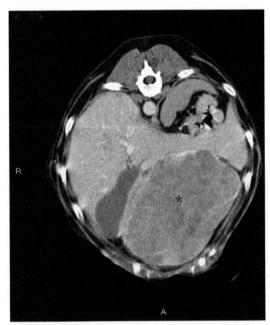

Fig. 1. Transverse computed tomography image of a dog with a hepatocellular carcinoma of the left medial liver lobe (*red asterisk*).

on the presence of such lesions because they could be benign, for example, owing to nodular hyperplasia. If further lesions are identified the appearance on imaging and sampling with cytology may be used to discern their relative importance. Studies have identified characteristics that more commonly occur with HCC including large size, heterogenous pattern with hyperintensity, isointensity, and hypointensity on arterial and portal phases central, and marginal contrast enhancement in the arterial phase.[40,41] One study found MRI has a high sensitivity and specificity for differentiation of malignant and benign focal liver masses.[42]

TREATMENT AND PROGNOSIS OF SELECTED TUMOR TYPES
Hepatocellular Tumors

Types of hepatocellular tumors that can arise include hepatic adenoma or hepatoma, HCC, and hepatoblastoma. Hepatoblastomas are very rare tumors with only 1 dog and 1 cat reported in the literature; these tumors arise from the putative pluripotent stem cells of the liver.[43,44] HCC is the most common primary hepatic tumor in the dog, whereas the benign tumor–hepatic adenoma is the most common hepatocellular tumor in the cat.[1,2,10] The massive morphology is the most common (61%), then nodular (29%), and diffuse (10%).[6]

Surgery is the treatment of choice for all liver tumors with massive morphology (**Fig. 2**). Ultrasound or advanced imaging techniques can help to assess the liver tumor location and relation to important anatomic structures, such as the caudal vena cava (**Fig. 3**). It is important that the surgeon has a good knowledge of the anatomy and techniques that can be used for liver lobectomy. Finger fracture, mass ligation, mattress sutures, bipolar vessel sealing device, surgical stapling device, and hilar dissection can be used to excise the affected liver lobe. The finger fracture technique uses digital fracture of the liver parenchyma to allow isolation and ligation of the liver blood vessels and bile ducts; this technique should only be attempted for small liver lesions. Mass ligation for complete lobectomy involves placement of a circumferential ligature around the liver hilus. This technique is not recommended for large dogs, or central or right divisional liver tumors because the hilus is large and vessels and bile ducts may not be attenuated sufficiently by this method increasing the risk of complications, such as hemorrhage or bile leakage. Surgical stapling devices are used

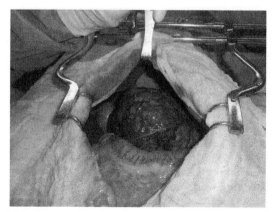

Fig. 2. Intraoperative photograph of dog (from **Fig. 1**) showing a hepatocellular carcinoma of the left medial liver lobe. The left medial liver lobe was removed using a surgical stapling device.

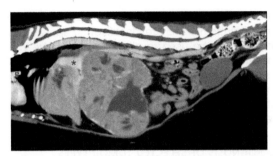

Fig. 3. Sagittal reconstructed computed tomography image of a cat with hepatocellular carcinoma of the caudate lobe. This image shows the relation of the massive hepatocellular carcinoma to the caudal vena cava and compression of the caudal vena cava (*red asterisks*).

commonly to perform complete liver lobectomy; these devices place overlapping rows of staples to attenuate vascular and biliary structures within the hilus of the liver lobe. Right-sided tumors can be more challenging to resect, requiring the surgeon to have a solid anatomic knowledge specifically of the relation of the right-sided liver lobes to the vena cava and the course of the vena cava.

In 1 case series evaluating 42 dogs with massive HCC treated with liver lobectomy, complications of surgery occurred in 28.6% of dogs and intraoperative mortality in 4.8%.[7] Complications of liver lobectomy that have been reported include perioperative hemorrhage (5% of cases), impairment of the adjacent liver lobe blood supply, transient hypoglycemia, portal hypertension, and liver dysfunction.[7,45–47] The prognosis for dogs with massive HCC was improved significantly with surgical resection of the affected liver lobe; the median survival time of dogs (n = 6) without surgery was 270 days and the median survival time was not reached at 1460 days in dogs that underwent surgery (n = 42).[7] Dogs with right-sided liver tumors had a greater likelihood of intraoperative death but a good prognosis if they survived the surgery.[7] Additional factors reported to be associated with poor likelihood of survival after liver lobectomy for primary liver tumors in dogs have included lethargy and tachypnea at presentation, experiencing anesthetic complications, and high serum alanine aminotransferase and aspartate aminotransferase activities.[7,48] These studies only represented fewer than 160 dogs with primary liver tumors and low numbers of dogs died of the disease so the clinical relevance of these prognostic factors is uncertain.

Overall, the prognosis for dogs with massive HCC is good with low reported recurrence rates (0%–13%).[1,7,22] The metastatic rates reported have been variable (0%–61%), with the lowest rates in clinical reports and the highest rates in necropsy reports, which likely represents selection bias with euthanasia of patients that were more symptomatic and had advanced disease.[1,7,21,22] The outcome in cats after liver lobectomy for HCC has only been reported in a few cases, so the benefit is unclear; however, the median survival time for 6 cats that had liver lobectomy in one study was prolonged at 2.4 years (range, 1.0–6.5).[5]

In the event that a massive primary liver tumor is unresectable, other treatments have been reported including chemoembolization, radiation therapy, and chemotherapy.[49–52] The biological behavior of diffuse and nodular forms is thought to be more aggressive compared with the massive form; with a higher metastatic rate seen with diffuse (100%) and nodular forms (93%) compared with massive (37%) in one necropsy study.[6] Treatment for diffuse or nodular forms could include surgical resection of liver nodules for nodular types if possible, chemoembolization or chemotherapy.[49,53] In human medicine, HCC is generally regarded as chemoresistant with low response rates of 25% or less to various single agent and multiagent protocols.[45,54] One study reported the use of gemcitabine for dogs with HCC with all morphologies. The dogs in this study experienced minimal toxicity, with median survival times in dogs with massive morphology (1339 days), nodular disease (983 days), and diffuse disease (113 days).[49]

Bile Duct Tumors

Bile duct tumors have been reported to be the most common primary hepatic tumors in cats (excluding lymphoma).[2,9,10] Bile duct adenomas can be present as massive lesions arising in a single liver lobe or as multifocal nodules. If the tumor is confined to 1 or 2 lobes, treatment with liver lobectomy can be performed in cats, resulting in a very good prognosis with no reports of recurrence or malignant transformation.[10,55] Bile duct carcinomas can be treated with liver lobectomy if they arise in 1 liver lobe (massive), but frequently they are multifocal or diffuse morphologies.[1,2,11] The outcome for this tumor is much worse, with median survival times of often less than 6 months.[10,56]

Neuroendocrine Tumors

Hepatic carcinoid tumors arise from the neuroectodermal cells or the amine precursor uptake and decarboxylation cells. Carcinoids in dogs and cats present most commonly with diffuse disease throughout the liver and, less commonly, nodular changes.[1,12,57] This tumor type is often associated with a high metastatic rate (up to 93%) in dogs, with metastases to the local lymph nodes and peritoneum being the most common sites.[1,12] With these factors present, surgical resection is rarely a treatment option and the efficacy of radiation therapy and chemotherapy is unknown.

Mesenchymal Tumors

Mesenchymal tumors only comprise up to 13% of all primary hepatic tumors in the dog.[1,21] Mesenchymal tumors may manifest as massive solitary liver masses and as such may be amenable for surgical resection with complete liver lobectomy (**Fig. 4**). However, hepatic sarcomas are often aggressive, either presenting with nodular or diffuse morphology at diagnosis or metastases at diagnosis (up to 57%).[1] The most common locations of metastases are the spleen, local lymph node, and lungs.[1] In cats, hemangiosarcoma has been reported as the most frequent sarcoma found in

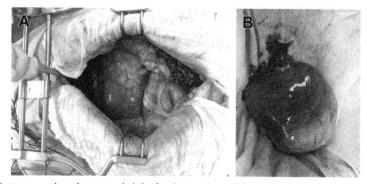

Fig. 4. Intraoperative photograph (*A*) of a dog with a left lateral liver lobe undifferentiated sarcoma. The left medial liver lobe was excised using a surgical stapling device. Image of excised tumor (*B*).

the liver and is most frequently seen as diffuse nodular disease with intraabdominal metastases or as multifocal disease, which is common (in up to 77% cats).[2,19] Thus, primary hepatic sarcoma is associated with a poor prognosis. The efficacy of chemotherapy for primary hepatic sarcoma has not been studied primarily, but the response of sarcomas to chemotherapy is generally poor.

MYELOLIPOMA

Myelolipomas are benign tumors that can arise in the liver in cats with chronic hypoxia proposed as an etiologic factor.[45] These tumors are composed of mature adipose tissue combined with hematopoietic elements.[45] Surgical resection results in an excellent prognosis with prolonged survival and no recurrence reported to date.[45]

SUMMARY

Hepatobiliary neoplasia is uncommon in dogs and cats. Metastatic neoplasia arises more commonly than primary hepatobiliary neoplasia. Older animals are generally affected and may show nonspecific clinical signs, which are often gastrointestinal in nature. Animals may have increased serum liver enzyme activities. Ultrasound imaging can help to characterize liver lesions and guide sampling with fine needle aspiration. Treatment for the massive liver tumor morphology involves liver lobectomy. The prognosis depends on the tumor morphology, type, and stage, but can be good for cats and dogs with massive hepatocellular tumors, with animals experiencing prolonged survival and low recurrence rates.

REFERENCES

1. Patnaik AK, Hurvitz AI, Lieberman PH. Canine hepatic neoplasms: a clinicopathologic study. Vet Pathol 1980;17(5):553–64.
2. Patnaik AK. A morphologic and immunocytochemical study of hepatic neoplasms in cats. Vet Pathol 1992;29(5):405–15.
3. Strombeck DR. Clinicopathologic features of primary and metastatic neoplastic disease of the liver in dogs. J Am Vet Med Assoc 1978;173(3):267–9.
4. Cullen JM, Popp JA. Tumors of the liver and gall bladder. In: Meuten DJ, editor. Tumors in domestic animals. 4th edition. Ames (IA): Iowa State Press; 2002. p. 483–508.
5. Goussev SA, Center SA, Randolph JF, et al. Clinical Characteristics of Hepatocellular Carcinoma in 19 cats from a Single Institution (1980-2013). J Am Anim Hosp Assoc 2016;52(1):36–41.
6. Patnaik AK, Hurvitz AI, Lieberman PH, et al. Canine hepatocellular carcinoma. Vet Pathol 1981;18(4):427–38.
7. Liptak JM, Dernell WS, Monnet E, et al. Massive hepatocellular carcinoma in dogs: 48 cases (1992-2002). J Am Vet Med Assoc 2004;225(8):1225–30.
8. Cortright CC, Center SA, Randolph JF, et al. Clinical features of progressive vacuolar hepatopathy in Scottish Terriers with and without hepatocellular carcinoma: 114 cases (1980-2013). J Am Vet Med Assoc 2014;245(7):797–808.
9. Post G, Patnaik AK. Nonhematopoietic hepatic neoplasms in cats: 21 cases (1983-1988). J Am Vet Med Assoc 1992;201(7):1080–2.
10. Lawrence HJ, Erb HN, Harvey HJ. Nonlymphomatous hepatobiliary masses in cats: 41 cases (1972 to 1991). Vet Surg 1994;23(5):365–8.
11. Patnaik AK, Hurvitz AI, Lieberman PH, et al. Canine bile duct carcinoma. Vet Pathol 1981;18(4):439–44.

12. Patnaik AK, Lieberman PH, Hurvitz AI, et al. Canine hepatic carcinoids. Vet Pathol 1981;18(4):445–53.

13. Marconato L, Albanese F, Viacava P, et al. Paraneoplastic alopecia associated with hepatocellular carcinoma in a cat. Vet Dermatol 2007;18(4):267–71.

14. Pascal-Tenorio A, Olivry T, Gross TL, et al. Paraneoplastic alopecia associated with internal malignancies in the cat. Vet Dermatol 1997;8:47–52.

15. Leifer CE, Peterson ME, Matus RE, et al. Hypoglycemia associated with nonislet cell tumor in 13 dogs. J Am Vet Med Assoc 1985;186(1):53–5.

16. Aronsohn MG, Dubiel B, Roberts B, et al. Prognosis for acute nontraumatic hemoperitoneum in the dog: a retrospective analysis of 60 cases (2003-2006). J Am Anim Hosp Assoc 2009;45(2):72–7.

17. Culp WT, Weisse C, Kellogg ME, et al. Spontaneous hemoperitoneum in cats: 65 cases (1994-2006). J Am Vet Med Assoc 2010;236(9):978–82.

18. Abrams-Ogg A. 191 Nonregenerative Anemia. In: Ettinger SJ, Feldman EC, editors. Textbook of veterinary internal medicine. St Louis (MO): Elsevier; 2010. p. 788–97.

19. Culp WT, Drobatz KJ, Glassman MM, et al. Feline visceral hemangiosarcoma. J Vet Intern Med 2008;22(1):148–52.

20. Badylak SF, Dodds WJ, Van Vleet JF. Plasma coagulation factor abnormalities in dogs with naturally occurring hepatic disease. Am J Vet Res 1983;44(12): 2336–40.

21. Trigo FJ, Thompson H, Breeze RG, et al. The pathology of liver tumours in the dog. J Comp Pathol 1982;92(1):21–39.

22. Kosovsky JE, Manfra-Marretta S, Matthiesen DT. Results of partial hepatectomy in 18 dogs with hepatocellular carcinoma. J Am Anim Hosp Assoc 1989;25:203–6.

23. Acheson MB, Patton RG, Howisey RL, et al. Histologic correlation of image-guided core biopsy with excisional biopsy of nonpalpable breast lesions. Arch Surg 1997;132(8):815–8 [discussion: 819–21].

24. Center SA, Slater MR, Manwarren T, et al. Diagnostic efficacy of serum alkaline phosphatase and gamma-glutamyl transferase in dogs with histologically confirmed hepatobiliary disease: 270 cases (1980-1990). J Am Vet Med Assoc 1992;201(8):1258–64.

25. Center SA, Baldwin BH, Erb HN, et al. Bile acid concentrations in the diagnosis of hepatobiliary disease in the dog. J Am Vet Med Assoc 1985;187(9):935–40.

26. Evans SM. The radiographic appearance of primary liver neoplasia in dogs. Vet Radiol 1987;28(6):192–6.

27. Wormser C, Reetz JA, Giuffrida MA. Diagnostic accuracy of ultrasound to predict the location of solitary hepatic masses in dogs. Vet Surg 2016;45(2):208–13.

28. Nyland TG, Koblik PD, Tellyer SE. Ultrasonographic evaluation of biliary cystadenomas in cats. Vet Radiol Ultrasound 1999;40(3):300–6.

29. Feeney DA, Johnston GR, Hardy RM. Two-dimensional, gray-scale ultrasonography for assessment of hepatic and splenic neoplasia in the dog and cat. J Am Vet Med Assoc 1984;184(1):68–81.

30. Voros K, Vrabely T, Papp L, et al. Correlation of ultrasonographic and pathomorphological findings in canine hepatic diseases. J Small Anim Pract 1991;32: 627–34.

31. Newell SM, Selcer BA, Girard E, et al. Correlations between ultrasonographic findings and specific hepatic diseases in cats: 72 cases (1985-1997). J Am Vet Med Assoc 1998;213(1):94–8.

32. Leveille R, Partington BP, Biller DS, et al. Complications after ultrasound-guided biopsy of abdominal structures in dogs and cats: 246 cases (1984-1991). J Am Vet Med Assoc 1993;203(3):413–5.

33. O'Brien RT, Iani M, Matheson J, et al. Contrast harmonic ultrasound of spontaneous liver nodules in 32 dogs. Vet Radiol Ultrasound 2004;45(6):547–53.

34. O'Brien RT. Improved detection of metastatic hepatic hemangiosarcoma nodules with contrast ultrasound in three dogs. Vet Radiol Ultrasound 2007;48(2):146–8.

35. Nakamura K, Takagi S, Sasaki N, et al. Contrast-enhanced ultrasonography for characterization of canine focal liver lesions. Vet Radiol Ultrasound 2010;51(1):79–85.

36. Ivancic M, Long F, Seiler GS. Contrast harmonic ultrasonography of splenic masses and associated liver nodules in dogs. J Am Vet Med Assoc 2009;234(1):88–94.

37. Barr F. Percutaneous biopsy of abdominal organs under ultrasound guidance. J Small Anim Pract 1995;36(3):105–13.

38. Bahr KL, Sharkey LC, Murakami T, et al. Accuracy of US-guided FNA of focal liver lesions in dogs: 140 cases (2005-2008). J Am Anim Hosp Assoc 2013;49(3):190–6.

39. Roth L. Comparison of liver cytology and biopsy diagnoses in dogs and cats: 56 cases. Vet Clin Pathol 2001;30(1):35–8.

40. Fukushima K, Kanemoto H, Ohno K, et al. CT characteristics of primary hepatic mass lesions in dogs. Vet Radiol Ultrasound 2012;53(3):252–7.

41. Kutara K, Seki M, Ishikawa C, et al. Triple-phase helical computed tomography in dogs with hepatic masses. Vet Radiol Ultrasound 2014;55(1):7–15.

42. Clifford CA, Pretorius ES, Weisse C, et al. Magnetic resonance imaging of focal splenic and hepatic lesions in the dog. J Vet Intern Med 2004;18(3):330–8.

43. Ano N, Ozaki K, Nomura K, et al. Hepatoblastoma in a cat. Vet Pathol 2011;48(5):1020–3.

44. Shiga A, Shirota K, Shida T, et al. Hepatoblastoma in a dog. J Vet Med Sci 1997;59(12):1167–70.

45. Liptak JM. Hepatobiliary tumors. In: Withrow SJ, Vail DM, Page RL, editors. Withrow & MacEwen's small animal clinical oncology. 5th edition. St Louis (Missouri): Saunders Elsevier; 2013. p. 405–10.

46. Mayhew PD, Weisse C. Liver and biliary system. In: Tobias KM, Johnson SA, editors. Veterinary surgery small animal. vol. 1. St Louis (MO): Elsevier; 2012. p. 1601–23.

47. May LR, Mehler SJ. Complications of hepatic surgery in companion animals. Vet Clin North Am Small Anim Pract 2011;41(5):935–48, vi.

48. Kinsey JR, Gilson SD, Hauptman J, et al. Factors associated with long-term survival in dogs undergoing liver lobectomy as treatment for liver tumors. Can Vet J 2015;56(6):598–604.

49. Elpiner AK, Brodsky EM, Hazzah TN, et al. Single-agent gemcitabine chemotherapy in dogs with hepatocellular carcinomas. Vet Comp Oncol 2011;9(4):260–8.

50. Weisse C, Clifford CA, Holt D, et al. Percutaneous arterial embolization and chemoembolization for treatment of benign and malignant tumors in three dogs and a goat. J Am Vet Med Assoc 2002;221(10):1430–6, 1419.

51. Iwai S, Okano S, Chikazawa S, et al. Transcatheter arterial embolization for treatment of hepatocellular carcinoma in a cat. J Am Vet Med Assoc 2015;247(11):1299–302.

52. Mori T, Ito Y, Kawabe M, et al. Three-dimensional conformal radiation therapy for inoperable massive hepatocellular carcinoma in six dogs. J Small Anim Pract 2015;56(7):441–5.
53. Weisse C. Hepatic chemoembolization: a novel regional therapy. Vet Clin North Am Small Anim Pract 2009;39(3):627–30.
54. Bartlett DI, Carr BI, Marsh JW. Cancer of the liver. In: DeVita VT Jr, Lawrence TS, Rosenberg SA, editors. DeVita, Hellman and Rosenberg's cancer: principles & practice of oncology. 8th edition. Philadelphia: Lippincott, Williams & Wilkins; 2008. p. 1124–50.
55. Trout NJ, Berg RJ, McMillan MC, et al. Surgical treatment of hepatobiliary cystadenomas in cats: five cases (1988-1993). J Am Vet Med Assoc 1995;206(4): 505–7.
56. Fry PD, Rest JR. Partial hepatectomy in two dogs. J Small Anim Pract 1993;34(4): 192–5.
57. Patnaik AK, Lieberman PH, Erlandson RA, et al. Hepatobiliary neuroendocrine carcinoma in cats: a clinicopathologic, immunohistochemical, and ultrastructural study of 17 cases. Vet Pathol 2005;42(3):331–7.

Index

Note: Page numbers of article titles are in **boldface** type.

Vet Clin Small Anim 47 (2017) 737–751
http://dx.doi.org/10.1016/S0195-5616(17)30018-9
0195-5616/17

Moving?

Make sure your subscription moves with you!

To notify us of your new address, find your **Clinics Account Number** (located on your mailing label above your name), and contact customer service at:

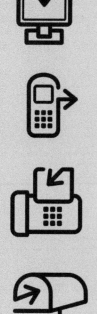

Email: journalscustomerservice-usa@elsevier.com

800-654-2452 (subscribers in the U.S. & Canada)
314-447-8871 (subscribers outside of the U.S. & Canada)

Fax number: 314-447-8029

Elsevier Health Sciences Division
Subscription Customer Service
3251 Riverport Lane
Maryland Heights, MO 63043

*To ensure uninterrupted delivery of your subscription, please notify us at least 4 weeks in advance of move.

Printed and bound by CPI Group (UK) Ltd, Croydon, CR0 4YY

03/10/2024

01040392-0005